10 0311391 0

UNIVER NOTTINGH

WITHDRAWN

LIBRA

F

D0241801

PROGRESS IN BRAIN RESEARCH

VOLUME 142

NEURAL CONTROL OF SPACE CODING AND ACTION PRODUCTION

Other volumes in PROGRESS IN BRAIN RESEARCH

Volume 114: The Cerebellum: From Structure to Control, by C.I. de Zeeuw, P. Strata and J. Voogd (Eds.) – 1997, ISBN 0-444-82313-1.

Volume 115: Brain Function in Hot Environment, by H.S. Sharma and J. Westman (Eds.) – 1998, ISBN 0-444-82377-8.

Volume 116: The Glutamate Synapse as a Therapeutical Target: Molecular Organization and Pathology of the Glutamate Synapse, by O.P. Ottersen, I.A. Langmoen and L. Gjerstad (Eds.) – 1998, ISBN 0-444-82754-4.

Volume 117: Neuronal Degeneration and Regeneration: From Basic Mechanisms to Prospects for Therapy, by F.W. van Leeuwen, A. Salehi, R.J. Giger, A.J.G.D. Holtmaat and J. Verhaagen (Eds.) – 1998, ISBN 0-444-82817-6.

Volume 118: Nitric Oxide in Brain Development, Plasticity and Disease, by R.R. Mize, T.M. Dawson, V.L. Dawson and M.J. Friedlander (Eds.) – 1998, ISBN 0-444-82885-0.

Volume 119: Advances in Brain Vasopressin, by I.J.A. Urban, J.P.H. Burbach and D. De Wied (Eds.) – 1999, ISBN 0-444-50080-4.

Volume 120: Nucleotides and their Receptors in the Nervous System, by P. Illes and H. Zimmermann (Eds.) – 1999, ISBN 0-444-50082-0.

Volume 121: Disorders of Brain, Behavior and Cognition: The Neurocomputational Perspective, by J.A. Reggia, E. Ruppin and D. Glanzman (Eds.) – 1999, ISBN 0-444-50175-4.

Volume 122: The Biological Basis for Mind Body Interactions, by E.A. Mayer and C.B. Saper (Eds.) – 1999, ISBN 0-444-50049-9.

Volume 123: Peripheral and Spinal Mechanisms in the Neural Control of Movement, by M.D. Binder (Ed.) – 1999, ISBN 0-444-50288-2.

Volume 124: Cerebellar Modules: Molecules, Morphology and Function, by N.M. Gerrits, T.J.H. Ruigrok and C.E. De Zeeuw (Eds.) – 2000, ISBN 0-444-50108-8.

Volume 125: Volume Transmission Revisited, by L.F. Agnati, K. Fuxe, C. Nicholson and E. Syková (Eds.) – 2000, ISBN 0-444-50314-5.

Volume 126: Cognition, Emotion and Autonomic Responses: The Integrative Role of the Prefrontal Cortex and Limbic Structures, by H.B.M. Uylings, C.G. Van Eden, J.P.C. De Bruin, M.G.P. Feenstra and C.M.A. Pennartz (Eds.) – 2000, ISBN 0-444-50332-3.

Volume 127: Neural Transplantation II. Novel Cell Therapies for CNS Disorders, by S.B. Dunnett and A. Björklund (Eds.) – 2000, ISBN 0-444-50109-6.

Volume 128: Neural Plasticity and Regeneration, by F.J. Seil (Ed.) – 2000, ISBN 0-444-50209-2.

Volume 129: Nervous System Plasticity and Chronic Pain, by J. Sandkühler, B. Bromm and G.F. Gebhart (Eds.) – 2000, ISBN 0-444-50509-1.

Volume 130: Advances in Neural Population Coding, by M.A.L. Nicolelis (Ed.) – 2001, ISBN 0-444-50110-X.

Volume 131: Concepts and Challenges in Retinal Biology, by H. Kolb, H. Ripps, and S. Wu (Eds.), – 2001, ISBN 0-444-506772.

Volume 132: Glial Cell Function, by B. Castellano López and M. Nieto-Sampedro (Eds.) – 2001, ISBN 0-444-50508-3.

Volume 133: The Maternal Brain. Neurobiological and neuroendocrine adaptation and disorders in pregnancy and post partum, by J.A. Russell, A.J. Douglas, R.J. Windle and C.D. Ingram (Eds.) – 2001, ISBN 0-444-50548-2.

Volume 134: Vision: From Neurons to Cognition, by C. Casanova and M. Ptito (Eds.) – 2001, ISBN 0-444-50586-5.

Volume 135: Do Seizures Damage the Brain, by A. Pitkänen and T. Sutula (Eds.) – 2002, ISBN 0-444-50814-7.

Volume 136: Changing Views of Cajal's Neuron, by E.C. Azmitia, J. DeFelipe, E.G. Jones, P. Rakic and C.E. Ribak (Eds.) – 2002, ISBN 0-444-50815-5.

Volume 137: Spinal Cord Trauma: Regeneration, Neural Repair and Functional Recovery, by L. McKerracher, G. Doucet and S. Rossignol (Eds.) – 2002, ISBN 0-444-50817-1.

Volume 138: Plasticity in the Adult Brain: From Genes to Neurotherapy, by M.A. Hofman, G.J. Boer, A.J.G.D. Holtmaat, E.J.W. Van Someren, J. Verhaagen and D.F. Swaab (Eds.) – 2002, ISBN 0-444-50981-X.

Volume 139: Vasopressin and Oxytocin: From Genes to Clinical Applications, by D. Poulain, S. Oliet and D. Theodosis (Eds.) – 2002, ISBN 0-444-50982-8.

Volume 140: The Brain's Eye, by J. Hyönä, D.P. Munoz, W. Heide and R. Radach (Eds.) – 2002, ISBN 0-444-51097-4.

Volume 141: Gonadotropin-releasing Hormone: Molecules and Receptors, by I.S. Parhar (Ed.) – 2002, ISBN 0-444-50979-8.

PROGRESS IN BRAIN RESEARCH

VOLUME 142

NEURAL CONTROL OF SPACE CODING AND ACTION PRODUCTION

EDITED BY

C. PRABLANC
D. PÉLISSON
Y. ROSSETTI

Unité 534, INSERM Espace et Action, 16 Avenue Doyen Lépine, 69500 Bron, France

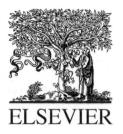

ELSEVIER

AMSTERDAM – BOSTON – LONDON – NEW YORK – OXFORD – PARIS
SAN DIEGO – SAN FRANCISCO – SINGAPORE – SYDNEY – TOKYO
2003

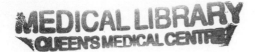

ELSEVIER SCIENCE B.V.
Sara Burgerhartstraat 25
P.O. Box 211, 1000 AE Amsterdam, The Netherlands

© 2003 Elsevier Science B.V. All rights reserved.

This work is protected under copyright by Elsevier Science, and the following terms and conditions apply to its use:

Photocopying
Single photocopies of single chapters may be made for personal use as allowed by national copyright laws. Permission of the Publisher and payment of a fee is required for all other photocopying, including multiple or systematic copying, copying for advertising or promotional purposes, resale, and all forms of document delivery. Special rates are available for educational institutions that wish to make photocopies for non-profit educational classroom use.

Permissions may be sought directly from Elsevier Science via their homepage (http://www.elsevier.com) by selecting 'Customer support' and then 'Permissions'. Alternatively you can send an e-mail to: permissions@elsevier.co.uk, or fax to: (+44) 1865 853333.

In the USA, users may clear permissions and make payments through the Copyright Clearance Center, Inc., 222 Rosewood Drive, Danvers, MA 01923, USA; phone: (+1) 978 7508400, fax: (+1) 978 7504744, and in the UK through the Copyright Licensing Agency Rapid Clearance Service (CLARCS), 90 Tottenham Court Road, London W1P 0LP, UK; phone: (+44) 207 631 5555, fax: (+44) 207 631 5500. Other countries may have a local reprographic rights agency for payments.

Derivative Works
Tables of contents may be reproduced for internal circulation, but permission of Elsevier Science is required for resale or distribution of such material.
Permission of the Publisher is required for all other derivative works, including compilations and translations.

Electronic Storage or Usage
Permission of the Publisher is required to store or use electronically any material contained in this work, including any chapter or part of a chapter.

Except as outlined above, no part of this work may be reproduced, stored in a retrieval system or transmitted in any form or by any means, electronic, mechanical, photocopying, recording or otherwise, without prior written permission of the Publisher.
Address permissions requests to: Elsevier Science Global Rights Department, at the mail, fax and e-mail addresses noted above.

Notice
No responsibility is assumed by the Publisher for any injury and/or damage to persons or property as a matter of products liability, negligence or otherwise, or from any use or operation of any methods, products, instructions or ideas contained in the material herein. Because of rapid advances in the medical sciences, in particular, independent verification of diagnoses and drugs dosages should be made.

First edition 2003

Library of Congress Cataloging-in-Publication Data
A catalog record from the Library of Congress has been applied for.

British Library Cataloguing in Publication Data
A catalogue record from the British Library has been applied for.

ISBN: 0-444-50977-1 (volume)
ISBN: 0-444-80104-9 (series)
ISSN: 0079-6123

⊗   The paper used in this publication meets the requirements of ANSI/NISO Z39.48-1992 (Permanence of Paper).
Printed in The Netherlands.

List of Contributors

A. Bergeron, Montreal Neurological Institute, McGill University, 3801 University Street, Montreal, QC H3A 2B4, Canada

J. Blouin, UMR 6152 Mouvement et Perception, CNRS and Université de la Méditerranée, Campus Scientifique de Luminy, F-13288 Marseille, Cedex 9, France

D. Boisson, Hôpital Neurologique Pierre Wertheimer, 59 Boulevard Pinel, 69003 Lyon, France

G. Bottini, Dipartimento di Psicologia, Università degli Studi di Pavia, Pavia, Italy

C. Bourdin, UMR 6152 Mouvement et Perception, CNRS and Université de la Méditerranée, Campus Scientifique de Luminy, F-13288 Marseille, Cedex 9, France

W.Y. Choi, Montreal Neurological Institute, McGill University, 3801 University Street, Montreal, QC H3A 2B4, Canada

J.D. Crawford, York Centre for Vision Research, York University, 4700 Keele Street, Toronto, ON M3J IP3, Canada

M. Desmurget, Espace et Action, INSERM Unité 534, 16 Avenue Doyen Lépine, 69676 Bron, France

H.C. Dijkerman, Psychological Laboratory, Helmholtz Research Institute, University of Utrecht, Heidelberglaan 2, 3584 CS Utrecht, The Netherlands

K.C. Engel, Department of Neuroscience, 6-145 Jackson Hall, 321 Church Street S.E., Minneapolis, MN 55455-0250, USA

A. Farnè, Dipartimento di Psicologia, Università di Bologna, Viale Berti Pichat 5 , 40127 Bologna, Italy

N.J. Gandhi, Division of Neuroscience, Baylor College of Medicine, 1 Baylor Plaza, Houston, TX 77030, USA

G. Gauthier, UMR 6152 Mouvement et Perception, CNRS and Université de la Méditerranée, Campus Scientifique de Luminy, F-13288 Marseille, Cedex 9, France

B. Gaymard, INSERM 289 and Service d'Explorations Fonctionnelles du Système Nerveux, Hôpital Salpêtrière, Paris, France

L. Goffart, Espace et Action, INSERM Unité 534, 16 Avenue Doyen Lépine, 69500 Bron, France

S.T. Grafton, Center for Cognitive Neuroscience, and the Department of Psychological and Brain Sciences, Dartmouth College, HB 6162 Moore Hall, Hanover, NH 03755, USA

H. Gréa, Espace et Action, INSERM Unité 534, 16 Avenue Doyen Lépine, 69676 Bron, France

A. Guillaume, UMR Mouvement et Perception, Université de la Méditerranée, CP 910, 163 Avenue de Luminy, 13288 Marseille, France

D. Guitton, Montreal Neurological Institute, McGill University, 3801 University Street, Montreal, QC H3A 2B4, Canada

K.-P. Hoffmann, Allgemeine Zoologie und Neurobiologie, Ruhr-Universität Bochum, D-44780 Bochum, Germany

G.W. Humphreys, Behavioural Brain Sciences Centre, School of Psychology, University of Birmingham, Birmingham, B15 2TT, UK

H. Imamizu, ATR Human Information Science Laboratories, 2-2-2, Hikaridai, Seika-cho, Soraku-gun, Kyoto 619-0288, Japan

S.H. Johnson, Center for Cognitive Neuroscience, and the Department of Psychological and Brain Sciences, Dartmouth College, HB 6162 Moore Hall, Hanover, NH 03755, USA

M. Kawato, ATR Human Information Science Laboratories, 2-2-2, Hikaridai, Seika-cho, Soraku-gun, Kyoto 619-0288, Japan

G. Kerkhoff, EKN – Clinical Neuropsychology Research Group, Department Neuropsychology, Hospital Bogenhausen, Dachauerstrasse 164, D-80992 Munich, Germany

E.M. Klier, York Centre for Vision Research, York University, 4700 Keele Street, Toronto, ON M3J IP3, Canada

T. Kuroda, JST/ERATO Kawato Dynamic Brain Project, 2-2-2, Hikaridai, Seika-cho, Soraku-gun, Kyoto 619-0288, Japan

W. Lindner, Allgemeine Zoologie und Neurobiologie, Ruhr-Universität Bochum, D-44780 Bochum, Germany

L. Lünenburger, Paraplegic Center of the University Hospital Balgrist, CH-8008 Zürich, Switzerland

J.C. Martinez-Trujillo, York Centre for Vision Research, York University, 4700 Keele Street, Toronto, ON M3J IP3, Canada

S. Matsuo, Montreal Neurological Institute, McGill University, 3801 University Street, Montreal, QC H3A 2B4, Canada

C. Maurer, Neurozentrum, Neurological University Clinic, Breisacher Strasse 64, 79106 Freiburg, Germany

R.D. McIntosh, Cognitive Neuroscience Research Unit, Wolfson Research Institute, University of Durham, Queen's Campus, University Boulevard, Stockton-on-Tees TS17 6BH, UK

W.P. Medendorp, York Centre for Vision Research, York University, 4700 Keele Street, Toronto, ON M3J IP3, Canada

T. Mergner, Neurozentrum, Neurological University Clinic, Breisacher Strasse 64, 79106 Freiburg, Germany

A.D. Milner, Cognitive Neuroscience Research Unit, Wolfson Research Institute, University of Durham, Queen's Campus, University Boulevard, Stockton-on-Tees TS17 6BH, UK

S. Miyauchi, Communications Research Laboratory, 588-2, Iwaoka, Iwaoka-cho, Nishi-ku, Kobe, Hyogo 651-2492, Japan

R.M. Müri, Eye Movement Research Laboratory and Department of Neurology, Inselspital, Bern, Switzerland

E. Nakano, ATR Human Information Science Laboratories, 2-2-2, Hikaridai, Seika-cho, Soraku-gun, Kyoto 619-0288, Japan

D. Pélisson, Espace et Action, INSERM Unité 534, 16 Avenue Doyen Lépine, 69500 Bron, France

R.J. Peterka, Neurological Sciences Institute, Oregon Health and Science University, 505 NW 185th Avenue, Beaverton, OR 97006, USA

C. Pierrot-Deseilligny, Service de Neurologie 1 (AP-HP), Hôpital de la Salpêtrière, 46 Bd. de l'Hôpital, 75671, Cedex 13, Paris, France

L. Pisella, Espace et Action, INSERM Unité 534, 16 Avenue Lépine, 69676 Bron, France

C.J. Ploner, Klinik für Neurologie, Charité, Berlin, Germany

C. Prablanc, Espace et Action, INSERM Unité 534, 16 Avenue Doyen Lépine, 69676 Bron, France

S. Rivaud-Péchoux, Service de Neurologie 1 (AP-HP), Hôpital de la Salpêtrière, 46 Bd. de l'Hôpital, 75671, Cedex 13, Paris, France

G. Rode, Service de Rééducation Neurologique, Hôpital Henry Gabrielle, Hospices Civils de Lyon, Lyon and Université Claude Bernard, Route de Vourles, BP 57, F-69565 St Genis-laval, France

Y. Rossetti, Espace et Action, Institut National de la Santé et de la Recherche Médicale, Unité 534, 16 Avenue Lépine, Case 13, 69676 Bron, France

F. Sarès, UMR 6152 Mouvement et Perception, CNRS and Université de la Méditerranée, Campus Scientifique de Luminy, F-13288 Marseille, Cedex 9, France

M.A. Smith, York Centre for Vision Research, York University, 4700 Keele Street, Toronto, ON M3J IP3, Canada

J.F. Soechting, Department of Neuroscience, 6-145 Jackson Hall, 321 Church Street S.E., Minneapolis, MN 55455-0250, USA

D.L. Sparks, Division of Neuroscience, Baylor College of Medicine, 1 Baylor Plaza, Houston, TX 77030, USA

R. Sterzi, Divisione Neurologica, Ospedale S. Anna, Como, Italy

M. Takagi, Divisions of Ophthalmology and Visual Science, Niigata University, Graduate School of Medical and Dental Sciences, and CREST, Japan Science and Technology, Niigata, 951-8510, Japan

R. Tamargo, Department of Neurosurgery, The Johns Hopkins University School of Medicine, Baltimore, MD 21287, USA

G. Vallar, Dipartimento di Psicologia, and Laboratorio di Neuroimmagini Cognitive e Cliniche, Università degli Studi di Milano-Bicocca, Edificio U6 Piazza dell'Ateneo, Nuovo 1, 20126, Milan, Italy

J.-L. Vercher, UMR 6152 Mouvement et Perception, CNRS and Université de la Méditerranée, Campus Scientifique de Luminy, F-13288 Marseille, Cedex 9, France

T. Yoshioka, ATR Human Information Science Laboratories, 2-2-2, Hikaridai, Seika-cho, Soraku-gun, Kyoto 619-0288, Japan

D.S. Zee, Departments of Neurology and Ophthalmology, The Johns Hopkins Hospital, Path 2-210, Baltimore, MD 21287, USA

Preface

The commonplace action of pointing or reaching and grasping the simplest object involves a complex series of neural processing, including object localization and identification, decision, and the sensorimotor transformations leading to the planning and control of action. The approach of such a problem has been initially divided into two main fields: perception and motor control.

Although visual perceptual integration and oculomotor control are commonly considered as hardly dissociable, the action per se has been considered as deriving from sensory input and very little the other way around. This book presents some new lines of research showing the sharp and fast reciprocal influences between the two systems (beyond the debate between gibsonian and motor theories of perception).

Another evolution of concepts has gone from the antagonist views of brain activity between neophrenology and widely distributed networks to an intermediate view integrating both specialized functional areas having multi-modal inputs and outputs and tightly interconnected with other areas. A simple example is that of the visual and posterior parietal structures, devoted to space perception, which integrate motor signals, whereas the limb premotor structures in turn integrate visual and oculomotor signals. The same intermingling occurs also within the brainstem: for instance whereas the superior colliculus was considered as a structure devoted only to eye and head movements, recent researches have shown that it includes hand movement related neurons.

In the same way the oversimplificative dichotomic association of conscious perception and action/cortical activity, versus unconscious perception and action/subcortical activity, has been strongly modulated.

More than fifteen years ago, in the same series of Progress in Brain Research, Freund, Büttner, Cohen and Noth compiled the main communications made in a symposium on the differences and similarities between the oculomotor and skeletal–motor systems. This book highlighted the main characteristics of those systems, including large differences in inertia and in degrees of freedom. At that time the concept of efference copy formalizing quantitatively the notion of corollary discharge, although very popular in the field of eye movements research, seemed inappropriate for the control of the upper limb and posture. This conceptual gap between the two fields has been partially overcome. The approach of animal behavior, as knowledge has become sharper, has led to concepts of multiple sources of influence and gone to the notion of cooperative networks, with functions scarcely reflected by single neuronal activity, but more often subserved by populations of neurons which give a new insight in the correlation between the average activity of a population and a behavioral variable. The neural basis of these networks has become possible through investigations of human brain activity, approached first by brain mapping evoked potentials and then by neuroimaging methods including PET and fMRI. In addition, the development of MEG associated with spatio-temporal EEG maps has allowed to follow the fast temporal evolution of cortical activity. Modeling sensory–motor adaptation and learning by neural networks compatible with known neurophysiological processes and especially those of the cerebellum has created a new fertilizing field. These theoretical advances allow tighter interactions between experimental and modeling approaches, which could be as fruitful as the metaphoric approach of control theory has been for the oculomotor neurophysiologists during more than twenty years. The field of neuropsychology, derived from the observation of specific dysfunctions in brain damaged patients, has been totally renewed by the association of sharp methodological approaches and neuroimaging allowing to observe the substitution processes that patients developed and the residual functions. Transient lesions achieved by transcranial magnetic stimulation have provided complementary information. Clinical neuropsychology has evolved by integrating in its field the knowledge derived from neuroanatomical, electrophysiological and psychophysical data, and has led to the development of more efficient rehabilitation tools.

If we have now a better understanding of the way the eye position signals modulate the visual response of neurons within cortical structures such as the parietal cortex, the premotor cortex, and in the subcortical brainstem and cerebellar circuitries where both arm movements and eye and head movements are encoded, we have not yet the key to the complex sensorimotor transformations for the control of the over-redundant degrees of freedom of the upper arm. However, some solutions are currently formalized by artificial neural networks making use of basic physiological principles.

In the field of visuomotor coordination, both the neuroanatomical pathways of fast feed-forward links between spatial vision and motor behavior and those of slower pathways, going through the temporal cortex for identification and frontal cortex for decision, have been revealed by the neuropsychological description of rare clinical cases. The discovered neuropsychological dissociations have allowed a better understanding of the link between perception and action.

The association of motor psychophysical techniques together with neuroimaging or transcranial stimulation of neural structures has also made feasible paradigms allowing the separation between planning and control phases. They have also revealed the powerful plasticity of the brain reorganization and their high dependence upon the active adaptation to sensorimotor conflicts. This adaptation has led to the surprising recovery of upper cognitive dysfunctions, suggesting that abstraction keeps tight links with sensorimotor processing. This hypothesis will stimulate new lines of research on the biological substrate of abstract levels of thinking and on their analogy with spatial representations.

The present book tries to link the new concepts and discoveries in the field of sensorimotor coordination. It puts together the main contributions of participants of an international symposium held in Lyon in 2001 and entitled "Neural Control of Space Coding and Action Production." The book emphasizes the reciprocal relationship between perception and action, and the essential role of active sensorimotor organization or reorganization in building up perceptual and motor representations of the self and of the external world.

C. Prablanc
D. Pélisson
Y. Rossetti
(Editors)

Acknowledgements

We greatly acknowledge the following institutions for the financial support of the symposium from which this book is issued : Institut National de la Santé et de la Recherche Médicale (INSERM), Université Claude Bernard, Centre National de la Recherche Scientifique (CNRS), Institut Fédératif des Neurosciences de Lyon (IFNL), Société des Neurosciences, Pôle Rhône-Alpes des Sciences Cognitives, Conseil Général du Rhône and Région Rhône-Alpes. We are also indebted to the following companies for their donations : Optique Peter, Ipsen, Synapsis, SMI-Gmbh, Crédit Mutuel Enseignants, Essilor, UCB-Pharma SA, John Benjamins, Jansen-Cilag.

We gratefully acknowledge the active contribution of the members of the INSERM Research Unit 534 Espace et Action to the organisation of the symposium, and especially the contribution of Mrs Soulier for the administrative part, and thank Mr Borach and Mr Prince for the illustrations. We also thank the reviewers for their helpful criticisms and for their contribution to the quality of the book.

Contents

List of Contributors v

Preface ix

Acknowledgements xi

Section I. Gaze Control

1. Cortical control of ocular saccades in humans: a model for motricity
    C. Pierrot-Descilligny, R.M. Müri, C.J. Ploner, B. Gaymard and
    S. Rivaud-Péchoux (Paris, France, Bern, Switzerland and Berlin,
    Germany) 3

2. Effects of lesions of the cerebellar oculomotor vermis on eye movements in
    primate: binocular control
    M. Takagi, R. Tamargo and D.S. Zee (Niigata, Japan and Baltimore,
    MD, USA) 19

3. Single cell signals: an oculomotor perspective
    D.L. Sparks and N.J. Gandhi (Houston, TX, USA)   35

4. On the feedback control of orienting gaze shifts made with eye and head
    movements
    D. Guitton, A. Bergeron, W.Y. Choi and S. Matsuo (Montreal, QC,
    Canada) 55

5. Control of saccadic eye movements and combined eye/head gaze shifts by the
    medio-posterior cerebellum
    D. Pélisson, L. Goffart and A. Guillaume (Bron, France)............ 69

6. Neural activity in the primate superior colliculus and saccadic reaction times in
    double-step experiments
    L. Lünenburger, W. Lindner, K.-P. Hoffmann (Bochum, Germany) .. 91

7. Neural control of 3-D gaze shifts in the primate
    E.M. Klier, J.C. Martinez-Trujillo, W.P. Medendorp, M.A. Smith and
    J.D. Crawford (Toronto, ON, Canada) 109

Section II. Motor Programming and Control

8. From 'acting on' to 'acting with': the functional anatomy of object-oriented
   action schemata
   S.H. Johnson and S.T. Grafton (Hanover, NH, USA) 127

9. Interactions between ocular motor and manual responses during two-dimensional
   tracking
   K.C. Engel and J.F. Soechting (Minneapolis, MN, USA) 141

10. Neural control of on-line guidance of hand reaching movements
    C. Prablanc, M. Desmurget and H. Gréa (Bron, France) 155

11. Internal forward models in the cerebellum: fMRI study on grip force and load
    force coupling
    M. Kawato, T. Kuroda, H. Imamizu, E. Nakano, S. Miyauchi and
    T. Yoshioka (Kyoto and Hyogo, Japan) 171

12. A multisensory posture control model of human upright stance
    T. Mergner, C. Maurer and R.J. Peterka (Freiburg, Germany and
    Portland, OR, USA) 189

13. Role of sensory information in updating internal models of the effector during
    arm tracking
    J.-L. Vercher, F. Sarès, J. Blouin, C. Bourdin and G. Gauthier
    (Marseille, France) 203

Section III. Normal and Pathological Spatial Representations

14. Delayed reaching and grasping in patients with optic ataxia
    A.D. Milner, H.C. Dijkerman, R.D. McIntosh, Y. Rossetti and L.
    Pisella (Stockton-on-Tees, UK, Utrecht, The Netherlands and Bron,
    France) 225

15. Conscious visual representations built from multiple binding processes: evidence
    from neuropsychology
    G.W. Humphreys (Birmingham, UK) 243

16. Modulation and rehabilitation of spatial neglect by sensory stimulation
    G. Kerkhoff (Munich, Germany) 257

17. Bottom-up transfer of sensory–motor plasticity to recovery of spatial cognition:
    visuomotor adaptation and spatial neglect
    G. Rode, L. Pisella, Y. Rossetti, A. Farnè and D. Boisson (Bron and
    Lyon, France) 273

18. Anosognosia for left-sided motor and sensory deficits, motor neglect and sensory
     hemiinattention: is there a relationship?
     G. Vallar, G. Bottini and R. Sterzi (Milan and Pavia, Italy) 289

Subject Index 303

Gaze Control

C. Prablanc, D. Pélisson and Y. Rossetti (Eds.)
Progress in Brain Research, Vol. 142
© 2003 Published by Elsevier Science B.V.

CHAPTER 1

Cortical control of ocular saccades in humans: a model for motricity

C. Pierrot-Deseilligny [1,*], R.M. Müri [2], C.J. Ploner [3], B. Gaymard [1,4] and
S. Rivaud-Péchoux [1]

[1] *INSERM 289 and Service de Neurologie 1 (AP-HP), Hôpital de la Salpêtrière, Paris, France*
[2] *Eye Movement Research Laboratory and Department of Neurology, Inselspital, Bern, Switzerland*
[3] *Klinik für Neurologie, Charité, Berlin, Germany*
[4] *Service d'Explorations Fonctionnelles du Système Nerveux, Hôpital Salpêtrière, Paris, France*

Abstract: Our knowledge of the cortical control of saccadic eye movements (saccades) in humans has recently progressed mainly thanks to lesion and transcranial magnetic stimulation (TMS) studies, but also to functional imaging. It is now well-known that the frontal eye field is involved in the triggering of intentional saccades, the parietal eye field in that of reflexive saccades, the supplementary eye field (SEF) in the initiation of motor programs comprising saccades, the pre-SEF in learning of these programs, and the dorsolateral prefrontal cortex (DLPFC) in saccade inhibition, prediction and spatial working memory. Saccades may also be used as a convenient model of motricity to study general cognitive processes preparing movements, such as attention, spatial memory and motivation. Visuo-spatial attention appears to be controlled by a bilateral parieto-frontal network comprising different parts of the posterior parietal cortex and the frontal areas involved in saccade control, suggesting that visual attentional shifts and saccades are closely linked. Recently, our understanding of the cortical control of spatial memory has noticeably progressed by using the simple visuo-oculomotor model represented by the memory-guided saccade paradigm, in which a single saccade is made to the remembered position of a unique visual item presented a while before. TMS studies have determined that, after a brief stage of spatial integration in the posterior parietal cortex (inferior to 300 ms), short-term spatial memory (i.e. up to 15–20 s) is controlled by the DLPFC. Behavioral and lesion studies have shown that medium-term spatial memory (between 15–20 s and a few minutes) is specifically controlled by the parahippocampal cortex, before long-term memorization (i.e. after a few minutes) in the hippocampal formation. Lastly, it has been shown that the posterior part of the anterior cingulate cortex, called the cingulate eye field, is involved in motivation and the preparation of all intentional saccades, but not in reflexive saccades. These different but complementary study methods used in humans have thus contributed to a better understanding of both eye movement physiology and general cognitive processes preparing motricity as whole.

Introduction

Eye movements serve vision and are either rapid or slow. Slow eye movements (ocular pursuit and

* Corresponding author. C. Pierrot-Deseilligny, Service de Neurologie 1, Hôpital de la Salpêtrière, 47 Bd de l'Hôpital, 75651 Paris cedex 13, France. Tel.: +33-14216-1828; Fax: +33-14424-5247;
E-mail: cp.deseilligny@psl.ap-hop-paris.fr

vestibulo-ocular reflex) stabilize images on the retina for vision, whereas rapid eye movements (i.e. ocular saccades) allow vision to change quickly the images which have to be seen. There are different types of saccades. Saccades may be reflexive, externally triggered by the sudden appearance of a visual target (reflexive visually guided saccade) (Fig. 1A) or intentional, internally triggered towards a target either already present (intentional visually guided saccade), not yet present (predictive saccade) or no

4

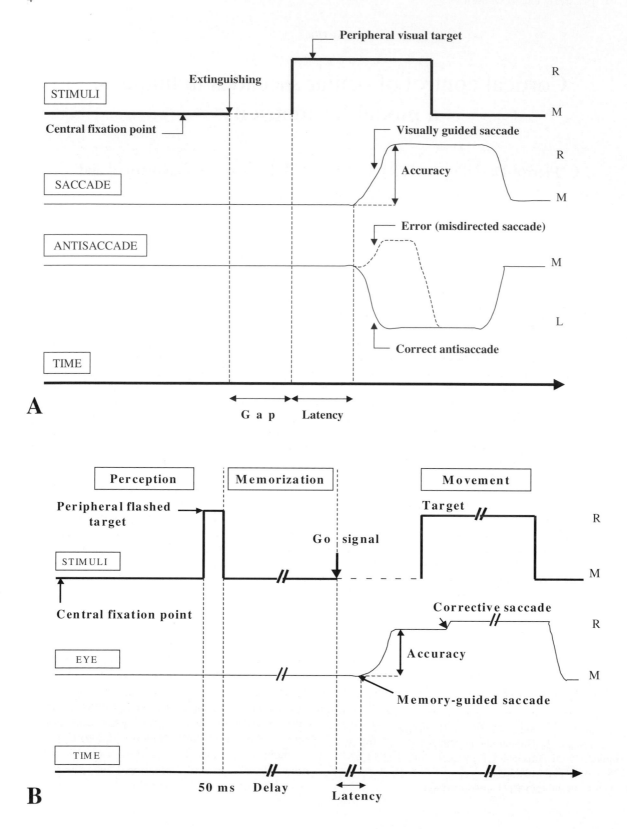

longer visible (memory-guided saccade) (Fig. 1B). Antisaccades, made in the opposite direction to a suddenly appearing visual target, are also intentional saccades (Fig. 1A). Lastly, there are spontaneous saccades, made for example at rest in darkness, and quick phases of nystagmus, which are also saccades.

Saccades are generated in the brainstem reticular formations, but are prepared and triggered by the cerebral cortex, except for the quick phases of nystagmus, which are entirely controlled in the brainstem. Between the cortical areas and the brainstem, a number of subcortical structures (basal ganglia and superior colliculus) are also involved in the control of saccades (see Pélisson et al., 2003, this volume), but this large field falls outside the scope of this chapter. In humans, several methods may be used to study the control of saccades at the cortical level. Lesion studies are required to determine which cortical areas are crucial to perform a saccade paradigm. However, lesion studies cannot tell us at what specific time in the execution of this paradigm each area plays a significant role. Transcranial magnetic stimulation (TMS), recently used in research to study different cerebral functions, can help to answer such questions. This technique, which inhibits or inactivates the stimulated areas for a few milliseconds, i.e. with the same effect as a brief functional lesion, has relatively good temporal resolution, but poor spatial resolution. Conversely, functional imaging, i.e. PET scan and functional magnetic resonance imaging (fMRI), has the best spatial resolution but relatively poor temporal resolution and at times false positive or negative activity. Functional imaging is therefore mainly useful to determine the precise locations of the ocular motor areas in humans, and other types of results obtained using this method

should be interpreted with caution. Finally, all these methods provide complementary information in the study of any human cerebral function, including the control of different types of saccades.

Saccades may be studied per se to improve our knowledge of eye movement physiology. However, saccades may also be used as a convenient model of motricity to understand complex neuropsychological processes such as attention, spatial integration, spatial memory, prediction and motivation. Therefore, after a brief review of our current knowledge of the cortical areas triggering or inhibiting saccades in humans, i.e. the movement taken here as a model, this chapter will focus on the study of the main neuropsychological processes preparing this movement as well as motricity in general.

Movement

In a sensory–motor act, i.e. a movement responding to a sensory stimulus, there are different stages of preparation and execution of the movement. At the cortical level, the movement is either triggered, the triggering marking the end of the preparation phase and the beginning of the execution phase (Fig. 2; 4), or inhibited.

Saccade triggering

Experimental studies have shown that three cerebral areas are capable of triggering saccades (Pierrot-Deseilligny et al., 1995b; Leigh and Zee, 1999): the frontal eye field (FEF), the supplementary eye field (SEF) and the parietal eye field (PEF). In humans, functional imaging suggests that the FEF, SEF and PEF are involved in the control of all saccade types.

Fig. 1. (A) Main saccade paradigms used. Reflexive visually guided saccade and antisaccade paradigms. In the saccade paradigm, the subject, fixating a central fixation point, has to make a reflexive visually guided saccade as soon as the peripheral visual target occurs. Latency is a reflection of the triggering mechanism of this reflexive saccade. Note that a gap is used, i.e. the central point is extinguished 200 ms before the appearance of the visual target, in order to facilitate the disengagement of fixation. In the antisaccade paradigm, the subject is instructed to make a saccade in the opposite direction to the visual target. A reflexive misdirected saccade to the target is an error and the percentage of errors is a reflection of inhibition mechanisms controlling saccades. Latency of correct antisaccades is a reflection of the triggering mechanisms of intentional saccades. (B) Memory-guided saccade paradigm. A peripheral visual target is flashed while the subject is fixating a central fixation point. After a delay (memorization), the central point is switched-off ('go signal') and the subject then has to make a saccade to the remembered position of the flash. Accuracy of this memory-guided saccade (or of the final eye position if there are several saccades) is a reflection of spatial memory. Latency is a reflection of the triggering mechanisms of intentional saccades. L, left; M, midline; R, right.

6

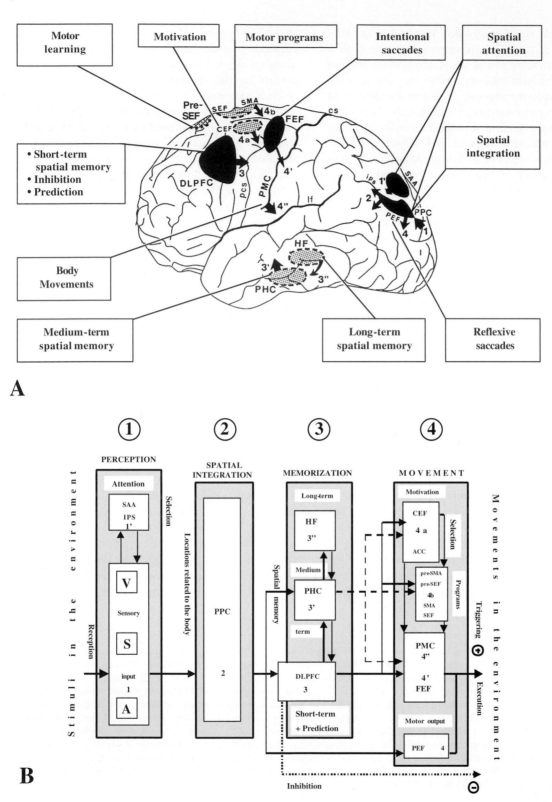

A

B

The FEF is located in the precentral gyrus and sulcus (Paus, 1996; Carter and Zee, 1997; Gaymard et al., 1999; Tehovnik et al., 2000; Lobel et al., 2001), anteriorly to the hand motor area and mainly around the intersection with the superior frontal sulcus (Fig. 2A). Complementing functional imaging studies, lesion studies have shown that the FEF is in particular involved in the control of intentional saccades, such as intentional visually guided saccades, correct antisaccades (Fig. 1A), memory-guided saccades (Fig. 1B) and predictive saccades (Pierrot-Deseilligny et al., 1991a,b, 1993; Rivaud et al., 1994; Israël et al., 1995; Heide and Kömpf, 1998; Gaymard et al., 1999; Ploner et al., 1999b). The increase in latency of such saccades observed in these studies and the eye displacements elicited by electrical stimulation of the FEF (Lobel et al., 2001) suggest that this area plays a significant role in the triggering process (Fig. 2; 4'). TMS studies of antisaccades (Müri et al., 1991) or memory-guided saccades (Wipfli et al., 2001) have confirmed that the FEF is more particularly involved in the triggering of such saccades. By contrast, the FEF does not appear to be crucial for the triggering of reflexive visually guided saccades (Pierrot-Deseilligny et al., 1991a), and furthermore was less activated for reflexive than for intentional saccades in a PET-scan study (Dorichi et al., 1997).

The human SEF is located anteriorly to the supplementary motor area (SMA) (Fig. 2A), namely in the upper part of the paracentral sulcus (Carter and Zee, 1997; Grosbras et al., 1999). The SEF, in particular on the left side, appears to be involved

in the control of motor programs comprising either several successive saccades (Gaymard et al., 1993), i.e. a sequence of saccades, or a saccade combined with a body movement (Pierrot-Deseilligny et al., 1993; Israël et al., 1995) (Fig. 2; 4b). TMS studies have shown that during sequences of saccades the SEF region could be crucial at two distinct times (Pierrot-Deseilligny et al., 1995b), i.e. during the learning phase (presentation of the visual targets) (Müri et al., 1995) and just after the go signal (Müri et al., 1994a), i.e. when the subject has to initiate the sequence of saccades. More recently, results of fMRI studies have suggested that the learning phase of a sequence of saccades could be controlled by a pre-SEF area, located just anteriorly to the SEF (Petit et al., 1996; Kawashima et al., 1998; Grosbras et al., 2001; Heide et al., 2001). Similarly, a pre-SMA exists anteriorly to the SMA for general motricity (Hikosaka et al., 1996). Thus, the learning phase and initiation of a sequence of saccades could be controlled by two close but distinctive areas in the SEF region.

The human PEF, which corresponds to area LIP (lateral intraparietal area) in the monkey, is located in the intraparietal sulcus, probably in its posterior part (Fig. 2A) (Müri et al., 1996a; Kawashima et al., 1996; Heide et al., 2001; Milea et al., 2001). This area appears to be mainly involved in the triggering of reflexive visually guided saccades, since, after a PEF lesion (but not after an FEF or an SEF lesion), latency of these saccades is significantly increased (Pierrot-Deseilligny et al., 1991a, Braun

Fig. 2. Cortical areas and pathways. Schematized representation of the cortical areas (A) and pathways (B) preparing movements in response to environmental stimuli. (1) At the perceptive stage, several areas (1) are involved in the reception of information (sensory input), depending upon the sensory modalities, and different attentional areas (1') contribute to the selection of salient information at this stage. (2) At the spatial integration stage, salient information is integrated in the PPC (2) to localize further the stimuli in relation to the body. (3) At the memorization stage, i.e. when information has not immediately been used, storage occurs in the DLPFC (3), PHC (3') and HF (3''), successively, for short-term, medium-term and long-term memorization, respectively. (4) At the movement stage, the motor areas will previously have been prepared for possible intentional forthcoming movements by motivation, i.e. by the ACC (body movements) and/or CEF (intentional saccades), with a selection of the useful corresponding areas by enhancing their basic activity (4a); if several movements are planned, their sequences will previously have been learned by the pre-SEF (saccades) and the pre-SMA (body movements), before an initiation of these sequences by the SEF (several successive saccades and/or a saccade with body movements) and/or SMA (body movements) (4b); movements (motor output) are triggered either immediately after spatial integration by the PEF (reflexive saccades) (4), or, after a delay, by the FEF (intentional saccades) (4') and/or the PMC (body movements) (4''). A, auditory areas; ACC, anterior cingulate cortex; CEF, cingulate eye field; cs, central sulcus; DLPFC, dorsolateral prefrontal cortex; FEF, frontal eye field; HF, hippocampal formation; ips and IPS, intraparietal sulcus; lf, lateral fissure; pcs, precentral sulcus; PEF, parietal eye field; PHC, parahippocampal cortex; PMC, primary motor cortex; PPC, posterior parietal cortex; pre-SEF, pre-supplementary eye field; S, somesthesic areas; SAA, spatial attentional area; SEF, supplementary eye field; SMA, supplementary motor area; V, visual areas.

et al., 1992), in particular when damage involves the right cerebral hemisphere (Fig. 2; 4). TMS over the posterior parietal cortex may also increase the latency of visually guided saccades (Elkington et al., 1992).

Therefore, three cortical areas contribute to the triggering of saccades, with apparently different roles depending upon the type of saccade to be performed: the PEF could mainly control reflexive saccades, whereas the FEF appears to be more involved in the control of the different modalities of intentional saccades and the SEF in the control of relatively more complex motor programs, comprising either several successive saccades or saccades combined with body movements. However, although the control exerted by the PEF and FEF, respectively, is relatively specialized in terms of the distinct types of saccades to be performed, these two areas also act complementarily in saccade triggering in general, since only bilateral lesions affecting both the PEF and the FEF result in a severe and long-lasting disturbance of saccade triggering (Michel et al., 1965; Pierrot-Deseilligny et al., 1988; Höllinger et al., 2001).

Saccade inhibition

Inhibition of saccades is useful when these eye movements might otherwise disturb another, more important task, such as relatively prolonged fixation. The antisaccade paradigm tests saccade inhibition, since, before performing a correct intentional antisaccade in the opposite direction to a suddenly appearing visual target, the subject has first to inhibit a reflexive visually guided saccade to the target (Fig. 1A). The percentage of errors (misdirected reflexive saccades made toward the target) is a reflection of saccade inhibition. We have shown that, at the cortical level, only patients with lesions affecting the dorsolateral prefrontal cortex (DLPFC) have an increased percentage of errors in this paradigm (Pierrot-Deseilligny et al., 1991a). In humans, the DLPFC is located in area 46 and the adjacent area 9 of Brodmann, namely in the middle frontal gyrus, anteriorly to the FEF (Fig. 2A) (Pierrot-Deseilligny et al., 1991b; Rajkowska and Goldman-Rakic, 1995; Petrides and Pandya, 1999; Heide et al., 2001). Our patients with a FEF lesion had a normal percentage

of errors (Pierrot-Deseilligny et al., 1991a; Rivaud et al., 1994; Gaymard et al., 1999), but, as seen above, an increase in the latency of intentional correct antisaccades. This suggests that the inhibitory role of the DLPFC is not mediated through the FEF, but is exerted directly upon the superior colliculus, via prefronto-collicular tracts (Fig. 2B). The role of the DLPFC in the antisaccade paradigm has also been shown using fMRI (Müri et al., 1998), and its more particular involvement in saccade inhibition was confirmed in a recent TMS study (Müri et al., 2000a). Therefore, the first stage in the execution of the antisaccade paradigm, i.e. inhibition of reflexive misdirected saccades, is under the control of the DLPFC, whereas the second stage, i.e. triggering of the intentional correct antisaccade, is controlled by the FEF.

Preparation of movements

A saccade is quite a simple motor act and relatively easy to record and interpret. This is why saccades have frequently been used as a convenient model of motricity to study the complex neuropsychological processes preparing these eye movements and body movements in general. Before a movement can be triggered, the main neuropsychological processes preparing the amplitude of the movement, which has to be adapted as accurately as possible to the target location, are firstly perception and spatial integration, followed by spatial memory, if the movement is delayed, and motivation, if the movement is intentional (Fig. 2).

Perception, attention and spatial integration

The perceptive areas are located in the parietal, temporal and occipital lobes, depending upon the stimulus modality (Fig. 2; 1). These perceptive areas are under the control of attentional processes selecting salient environmental information (Fig. 2; 1'). Visuo-spatial attention appears to be controlled by a bilateral parieto-frontal network comprising different parts of the posterior parietal cortex (PPC) and the frontal areas involved in saccade control (i.e. the FEF and SEF), suggesting that visual attentional shifts and saccades are closely linked (Nobre et al., 1997; Buchel et al., 1998; Corbetta et al., 1998; Perry and Zeki, 2000; Craighero et al., 2001). In the PPC, the posterior part of the superior parietal lobule, the intraparietal sulcus, and maybe also some parts of the inferior parietal lobule (Mort et al., 2000; Perry and Zeki, 2000; Heide et al., 2001) are activated during visually guided saccades (Fig. 2A): although these different parts of the superior and inferior parietal lobules located outside the intraparietal sulcus appear to be more specifically involved in purely attentional processes, it remains to be determined whether the active area in the intraparietal sulcus is the PEF alone or two separate areas (i.e. the PEF and another attentional area) within this sulcus are involved.

After perception, modulated by attentional processes, spatial integration is needed to know more precisely the locations of targets in respect to the body, and not simply to a part of it (eyes or ears) (Fig. 2; 2). When saccades are used as a model of motricity, their amplitude reflects the accuracy of spatial integration. This is particularly marked in paradigms comprising two or more successive saccades, since calculation of the amplitude of the second saccade requires a knowledge of the position reached by the eyes in the orbit after the first saccade (double-step paradigm). Lesion studies using memory-guided saccades (Pierrot-Deseilligny et al., 1991b) or a double-step saccade paradigm (Heide et al., 1995), as well as fMRI studies using a double-step (Tobler et al., 2001) or a triple-step saccade paradigm (Heide et al., 2001), suggest that an area located in the posterior part of the intraparietal sulcus is involved in spatial integration. However, the precise location of such an area within the intraparietal sulcus, in particular related to the PEF, is not yet known: the area involved in spatial integration in humans could be the equivalent of area 7a in the monkey, which is close to but distinct from area LIP, i.e. the equivalent of the PEF in humans; therefore, in humans, two areas could either be separate or could share the same location, with two types of intermingled cells, involved in spatial integration and saccade triggering, respectively. It should be noted that a spatial integrative area for the hand, equivalent to the area for saccades, is located in the anterior part of the intraparietal sulcus, namely anteriorly to the area for saccades (Kawashima et al., 1996; Binkofski et al., 1998).

Spatial memory

Spatial memory is another essential cognitive function preparing motricity, whether for eye movements or other body movements, when such movements are delayed. In animals and humans, spatial memory has been extensively studied either for short delays (of a few seconds) or long delays (more than a few minutes), but little is known about intermediate delays, i.e. between a few seconds and a few minutes. To study spatial memory, the visuo-oculomotor model, represented by the memory-guided saccade (MGS) paradigm (Fig. 1B), has frequently been used because of its simplicity. A simple visual item is first flashed and memorized. Then, after a delay, a single MGS is made to the remembered location of the visual item. The accuracy of this saccade is a reflection of spatial memory, provided that perceptive and oculomotor deficits have been ruled out. The results relating to short-term, medium-term and long-term spatial memory will be reviewed in turn.

Short-term spatial memory

Short-term spatial memory is the working memory used for current, on-going behavior (Fig. 2; 3). In monkeys, single-neuron recordings have shown that the DLPFC is involved in MGS (Goldman-Rakic, 1996). In humans, lesion studies (Pierrot-Deseilligny et al., 1991b, 1993; Gaymard et al., 1993, 1999; Rivaud et al., 1994; Israël et al., 1995) have shown that several cortical areas — such as the DLPFC, the FEF and the posterior parietal cortex (PPC), but not the SEF — control MGS. The PPC, i.e. the equivalent of area 7a involved in spatial integration in the monkey, is probably located in the vicinity of the PEF (see above). Functional imaging also suggests the involvement of various parieto-frontal areas in MGS, including the DLPFC (O'Sullivan et al., 1995; Sweeney et al., 1996). In fact, the MGS paradigm comprises three successive physiological phases after the visual target presentation, namely spatial integration, memorization and saccade triggering. To determine the specific role(s) played by the different cortical areas involved in the control of MGS, a method other than lesion studies (or functional imaging) is needed. Several TMS studies have allowed us to resolve this question. TMS applied

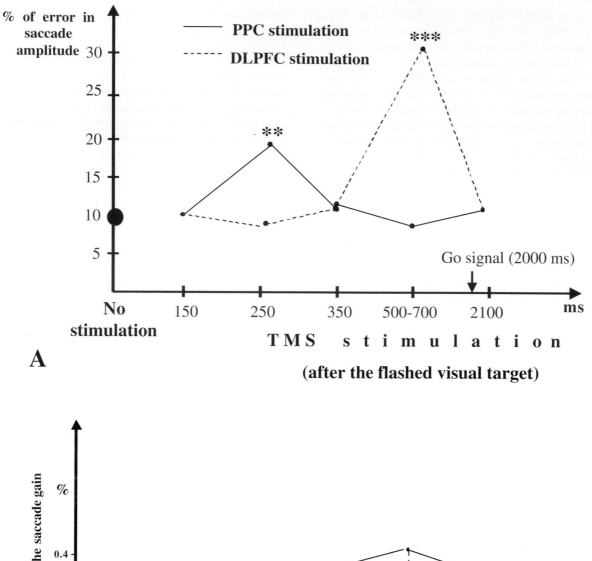

A

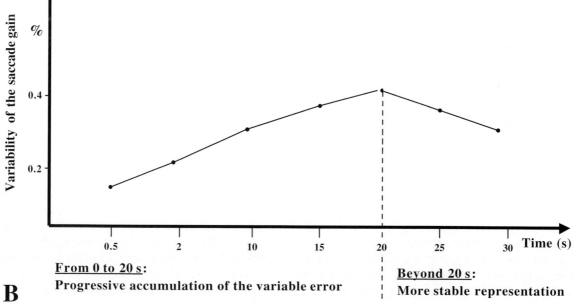

B

over the PPC or DLPFC showed that (1) the right PPC (but not the left PPC) is involved at 260 ms after the target presentation (Müri et al., 1996b, 2000b), but not later in the paradigm, and (2) both DLPFC are involved during the memorization phase (around 1 s after the target presentation), but not earlier in the paradigm (Müri et al., 1996b; Brandt et al., 1998) (Fig. 3A). Furthermore, other TMS studies have suggested that the FEF is involved in MGS triggering (Wipfli et al., 2001), with also a possible contribution of the PEF at this stage (Müri et al., 1996a,b, 2000a,b).

Overall, these different results suggest that: (1) the right PPC is involved in the control of saccade accuracy during the brief initial visuo-spatial integration stage, immediately after the stimulus presentation, but not later during the memorization phase of the paradigm, and is not, therefore, crucial in the control of short-term spatial memory; (2) the left PPC is either uninvolved or less involved than the right PPC in the control of saccade accuracy, a result which is probably related to the well-known dominance in humans of the right cerebral hemisphere for visuo-spatial functions; (3) by contrast, both the right and the left DLPFC control saccade accuracy during the memorization phase of this paradigm, i.e. short-term spatial memory; and (4) lastly, the FEF is mainly involved in MGS triggering, to which the PPC may also contribute. Thus, these TMS studies succeeded in determining the chronology of the cortical control of MGS (Fig. 2). In the monkey, the DLPFC is reciprocally connected with both the PPC and the FEF (Chafee and Goldman-Rakic, 2000), with, therefore, the existence of an anatomical substrate for such cortical control. Lastly, it should also be noted that, according to the results of our recent lesion studies, the FEF may be prepared by short-term memorized information maintained in the DLPFC, in order to perform possible forthcoming ocular saccades corresponding to such salient information (Gaymard et al., 1999; Ploner et al., 1999b).

Medium-term spatial memory

How long the transient DLPFC control of spatial memory lasts was the next question to be resolved. Accuracy of MGS decreases during the first seconds of the memory delay (White et al., 1994). This is mainly reflected in an increase in variable targeting errors, i.e. scatter of MGS endpoints around the to-be-remembered target position, and probably represents information loss in short-term spatial memory (White et al., 1994; Wang, 2001). In a recent study, we used this delay-dependency of targeting errors to investigate possible temporal limits for short-term spatial memory (Ploner et al., 1998). Normal subjects performed an MGS task with unpredictable varied memory delays of 0.5 to 30 s. The results confirmed that variable targeting errors initially increased linearly with delay length (Fig. 3B). Surprisingly, after a maximum error around delays of 20 s, this process did not stabilize, but reverted partially, and MGS accuracy improved significantly with longer delays. This time-limited decay of spatial information strongly suggests involvement of a more stable memory system at longer delays and thus allows for the hypothesis of an upper temporal limit of about 20 s for short-term spatial memory in humans. This temporal limit fits remarkably well with the limited temporal stability of spatially selective neuronal activity in the monkey DLPFC and the known temporal properties of short-term plasticity in prefrontal neurons (Goldman-Rakic, 1996; Wang, 2001).

Fig. 3. Spatial memory results. (A) Results of a transcranial magnetic stimulation (TMS) study on the right hemisphere in 8 normal subjects performing memory-guided saccades (with a 2-s delay) (Müri et al., 1996b): results with TMS are compared to those without stimulation; note that (1) after PPC stimulation, saccade accuracy was significantly impaired when stimulation was performed 260 ms after the flashed peripheral target ($p < 0.01$), (2) after DLPFC stimulation, saccade accuracy was impaired when stimulation was performed during the memorization period (i.e. beyond 500 ms) ($p < 0.001$), and (3) after the go signal (2 s), accuracy was normal in both cases. DLPFC, dorsolateral prefrontal cortex; PPC, posterior parietal cortex. (B) Delay-dependency of variable targeting errors of memory-guided saccades in 16 normal subjects (Ploner et al., 1998). The delay varied from 0.5 to 30 s. Only the group results are shown. Note that the variability of the gain increased up to a 20-s delay, but, surprisingly, significantly improved (i.e. decreased) after 20 s. This means that after 20 s a more stable representation is involved. Therefore, probably two different structures, working in parallel, control spatial memory, before and after 20 s, respectively.

This new finding of improvement of spatial memory at delays longer than 20 s then led us to determine which cerebral structure could be involved in such medium-term spatial memory. Previous lesion studies in humans have suggested that the medial temporal lobe (MTL) is the region containing the neuronal substrate of the putative medium-term memory, since spatial memory was deficient at delays of about 20 s but normal at shorter delays (Sidman et al., 1968; Rains and Milner, 1994). However, the MTL is a complex anatomical region, consisting of the hippocampal formation (HF) (i.e. hippocampus and entorhinal cortex), the perirhinal cortex (PRC) and the parahippocampal cortex (PHC) (Amaral and Insausti, 1990). The HF is directly connected with both cortices, but it is mainly the PHC which is reciprocally connected with neocortical areas involved in spatial cognition, i.e. the PPC and DLPFC (Fig. 2) (Goldman-Rakic et al., 1984; Carter and Zee, 1997), and motor areas such as the FEF (Barbas and Mesulam, 1981). In two recent studies, we investigated the question of possible differential contributions of MTL subregions to spatial memory in humans with postsurgical lesions of the right MTL (Ploner et al., 1999a, 2000). The results showed that only patients with PHC involvement exhibited a significant inaccuracy of MGS at delays longer than 20 s contralateral to the lesion side. MGS with short delays (i.e. inferior to 20 s) were normal, a result confirming the findings of our previous study of patients with large lesions of the right MTL (Müri et al., 1994b). Thus, these results show that the right PHC contributes to spatial memory at delays beyond DLPFC-based short-term spatial memory, and, therefore, that the PHC, and not the HF or the PRC, is a likely neuronal substrate for medium-term spatial memory of single visual items in humans (Fig. 2; 3′).

Long-term spatial memory

What is the next structure involved in spatial memory, i.e. in long-term spatial memory, and at which critical time? There is ample evidence, both from single-neuron recordings and lesion studies in monkeys, that the HF is involved in spatial memory processes (Rolls, 1999). The HF is situated, by virtue of its extensive direct and indirect connections with areas involved in spatial processing and object recognition (Amaral and Insausti, 1990; Suzuki and Amaral, 1994), at the highest level of integration of perceptual information, and is thus in a privileged position to bind together information from different sensory modalities and spatial coordinate frames into a spatial memory map of the environment (Fig. 2; 3″).

Furthermore, previous studies with patients with verified lesions (necropsy) restricted to the HF have shown that memory for locations of a simple spatial array of objects is impaired with delays of 5 min (Cave and Squire, 1991; Rempel-Clower et al., 1996). Thus, it appears that at delays of some minutes the hippocampus may be actively involved in spatial memory, at least for largely non-relational spatial information. This interpretation would parallel the known delay-dependent memory deficits for non-relational object information seen in monkeys with lesions to the HF, where memory is normal at delays of 60 s, but impaired at delays of 10 min (Alvarez et al., 1995; Leonard et al., 1995). Thus, the HF is a likely candidate region for a long-term spatial memory system, subserving spatial memory formation beyond PHC-based medium-term spatial memory.

Taken together, the results of the different studies using such a simple visuo-oculomotor model allow us to suggest that, after a brief initial visuo-spatial integration stage under the control mainly of the right PPC (up to about 300 ms), spatial memory is controlled, successively, by the DLPFC for its short-term component (up to 15–20 s), the PHC for its medium-term component (between 15–20 s and probably a few minutes) and, lastly, the HF for its long-term component (after a few minutes) (Fig. 4). It should be noted that such an organization of spatial memory involves a new concept, namely an intermediary link between short-term and long-term memorizations, with the involvement of the PHC in medium-term memorization. It remains, however, to be determined how memorized information is coordinated between the different structures successively involved in spatial memory: in parallel, according to certain behavioral results (Ploner et al., 1998) (see above), serially according to other preliminary TMS results (Nyffeler et al., 2002), or, as it seems more likely, by a combination of the two. Furthermore, is this simple visuo-oculomotor model of spatial memory applicable to the memorization of

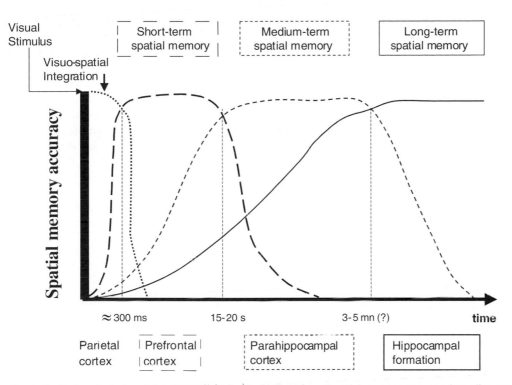

Fig. 4. Cortical control of spatial memory. Schematic representation of spatial memory accuracy depending upon time. During the first 300 ms, the (posterior) parietal cortex controls visuo-spatial integration, then short-term spatial memory (up to 15–20 s), medium-term spatial memory (probably up to a few minutes), and long-term spatial memory (after a few minutes) are controlled, successively, by the (dorsolateral) prefrontal cortex, the parahippocampal cortex and the hippocampal formation, respectively, with, therefore, a different structure crucially involved for each of these 4 periods of time.

other types of stimuli (i.e. more complex visual, auditory and somesthesic stimuli) and the rest of body motricity? Although this appears probable — since the DLPFC, the PPC and the HF are involved for other types of stimuli and the preparation of other movements (Goldman-Rakic et al., 1992; Rains and Milner, 1994; Culham and Kanwisher, 2001) — the demonstration of such general mechanisms and of the systematic involvement of the PHC requires other studies.

Motivation

Motivation is a neuropsychological process preparing motor areas to perform forthcoming intentional motor acts (Fig. 2; 4a). The anterior cingulate cortex (ACC) could be involved in this process (Colby and Goldberg, 1999; Kastner and Ungerleider, 2000). In a PET-scan study (Petit et al., 1993), it has been

shown that the posterior part of the ACC (Fig. 2A), which may be called the 'cingulate eye field' (CEF) (Gaymard et al., 1998), is involved in voluntary saccades made in darkness, i.e. a type of intentional saccades. We have shown that small lesions affecting the same area result in deficits (increased latency and decreased accuracy) of different types of intentional saccades, whereas reflexive saccades remain normal (Gaymard et al., 1998). Since the ACC appears to be involved well before a motor act (Shima et al., 1991) and is connected with the motor areas (Paus, 2001), whereas the CEF is strongly connected with all frontal ocular motor areas and the brainstem (Paus, 2001), the role of the ACC (in general motricity) and the CEF (in eye movements) could be to enhance the basic activity of the motor areas involved in the control of the forthcoming intentional motor acts, in order to facilitate their triggering at the appropriate time. It should also be noted that the

ACC is reciprocally connected with the DLPFC and the parahippocampal cortex (see above) (Gaymard et al., 1998), and could, therefore, contribute both to maintaining the salience of memorized information and to facilitating its transmission to the motor areas. This could represent the physiological mechanisms by which motivation is expressed at the neuronal level, for eye movements in the CEF as well as for general motricity in the remainder of the ACC.

Conclusions

The brain is continuously organizing possible multiple accurate motor responses to a number of sensory stimuli occurring in the environment. A visuo-oculomotor model comprising a simple visual item as the stimulus and a single saccade as the motor response appears to be convenient to understand the multiplicity of possible movements and the relatively complex neuropsychological processes preparing them. As early as the perceptive stage, different attentional processes select salient information (Colby and Goldberg, 1999; Kastner and Ungerleider, 2000; Ploner et al., 2001) (Fig. 2; 1 and 1'). This information is then spatially integrated in the PPC in order to know the location of the stimulus related to the whole body and not simply to a part of it (Fig. 2; 2). Just after this stage, a reflexive saccadic response without any delay may be triggered in the motor part of the parietal lobe (PEF) towards a suddenly (possibly interesting and/or threatening) occurring stimulus (Fig. 2; 4). By contrast, if reflexive saccades have to be inhibited, the DLPFC (but not the FEF) plays a major role. When the motor response is planned but not immediately made, salient memorized information is stored, successively, in the DLPFC (short-term memory) (Kastner and Ungerleider, 2000), the PHC (medium-term memory) and the HF (long-term memory) depending upon the time of the delayed response (Fig. 2; 3, 3' and 3''). When the response is predicted (predictive saccade) to a specific location before the appearance of the target, the DLPFC also appears to be involved (Pierrot-Deseilligny et al., 1995b, 2003). Therefore, with these multiple functions (short-term spatial memory, inhibition and prediction), the DLPFC appears to play a crucial role in the decisional processes preparing movements. At the memorization stage, the ACC

and CEF could already select and prepare the motor areas which might have to respond (Fig. 2; 4a). If several movements are planned, the SMA and SEF are involved in the preparation of motor programs, previously learned thanks to the pre-SMA and pre-SEF (Fig. 2; 4b). Finally, the responses are executed by the primary motor cortex and/or the FEF if body movements and/or intentional saccades, respectively, are required (Fig. 2; 4' and 4'').

References

Alvarez, A., Zola-Morgan, S. and Squire, L.R. (1995) Damage limited to the hippocampal region produces long-lasting memory impairment in monkeys. *J. Neurosci.*, 15: 5637–5807.

Amaral, D.G. and Insausti, R. (1990) The hippocampal formation. In: G. Paxinos (Ed.), *The Human Nervous System*. Academic Press, San Diego, CA.

Barbas, H. and Mesulam, M.M. (1981) Organization of afferent input to subdivisions of Area 8 in the rhesus monkey. *J. Comp. Neurol.*, 200: 407–431.

Binkofski, F., Dohle, C., Posse, S., Stephan, K.M., Hefter, H., Seitz, R.J. and Freund, H.J. (1998) Human anterior intraparietal area subserves prehension. A combined lesion and functional MRI activation study. *Neurology*, 50: 1253–1259.

Brandt, S.A., Ploner, C.J., Meyer, B.U., Leistner, S. and Villringer, A. (1998) Effects of repetitive transcranial magnetic stimulation over dorsolateral prefrontal and posterior parietal cortex on memory-guided saccades. *Exp. Brain Res.*, 118: 197–204.

Braun, D., Weber, H., Mergner, T.H. and Schulte-Montig, J. (1992) Saccadic reaction times in patients with frontal and parietal lesions. *Brain*, 115: 1359–1386.

Buchel, C., Josephs, O., Rees, G., Turner, R., Frith, C.D. and Friston, K.J. (1998) The functional anatomy of attention to visual motion. A functional MRI study. *Brain*, 121: 1281–1294.

Carter, N. and Zee, D.S. (1997) The anatomical localization of saccades using functional imaging studies and transcranial magnetic stimulation. *Curr. Opin. Neurol.*, 10: 10–17.

Cave, C.B. and Squire, L.R. (1991) Equivalent impairment of spatial and nonspatial memory following damage to the human hippocampus. *Hippocampus*, 1: 329–340.

Chafee, M.V. and Goldman-Rakic, P.S. (2000) Inactivation of parietal and prefrontal cortex reveals interdependence of neural activity during memory-guided saccades. *J. Neurophysiol.*, 83: 1550–1566.

Colby, C.L. and Goldberg, M.E. (1999) Space and attention in parietal cortex. *Annu. Rev. Neurosci.*, 22: 319–349.

Corbetta, M., Akbudak, E., Conturo, T.E., Snyder, A.Z., Ollinger, J.M., Drury, H.A., Linenweber, M.R., Petersen, S.E., Raichle, M.E., Van Essen, D.C. and Shulman, G.L. (1998) A common network of functional areas for attention and eye movements. *Neuron*, 21(4): 761–773.

Craighero, L., Carta, A. and Fadiga, L. (2001) Peripheral oculomotor palsy affects orienting of visuospatial attention. *Neuroreport*, 12: 3283–3286.

Culham, J.C. and Kanwisher, N.G. (2001) Neuroimaging of cognitive functions in human parietal cortex. *Curr. Opin. Neurobiol.*, 11: 157–163.

Doricchi, F., Perani, D., Incoccia, C., Grassi, F., Cappa, S.F., Bettinardi, V., Galati, G., Pizzamiglio, L. and Fazio, F. (1997) Neural control of fast-regular saccades and antisaccades: an investigation using positron emission tomography. *Exp. Brain Res.*, 116: 50–62.

Elkington, P.T., Ker, G.K. and Stein, J.S. (1992) The effect of electromagnetic stimulation of the posterior parietal cortex on eye movements. *Eye*, 6: 510–514.

Gaymard, B., Rivaud, S. and Pierrot-Deseilligny, C. (1993) Role of the left and right supplementary motor areas in memory-saccade sequences. *Ann. Neurol.*, 34: 404–406.

Gaymard, B., Rivaud, S., Cassarini, J.F., Ploner, C. and Pierrot-Deseilligny, C. (1998) Effects of anterior cingulate cortex lesions on ocular saccades in humans. *Exp. Brain Res.*, 120: 173–183.

Gaymard, B., Ploner, C.J., Rivaud-Péchoux, S. and Pierrot-Deseilligny, C. (1999) The frontal eye field is involved in spatial short-term memory but not in reflexive saccade inhibition. *Exp. Brain Res.*, 129: 288–301.

Goldman-Rakic, P.S. (1996) Regional and cellular fractionation of working memory. *Proc. Natl. Acad. Sci. USA*, 93: 13473–13480.

Goldman-Rakic, P.S., Selemon, L.D. and Schwartz, M.L. (1984) Dual pathways connecting the dorsolateral prefrontal cortex with the hippocampal formation and parahippocampal cortex in the rhesus monkey. *Neuroscience*, 12: 719–743.

Goldman-Rakic, P.S., Bates, J.F. and Chafee, M.V. (1992) The prefrontal cortex and internally generated motor acts. *Curr. Opin. Neurobiol.*, 2: 830–835.

Grosbras, M.H., Lobel, E., Van de Moortele, P.F., Le Bihan, D. and Berthoz, A. (1999) An anatomical landmark for the supplementary eye fields in human revealed with functional magnetic resonance imaging. *Cereb. Cortex*, 9: 705–711.

Grosbras, M.H., Leonards, U., Lobel, E., Poline, J.B., Le Bihan, D. and Berthoz, A. (2001) Human cortical networks for new and familiar sequences of saccades. *Cereb. Cortex*, 11: 606–618.

Heide, W. and Kömpf, D. (1998) Combined deficits of saccades and visuo-spatial orientation after cortical lesions. *Exp. Brain Res.*, 123: 164–171.

Heide, W., Blankenburg, M., Zimmermann, E. and Kömpf, D. (1995) Cortical control of double-step saccades — Implications for spatial orientation. *Ann. Neurol.*, 38: 739–748.

Heide, W., Binkofski, F., Seitz, R.J., Posse, S., Nitschke, M.F., Freund, H.J. and Kömpf, D. (2001) Activation of frontoparietal cortices during memorized triple-step sequences of saccadic eye movements: an fMRI study. *Eur. J. Neurosci.*, 13: 1177–1189.

Hikosaka, O., Sakai, K., Miyauchi, S., Takino, R., Sasaki, Y. and Pütz, B. (1996) Activation of human presupplementary area in learning of sequential procedures: a functional MRI study. *J. Neurophysiol.*, 76: 617–621.

Höllinger, P., Zenhäusern, R., Schroth, G. and Mattle, H.P. (2001) MR findings in Balint's syndrome following intrathecal methotrexate and cytarabine therapy in adult acute lymphoblastic leukemia. *Eur. Neurol.*, 46: 166–167.

Israël, I., Rivaud, S., Gaymard, B., Berthoz, A. and Pierrot-Deseilligny, C. (1995) Cortical control of vestibular-guided saccades in man. *Brain*, 118: 1169–1183.

Kastner, S. and Ungerleider, L.G. (2000) Mechanisms of visual attention in the human cortex. *Annu. Rev. Neurosci.*, 23: 315–341.

Kawashima, R., Naitoh, E., Matsumura, M., Itoh, H., Ono, S., Satoh, K., Gotoh, R., Koyama, M., Inoue, K., Yoshioka, S. and Fukuda, H. (1996) Topographic representation in human intraparietal sulcus of reaching and saccade. *Neuroreport*, 7: 1253–1256.

Kawashima, R., Tanji, J., Okada, K., Sigiura, M., Sato, K., Kinomura, S., Inoue, K., Ogawa, A. and Fukuda, H. (1998) Oculomotor sequence learning: a positron emission tomography study. *Exp. Brain Res.*, 122: 1–8.

Leigh, R.J. and Zee, D.S. (1999) *The Neurology of Eye Movements*. Oxford University Press, New York.

Leonard, B.W., Amaral, D.G., Squire, L.R. and Zola-Morgen, S. (1995) Transient memory impairment in monkeys with bilateral lesions of the entorhinal cortex. *J. Neurosci.*, 15: 5637–5659.

Lobel, E., Kahane, P., Leonards, U., Grosbras, M.H., Lehéricy, S., Le Bihan, D. and Berthoz, A. (2001) Localization of the human frontal eye fields: anatomical and functional findings from fMRI and intracerebral electrical stimulation. *J. Neurosurg.*, 95: 804–815.

Luna, B., Thulborn, K.R., Stojwas, M.H., McCurtain, B.J., Berman, R.A., Genovese, C.R. and Sweeney, J.A. (1998) Dorsal cortical regions subversing visually guided saccades in humans: an fMRI study. *Cereb. Cortex*, 8: 40–47.

Michel, F., Jeannerod, M. and Devic, M. (1965) Troubles de l'orientation visuelle dans les 3 dimensions de l'espace. *Cortex*, 1: 441–446.

Milea, D., Lobel, E., Lehericy, S., Berthoz, A. and Pierrot-Deseilligny, C. (2001) Functional MRI mapping of parietal and cingular activity during voluntary saccades. *Soc. Neurosci. Abstr.*: 71.27

Mort, D.J., Mannan, S.K., Hodgson, T.L., Anderson, E., Husain, M. and Kennard, C. (2000) An event-related fMRI study contrasting exogenous and endogenous saccades in humans. *Soc. Neurosci. Abstr.*, 26: 967.

Müri, R.M., Hess, C.W. and Meienberg, O. (1991) Transcranial stimulation of the human frontal eye field by magnetic pulses. *Exp. Brain Res.*, 86: 219–223.

Müri, R.M., Roesler, K.M. and Hess, C.W. (1994a) Influence of transcranial magnetic stimulation on the execution of memorized sequences of saccades in man. *Exp. Brain Res.*, 101: 521–524.

Müri, R.M., Rivaud, S., Timsit, S., Cornu, P. and Pierrot-Deseilligny, C. (1994b) The role of the right medial temporal lobe in the control of memory-guided saccades. *Exp. Brain Res.*, 101: 165–168.

Müri, R.M., Rivaud, S., Vermersch, A.I., Léger, J.M. and Pier-

16

rot-Deseilligny, C. (1995) Effects of transcranial magnetic stimulation on the supplementary motor area region during sequences of memory-guided saccades. *Exp. Brain Res.*, 104: 163–166.

Müri, R.M., Iba-Zizen, M.T., Derosier, C., Cabanis, E. and Pierrot-Deseilligny, C. (1996a) Location of the human posterior eye field with functional magnetic resonance imaging. *J. Neurol. Neurosurg. Psychiatry*, 6: 445–448.

Müri, R.M., Vermersch, A.I., Rivaud, S., Gaymard, B. and Pierrot-Deseilligny, C. (1996b) Effects of single-pulse transcranial magnetic stimulation over the prefrontal and posterior parietal cortices during memory-guided saccades in humans. *J. Neurophysiol.*, 76: 2102–2106.

Müri, R.M., Heid, O., Nirkko, A.C., Ozdoba, C., Felblinger, J., Schroth, G. and Hess, C.W. (1998) Functional organisation of saccades and antisaccades in the frontal lobe in humans: a study with echo planar functional magnetic resonance imaging. *J. Neurol. Neurosurg. Psychiatry*, 65: 374–377.

Müri, R.M., Felblinger, J., Ottiger, Y., Mosimann, U.P. and Hess, C.W. (2000a) Transcranial magnetic stimulation of the dorsolateral prefrontal cortex reduces antisaccade performance. *Soc. Neurosci. Abstr.*, 26: 1076.

Müri, R.M., Gaymard, B., Rivaud, S., Cassarini, J., Hess, C.W. and Pierrot-Deseilligny, C. (2000b) Hemispheric asymmetry in cortical control of memory-guided saccades. A transcranial magnetic stimulation study. *Neuropsychology*, 38: 1105–1111.

Nobre, A.C., Sebestyen, G.N., Gitetlman, D.R., Mesulam, M.M., Frackowiak, R.S.J. and Frith, C.D. (1997) Functional localization of the system for visuospatial attention using positron emission tomography. *Brain*, 120: 515–533.

Nyffeler., T, Pierrot-Deseilligny, C., Felblinger, J., Mosimann, U.P., Hess, C.W. and Muri, R.M. (2002) Time-dependent hierarchical organization of spatial working memory: a transcranial magnetic stimulation study. *Eur. J. Neurosci.*, 16: 1823–1827.

O'Sullivan, E.P., Jenkins, I.H., Henderson, L., Kennard, C. and Brooks, D.J. (1995) The functional anatomy of remembered saccades: a PET study. *Neuroreport*, 6(44): 2141–2144.

Paus, T. (1996) Location and function of the human frontal eye field: a selective review. *Neuropsychology*, 734: 475–483.

Paus, T. (2001) Primate anterior cingulate cortex: where motor control, drive and cognition interface. *Nat. Rev. Neurosci.*, 2: 417–424.

Pélisson, D., Goffart, L. and Guillaume, A. (2003) Control of saccadic eye movements and combined eye/head gaze shifts by the medio-posterior cerebellum. In: C. Prablanc, D. Pélisson and Y. Rossetti (Eds.), *Neural Control of Space Coding and Action Production. Progress in Brain Research*, Vol. 142. Elsevier, Amsterdam, pp. 69–89 (this volume).

Perry, R.J. and Zeki, S. (2000) The neurology of saccades and covert shifts in spatial attention. An event-related fMRI study. *Brain*, 123: 2273–2288.

Petit, L., Orsaud, C., Tzourio, N., Salamon, G., Mazoyer, B. and Berthoz, A. (1993) PET study of voluntary saccadic eye movements in humans: basal ganglia–thalamocortical system and cingulate cortex involvement. *J. Neurophysiol.*, 69: 1009–1017.

Petit, L., Orsaud, C., Tzourio, N., Crivello, F., Berthoz, A. and Mazoyer, B. (1996) Functional anatomy of prelearned sequence of horizontal saccades in humans. *J. Neurosci.*, 16: 3714–3726.

Petrides, M. and Pandya, D.N. (1999) Dorsolateral prefrontal cortex: comparative cytoarchitectonic analysis in the human and the macaque brain and corticocortical connection patterns. *Eur. J. Neurosci.*, 11: 1011–1036.

Pierrot-Deseilligny, C., Gautier, J.C. and Loron, P. (1988) Acquired ocular motor apraxia due to bilateral frontoparietal infarcts. *Ann. Neurol.*, 23: 199–202.

Pierrot-Deseilligny, C., Rivaud, S., Gaymard, B. and Agid, Y. (1991a) Cortical control of reflexive visually guided saccades in man. *Brain*, 114: 1473–1485.

Pierrot-Deseilligny, C., Rivaud, S., Gaymard, B. and Agid, Y. (1991b) Cortical control of memory-guided saccades in man. *Exp. Brain Res.*, 83: 607–617.

Pierrot-Deseilligny, C., Israël, I., Berthoz, A., Rivaud, S. and Gaymard, B. (1993) Role of the different frontal lobe areas in the control of the horizontal component of memory-guided saccades in man. *Exp. Brain Res.*, 95: 166–171.

Pierrot-Deseilligny, C., Müri, R.M., Rivaud, S. and Gaymard, B. (1995a) Eye movement disorders after prefrontal cortex lesions in humans. *Soc. Neurosci. Abstr.*, 21: 1270.

Pierrot-Deseilligny, C., Rivaud, S., Gaymard, B., Müri, R.M. and Vermersch, A.I. (1995b) Cortical control of saccades. *Ann. Neurol.*, 37: 557–567.

Pierrot-Deseilligny, C., Ploner, C., Müri, R.M., Gaymard, B. and Rivaud-Péchoux, S. (2002) Cortical control of spatial memory in humans: the visuo-oculomotor model. *Ann. Neurol.*, 52: 10–19..

Pierrot-Deseilligny, Müri, R.M., C., Ploner, C.J., Gaymard, B. and Rivaud-Péchoux, S. (2003) Decisional role of the dorsolateral prefrontal cortex in ocular motor behaviour. *Brain*, in press.

Ploner, C.J., Gaymard, B., Rivaud, S., Agid, Y. and Pierrot-Deseilligny, C. (1998) Temporal limits of spatial working memory in humans. *Eur. J. Neurosci.*, 10: 794–797.

Ploner, C.J., Gaymard, B., Ehrlé, N., Rivaud-Péchoux, S., Baulac, M., Brandt, S.A., Clémenceau, S., Samson, S. and Pierrot-Deseilligny, C. (1999a) Spatial memory deficits in patients with lesions affecting the medial temporal neocortex. *Ann. Neurol.*, 45: 312–319.

Ploner, C.J., Rivaud-Péchoux, S., Gaymard, B., Agid, Y. and Pierrot-Deseilligny, C. (1999b) Errors of memory-guided saccades in humans with lesions of the frontal eye field and the dorsolateral prefrontal cortex. *J. Neurophysiol.*, 82: 1086–1090.

Ploner, C.J., Gaymard, B., Rivaud-Pechoux, S., Baulac, M., Clémenceau, S., Samson, S. and Pierrot-Deseilligny, C. (2000) Lesions affecting the parahippocampal cortex yield spatial memory deficits in humans. *Cereb. Cortex*, 10: 1211–1216.

Ploner, C.J., Ostendorf, F., Brandt, S.A., Gaymard, B., Rivaud-Péchoux, S., Ploner, M., Villringer, A. and Pierrot-Deseilligny, C. (2001) Behavioral relevance modulates access to spatial working memory in humans. *Eur. J. Neurosci.*, 13: 357–363.

Rains, G.D. and Milner, B. (1994) Right-hippocampal contralateral-hand effect in the recall of spatial location in the tactual modality. *Neuropsychology*, 32: 1233–1242.

Rajkowska, G. and Goldman-Rakic, P.S. (1995) Cytoarchitectonic definition of prefrontal areas in the normal human cortex. II. Variability in locations of area 9 and 46 and relationship to the Talairach coordinate system. *Cereb. Cortex*, 5: 323–337.

Rempel-Clower, N.L., Zola, S.M., Squire, L.R. and Amaral, D.G. (1996) Three cases of enduring memory impairment after bilateral damage limited to the hippocampal formation. *J. Neurosci.*, 16: 5233–5255.

Rivaud, S., Müri, R.M., Gaymard, B., Vermersch, A.I. and Pierrot-Deseilligny, C. (1994) Eye movement disorders after frontal eye field lesions in humans. *Exp. Brain Res.*, 102: 110–120.

Rolls, E.T. (1999) Spatial view cells and the representation of place in the primate hippocampus. *Hippocampus*, 9: 467–480.

Shima, K., Aya, K., Mushiake, H., Inase, M., Aizawa, H. and Tanji, J. (1991) Two movement-related foci in the primate cingulate cortex observed in signal-triggered and self-paced forelimb movements. *J. Neurophysiol.*, 65: 188–202.

Sidman, M., Stoddard, L.T. and Mohr, J.P. (1968) Some additional observations of immediate memory in a patient with bilateral hippocampal lesions. *Neuropsychology*, 6: 245–254.

Suzuki, W.A. and Amaral, D.G. (1994) Perirhinal and parahippocampal cortices of the macaque monkey: Cortical afferents. *J. Comp. Neurol.*, 350: 497–533.

Sweeney, J.A., Mintun, M.A., Kwee, M., Wiseman, M.B., Brown, D.L., Rosenberg, D.R. and Carl, J.R. (1996) Positron emission tomography study of voluntary saccadic eye movements and spatial working memory. *J. Neurophysiol.*, 75: 454–468.

Tehovnik, E.J., Sommer, M.A., Chou, I.H., Slocum, W.M. and Schiller, P.H. (2000) Eye fields in the frontal lobes of primates. *Brain Res. Rev.*, 32: 413–448.

Tobler, P.N., Felblinger, J., Bürki, M., Nirkko, A.C., Ozdoba, C. and Müri, R.M. (2001) Functional organisation of the saccadic reference system processing extraretinal signals in humans. *Vis. Res.*, 41: 1351–1358.

Wang, X.J. (2001) Synaptic reverberation underlying mnemonic persistent activity. *Trends Neurosci.*, 24: 455–463.

White, J.M., Sparks, D.L. and Stanford, T.R. (1994) Saccades to remembered target locations: An analysis of systematic and variable errors. *Vis. Res.*, 34: 79–92.

Wipfli, M., Felblinger, J., Mosimann, U.P., Hess, C.W., Schlaepfer, T.F. and Müri, R.M. (2001) Double pulse transcranial magnetic stimulation over the frontal eye field facilitates triggering of memory-guided saccades. *Eur. J. Neurosci.*, 14: 571–575.

C. Prablanc, D. Pélisson and Y. Rossetti (Eds.)
Progress in Brain Research, Vol. 142
© 2003 Elsevier Science B.V. All rights reserved

CHAPTER 2

Effects of lesions of the cerebellar oculomotor vermis on eye movements in primate: binocular control

Mineo Takagi [1], Rafael Tamargo [2] and David S. Zee [3,*]

[1] *Divisions of Ophthalmology and Visual Science, Niigata University, Graduate School of Medical and Dental Sciences, and CREST,
Japan Science and Technology, Niigata, 951-8510, Japan*
[2] *Department of Neurosurgery, The Johns Hopkins University School of Medicine, Baltimore, MD 21287, USA*
[3] *Departments of Neurology and Ophthalmology, The Johns Hopkins University School of Medicine, Baltimore, MD 21287, USA*

Abstract: The effects of lesions of the dorsal 'oculomotor' cerebellar vermis on binocular oculomotor functions in three monkeys were examined. Prominent findings included (1) a convergence bias during monocular fixation, i.e., an 'esodeviation' in the absence of disparity cues, (2) a loss of comitancy, i.e., alignment varies more with orbital position, (3) abnormal saccade yoking producing saccade disconjugacy, and (4) defects in prism-induced phoria adaptation. There was also a suggestion of a disturbance in the dynamic properties of disparity-induced vergence. These findings point to a role for the 'oculomotor' vermis in binocular aspects of the control of eye movements.

Introduction

Our understanding of the role of the dorsal vermis (lobules V–VII) or 'oculomotor vermis' of the cerebellum in the control of conjugate eye movements has grown considerably in the past few decades, but much less is known about its role in binocular aspects of eye movement control (Robinson and Fuchs, 2001). The dorsal vermis of the cerebellum has been directly implicated in the control of saccades and pursuit eye movements (Takagi et al., 1998, 2000; Barash et al., 1999; Pélisson et al., 2003, this volume) but not directly in binocular aspects of ocular motor control, such as vergence and alignment. Clinical studies hint at a role for the cerebellum in the control of vergence and eye alignment (Holmes, 1922; Versino et al., 1996; Mossman and Halmagyi,

1997; Kono et al. 2002), and experimental lesion studies, too, support this idea (Westheimer and Blair, 1973; Burde et al., 1975; Vilis et al., 1983; Gamlin and Zhang, 1996; Scheurer et al., 2001). There is some evidence that the oculomotor vermis should be one region within the cerebellum that does contribute to the control of vergence, eye alignment and other aspects of binocular ocular motor control. Humans performing disparity discrimination tasks show an increase in activity in the dorsal cerebellum (Gulyás and Roland, 1994). There are also anatomical connections between the brainstem areas that carry vergence signals and the dorsal vermis and the underlying fastigial nuclei of the cerebellum (May et al., 1992; Gamlin and Clarke, 1995; Gamlin et al., 1996; Zhang and Gamlin, 1997). Lesions within the projection site of the dorsal vermis — the posterior portion of the fastigial nucleus called the FOR (fastigial oculomotor region) — lead to abnormalities of vergence (Gamlin and Zhang, 1996).

To clarify the role of the dorsal vermis in disconjugate ocular motor control, we studied the effects of lesions in the dorsal cerebellar vermis on vergence,

* Corresponding author: D.S. Zee, Path 2-210, The Johns Hopkins Hospital, Baltimore, MD 21287, USA. Tel.: +1-410-955-3319; Fax: +1-410-614-1746; E-mail: dzee@dizzy.med.jhu.edu

static eye alignment, the yoking of the eyes during saccades, and some aspects of vergence adaptation. Preliminary aspects of some of this data have been published (Takagi et al., 2001).

Methods

General experimental procedures

The three monkeys reported here are the same animals in which the effects of surgical ablations in the dorsal vermis on conjugate eye movements have been reported previously (Takagi et al., 1998; Takagi et al., 2000). The general experimental procedures, methods of recording eye movements and detailed description of the method and extent of surgical lesions, are described in those papers. For *monkey 1 (M1)*, the lesion was nearly symmetrical, being deepest in the midline where lobules VII and VIII were completely lesioned; lobules VI and IX were partially involved. For *monkey 2 (M2)*, lobules VI–VIII were lesioned on both sides although the lesion was deeper on the right. For *monkey 3 (M3)*, lobule VII was completely lesioned but there was mild sparing in lobule VI and moderate sparing in lobule VIII. In all three monkeys the cerebellar deep nuclei were completely spared including the posterior portion of the fastigial nucleus.

Eye movements were recorded with the magnetic field search coil technique as described previously (Takagi et al., 1998; Takagi et al., 2000). Saccades were marked using the criteria for the beginning of saccades when eye velocity reached $40°/s$ and the end of saccades when eye velocity dropped below $45°/s$.

Measures of static alignment

To measure static eye alignment, the monkeys were required to fix upon a 1.8×1.8 mm target presented on a video monitor placed at 33 cm from the eye. The target jumped to one of 25 target positions separated by $5°$ in a $25 \times 25°$ rectangular grid. For some of the analysis the data from the inner 9 and outer 16 positions were analyzed separately. Viewing was either monocular to test alignment (phoria) in the absence of disparity cues, or binocular to test alignment (tropia) in the presence of disparity cues.

An opaque occluder was attached to the head holder in front of one eye to assure monocular viewing. The horizontal and vertical angles of ocular misalignment were calculated as the difference in the respective positions of the right and left eyes. The position of the eye at each fixation point was taken just before the saccade in response to the target jump to the next position. A median value of the phoria at each eye position was calculated by averaging the right and left eye viewing data.

Binocular yoking during saccades

Binocular yoking during horizontal and vertical saccades was assessed by comparing the difference between the sizes of the pulse portion of the saccades made by each eye. Measurements were made during binocular viewing of visual targets (1.8×1.8 mm on a video display 33 cm away) since our animals had no static ocular misalignment with both eyes viewing.

Vergence

Pure vergence eye movements were elicited using small light-emitting diodes (2 mm diameter LEDs) on a bar aligned on the animal's mid-sagittal plane. From a center position the target jumped non-predictably to closer or farther positions to induce convergence or divergence, respectively. The amplitude of disparity was either 0.5 or $1.0°$. In all experiments with vergence there were no other lights on in the room apart from those on the stimulus array.

Phoria adaptation

Phoria adaptation was first tested with the animal wearing a laterally displacing Fresnel, paste-on prism. Five types of prisms were used: three for horizontal phoria adaptation (4Δ (prism diopters) base out, 10Δ base out, and 3Δ base in); and two for vertical phoria adaptation (2Δ base down and 2Δ base up). The prism adhered to a translucent piece of Plexiglas attached to the monkey's head holder and was positioned to cover the entire visual field of one eye. During binocular viewing these prisms called for convergence of about 2 or $5°$, divergence of $1.5°$, or a vertical hypertropia or hypotropia of $1°$, respectively. Before wearing the prism, eye alignment under binocular viewing and monocular viewing were measured. The monkey looked between a straight-ahead target and left and right 10°. The phoria was measured when the monkey fixed upon a distant (vergence angle of 1.0°) straight-ahead target (mean based upon 20 fixation periods). After the prism was placed, eye alignment was again measured with both eyes viewing to confirm that the prism had the desired effect on ocular alignment. Monkeys were then relieved of their head restraint but kept in their primate chair so they could look around the room (all lights were turned on) for 30 min with both eyes viewing while wearing the prism. The head of the animal was briefly restrained and the phoria measured three times, at 10-min intervals (10, 20, and 30 min) with the eye wearing the prism occluded. It took 1 min to make these measures. After the measurement was taken at 30 min, the prism was removed and the animal viewed binocularly for 5 more minutes. Eye alignment was then measured again to look for any sustained aftereffect. No more than one prism adaptation experiment was performed on a given day. No aftereffects were noted on the next day following a prism adaptation experiment.

Disconjugate, 'non-concomitant' phoria adaptation was elicited with a 2Δ Fresnel prism positioned to cover about one half of the visual field with the edge of the prism located near the midpoint of the orbit (Oohira and Zee, 1992). The prism was always placed on the temporal side of the visual field. The monkey wore the prism for 2 days. The prism was oriented to produce a relative divergence (exo prism) or convergence (eso prism), horizontally, or a relative hyperdeviation, vertically. Pre- and post-adaptation data were obtained with monocular viewing (the eye with the prism was transiently occluded during testing). Using a static alignment paradigm with targets at 5° intervals across a range of ±25°, the phoria was measured. The position of the eye was taken just before the saccade in response to each target displacement. The collection period for these two paradigms took about 10 min. Pre-adaptation, with both eyes viewing, eye alignment was measured to confirm that the prism was properly positioned. The monkey was then returned to its cage wearing the prism with both eyes viewing. 48 h later, alignment was measured again. Before any further testing of

adaptation the monkey was given 4 days of normal viewing, and alignment was re-tested to confirm that it had returned to normal.

The Johns Hopkins University committee on animal experimentation approved all surgical and experimental protocols, and all aspects of their care complied with the guidelines for veterinary care of The Johns Hopkins School of Medicine and of the National Institutes of Health Guide for the Care and Use of Animals including the appropriate use of analgesia after surgical procedures.

Results

Static alignment (phoria and tropia)

Fig. 1 plots the horizontal phoria, pre- and post-lesion. The median values of the phoria at the 25 different eye positions are plotted. Data were obtained before, in the first few weeks, and several months after the lesion. All three monkeys developed a relative esodeviation after the lesion. M1 developed an average esophoria of 1.7° over the 25 eye positions. It persisted even 3 months after the lesion. The pre-lesion exophoria of about 1.7° for M2 disappeared after the lesion and then reappeared when tested 4 months later. M3 developed an increase in its esophoria by about 1.6°. The phoria returned to its baseline value in 3 months. In contrast, no animal developed a tropia after the lesion. There were no changes in vertical alignment (phoria or tropia) after these vermal lesions.

We also examined the relative comitancy, i.e., how alignment varies with orbital position, pre- and post-lesion. Table 1 shows that the variability in phoria values, as reflected in the standard deviation of the phoria values over the range of eye positions tested, increased in all three animals following the lesion. Using the F-test for differences between variances the changes were statistically significant in M1 ($p < 0.05$) and close to being significant in the other two animals ($p = 0.07$). The variability returned to pre-lesion values only in the two animals (M2 and M3) in which the phoria reverted back to its pre-lesion value. We also compared changes in the phoria between the less eccentric, 'inner' fixation positions ($n = 9$) and the more eccentric 'outer' fixation positions ($n = 16$). In two animals (M1 and M3), the

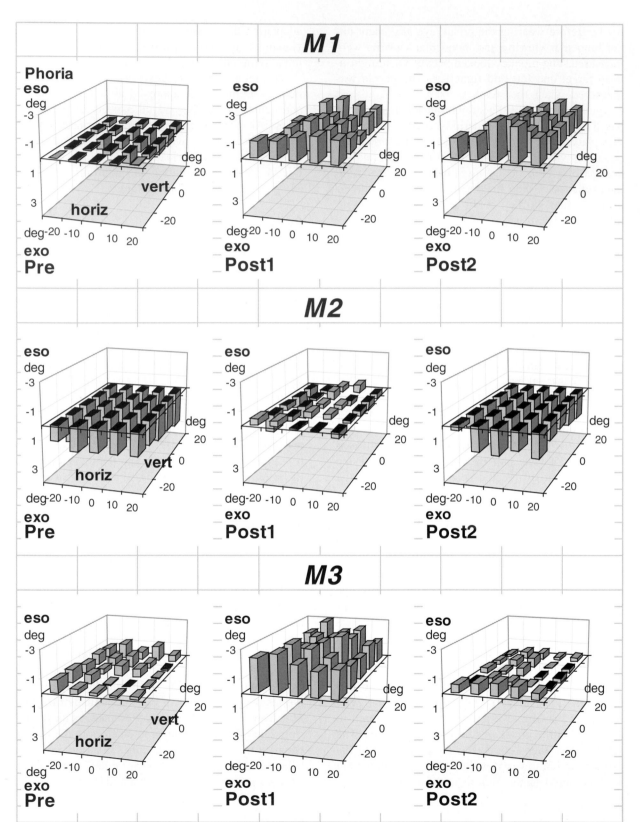

TABLE 1

Mean values of horizontal phoria and standard deviation across the 25 fixation positions (all), 9 inner fixation positions (inner) and 16 outer fixation positions (outer)

		Pre			Post1			Post2		
		outer	inner	all	outer	inner	all	outer	inner	all
M1	Mean	0.28	0.59	0.39	−1.26	−1.46	−1.33	−1.36	−1.58	−1.44
	SD	0.29	0.26	0.32	0.57	0.35	0.50	0.76	0.42	0.66
M2	Mean	1.70	1.62	1.67	0.23	−0.03	0.14	1.59	1.36	1.50
	SD	0.44	0.27	0.38	0.52	0.49	0.52	0.49	0.21	0.42
M3	Mean	−0.51	−0.47	−0.50	−1.99	−2.43	−2.15	−0.32	−0.27	−0.30
	SD	0.39	0.30	0.36	0.48	0.34	0.48	0.36	0.29	0.33

These data correspond to Fig. 1. Negative values are esophoria, positive values exophoria.

standard deviations of the phoria values increased more for the outer positions, in the third (*M2*), the opposite.

Dynamic alignment during saccades

Fig. 2 shows the difference in amplitude between the pulse portion of saccades for the two eyes, pre- and post-lesion. Viewing distance was 33 cm. For horizontal saccades (Fig. 2A), before the lesion, there was a small difference between the two eyes (usually <1.0°). For vertical saccades (Fig. 2B), binocular yoking was tighter, with the difference between the two eyes being <0.5°. The effects of the lesion were clear but relatively small for *M2* and *M3*, with some increase in the pulse–pulse difference, especially for rightward saccades. In *M1*, however, there was a marked change in saccade yoking; the pulse–pulse difference increased for some leftward saccades to values as high as 2.5° (compare filled and open symbols, Fig. 2A). The yoking of vertical saccades was little affected by the lesion in *monkeys 1* and *3*, but *monkey 2* showed a change for downward saccades and for large upward saccades (compare filled (pre-lesion) and open (post-lesion) symbols (Fig. 2B).

Pure vergence

The vergence response to small disparities (up to 1.0° only) was examined and there was little difference pre- and post-lesion for *M2* and *M3*. In *M1*, however, there was a clear change following the lesion. Average velocity traces were calculated for both divergence and convergence and are plotted for *M1* in Fig. 3. The main finding was a change in the dynamics of divergence. While slightly delayed, the first 50 ms or so of the divergence response appeared unchanged. In the next epoch, however, there was a decrease in divergence acceleration (compare slopes of black (pre-lesion) and gray (post-lesion) lines). Likewise, the peak value of vergence velocity for the larger disparity stimulus was diminished by about 25% post-lesion. The initial (first 25–40 ms) response to a convergence stimulus was similar pre and post-lesion, but immediately following, in the post-lesion trace (gray), there was some increase in convergence velocity. The increase in convergence velocity at 200 ms reflects a boost in vergence velocity because of associated saccades which is a normal phenomenon.

Fig. 1. Horizontal phoria (right eye minus left eye during monocular viewing): pre-lesion, and early and late post-lesion, in three monkeys. The median values of 10 phoria measurements at the 25 different eye positions are plotted. Horizontal eye positions of the fixing eye are shown on the bottom axis and vertical eye positions on the right hand axis. Data were obtained before the lesion (Pre), just after lesion (Post1: 7, 13 and 4 days after lesion for *M1*, *M2* and *M3*, respectively), and around 3 months after the lesion (Post2: 91, 121 and 81 days after lesion for *M1*, *M2* and *M3*, respectively). Note the relative esophoria that develops after lesions in the oculomotor vermis. (Modified from Takagi et al., 2001, with permission.)

PULSE-PULSE DIFFERENCE (Horizontal)

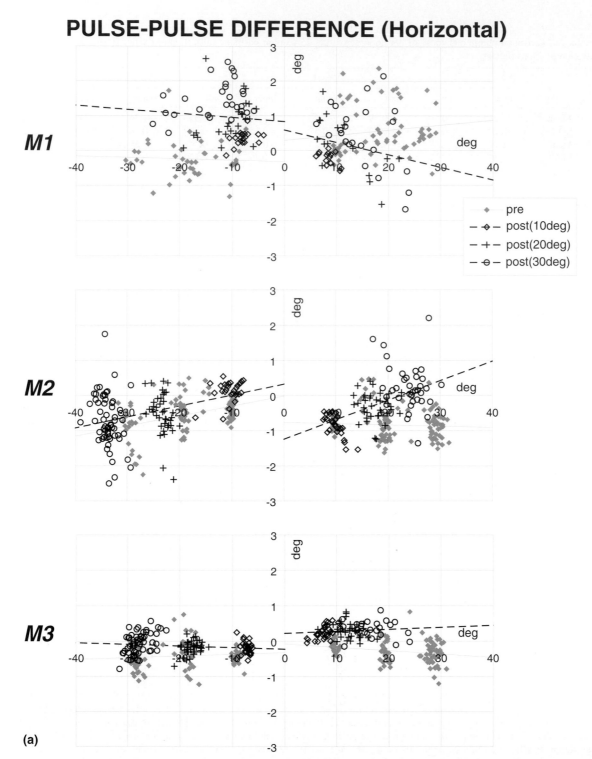

(a)

Fig. 2. Binocular yoking during horizontal (a) and vertical (b) saccades. Difference in the amplitudes (right minus left) of saccades between the two eyes (pulse–pulse difference) was plotted as a function of conjugate (average of right and left eye) saccade amplitude (abscissa). Measurements were made during binocular viewing. Pre-lesion and early post-lesion (first 2 weeks) results are shown. Regression lines were applied to the data. Symbols indicate target displacement. Note the difference between filled (pre-lesion) and open (post-lesion) data points, especially for *M1* for horizontal saccades and *M2* for vertical saccades.

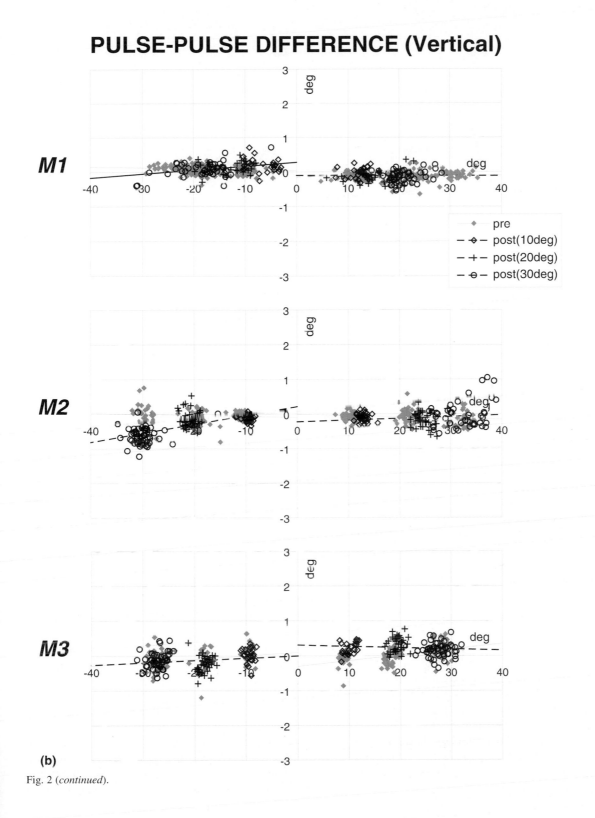

PULSE-PULSE DIFFERENCE (Vertical)

Fig. 2 (*continued*).

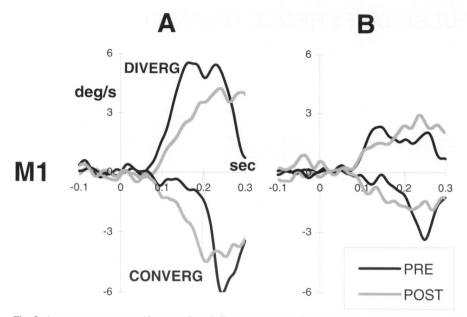

Fig. 3. Average convergence (downward) and divergence (upward) velocity traces for 20 trials for *M1*. Vergence responses were recorded 64 days after the lesion. Stimulus disparities are 1° (A) and 0.5° (B). Pre-lesion data are shown by darker traces. Note the increase in latency and decrease in rate of rise and peak value of divergence velocity for the larger disparity (A), post-lesion. There were subtler changes in the convergence response with perhaps some increase in vergence velocity post-lesion. Since saccades occurred at around 200 ms (thin dashed vertical line), changes in the velocity of pure vergence after this point cannot be evaluated.

Phoria adaptation

The time course of horizontal phoria adaptation to a prism placed in front of one eye, pre- and post-lesion, is shown in Fig. 4. Plotted are the phoria before adaptation, 10, 20 and 30 min after adaptation, and 5 min after exposure to normal binocular viewing. In all cases, the monkeys were able to fuse the disparities induced by the prisms and the vergence angle with binocular viewing was as predicted from the power of the prisms.

Pre-lesion, for the 10Δ base-out prism, the amount of adaptation gradually increased during the session. For the 4Δ base-out prisms there was a steep increase in the phoria during the first 10 min of adaptation, then little change thereafter. For the 3Δ base-in prism, adaptation reached a plateau within the first 10 min. The amount of phoria adaptation to the same prism varied among monkeys. Thus, *M1* had a strong tendency to develop esophoria. In a few cases, the amount of phoria adaptation in response to a base-out prism was larger than expected based upon the power of the prism.

Post-lesion, phoria adaptation by *M1* and *M2* was impaired for the large, 10Δ base-out prism even though they were able to overcome the prism-induced disparity and fuse the images of the target during the period they were wearing the prism. The change in phoria after 30 min of adaptation decreased to 38% for *M1* and 44% for *M2*. There was no change for *M3*. *M2* also showed a diminished adaptation to the 3Δ base-in prism. Little or no change was seen for the smaller, 4Δ base-out prism. Vertical phoria adaptation to a 2Δ base-up or base-down prism showed no change following the vermal lesions.

We also measured disconjugate, 'noncomitant' changes in alignment in response to wearing a prism that covered one-half (temporal side) of the visual field in front of one eye for 48 h. Fig. 5 shows the change in static alignment (phoria) in different orbital positions along the horizontal meridian for *M2*. Data before (Pre) and 2 days after (Post) adaptation wearing the 0–2Δ base-in ('exo') prism combination are shown. Before the lesion the monkey had little phoria in each position at this viewing distance. One

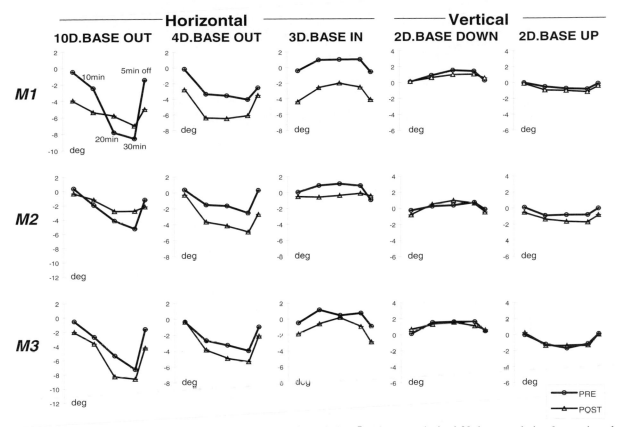

Fig. 4. The time course of horizontal phoria adaptation, pre- and post-lesion. Results were obtained 30 days post-lesion for *monkeys 1* and *2* (*M1* and *M2*), and >40 days after the lesion for *monkey 3* (*M3*). Animals wore a 10Δ base-out, 4Δ base-out, 3Δ base-in, 2Δ base-down and 2Δ base-up, Fresnel, paste-on displacing prism that covered the entire visual field of one eye. Measures of the phoria (right eye minus left eye under monocular viewing) were made before wearing the prism (0 min), at 10-min intervals up to 30 min with the prism, and then 5 min after binocular vision without the prism. Pre-lesion (open circles), the amount of adaptation showed a gradual increase during the session. Changes post-lesion were greatest in *monkey 1* (*M1*) and for the largest prism (10Δ base out). (Left hand panel is modified from Takagi et al., 2001, with permission.)

day and two days after wearing the prism, the phoria shifted in the direction appropriate to the demands of the prism (the dashed horizontal line) in the leftward eye positions. The change in phoria was gradual from right 7.5° to left 7.5°. Post-lesion, the monkey showed 1–2° of relative esophoria that was relatively noncomitant, compared to the pre-lesion data. There was some preservation of disconjugate phoria adaptation as the phoria shifted in a direction appropriate to the demands of the prism in the leftward eye positions. Post-lesion, however, there were also changes in rightward positions (where there should not have been) and adaptation occurred more slowly. Furthermore, compared to pre-lesion performance, the overall pattern of phoria adaptation post-lesion

was not tailored as precisely to the demands of the prism.

To see the effects of the disconjugate prism combination more clearly, independent of any baseline phoria, we plotted the difference between the post- and pre-adaptation values for the phoria at each orbital position, pre- and post-lesion (Fig. 6). Pre-lesion, the adaptation was complete within 1 day and thereafter there was little development of phoria. This was also true for most cases post-lesion, but for *monkey 3* with the 0–2Δ base-in (exo) prism, there was less phoria on the first day of wearing the prism. In the data for *M1* and *M3* with the 0–2Δ base-out (eso) prism, an esophoria developed with an appropriate amount and direction, both pre- and

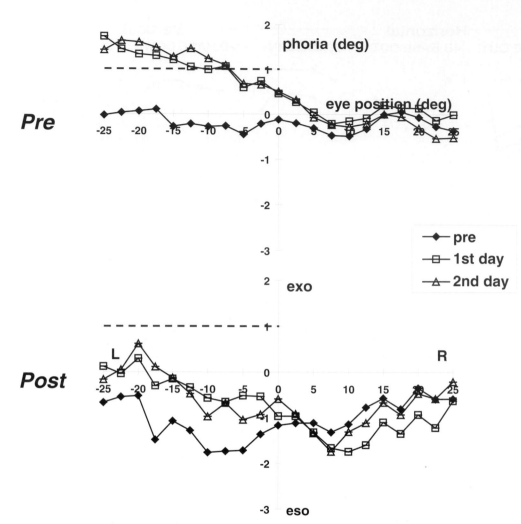

Fig. 5. The change in static alignment (phoria) in different orbital positions along the horizontal meridian from *M2*, with the 0–2Δ (exo) prism combination, pre-lesion. The phoria in each direction before, 1 day and 2 days after wearing the prism combination are shown. Upper panel shows pre-lesion, lower panel post-lesion. Horizontal dashed line indicates expected phoria required from 0 to 2Δ (exo) prism combination. Note that post-lesion there was some loss in the precision to which the phoria change was tailored to the demands of the prism.

post-lesion. Post-lesion, however, the phoria shifted to esophoria in the range where there was no prism. Similarly, with the 0–2Δ vertical prism, a hyperphoria of the appropriate amount and direction developed both pre- and post-lesion. In *M2*, however, the phoria shifted in the range where there was no prism (in downward orbital positions), post-lesion. Thus, while there were still adaptive changes in phoria as a function of eye position, post-lesion, the responses were less well tailored to the prism demand.

Discussion

The main implication of our study is that the dorsal 'oculomotor' vermis plays a role in the control of both static and dynamic aspects of maintaining the alignment of the eyes. This conclusion is not surprising since the fastigial oculomotor region (FOR), to which the dorsal vermis projects, has been implicated in the control of vergence. Zhang and Gamlin (1996) found neurons within the FOR that modulated with convergence alone or with convergence and saccades. Inactivation of this region with muscimol produced a decrease in convergence velocity and 'convergence insufficiency' (Gamlin and Zhang, 1996) and a relative exodeviation (Scheuerer et al., 2001). Both the dorsolateral pontine nucleus and the nucleus reticularis tegmenti pontis have neurons that discharge in relation to vergence and by virtue of projections directly to the FOR or via the oculomotor vermis, could provide the signals needed by the FOR to mediate its vergence function (Gamlin et al., 1996; Zhang and Gamlin, 1997). Moreover the oculomotor vermis is richly supplied with sensory information including orbital proprioception (Baker et al., 1972) as well as efferent copies of premotor oculomotor commands (Yamada and Noda, 1987; Ohtsuka and Noda, 1992). Thus, there is a rich anatomical and physiological substrate for a role for the oculomotor vermis in binocular eye movement control.

Disorder of static alignment

The most striking finding and consistent finding in our study was the development of a relative 'esophoria' following the lesion in each animal. This was enduring in one animal (*M1*), and resolved after several months in the other two. What might be the mechanism underlying such a change in phoria? First, there simply could be a change in tone, i.e., development of a bias towards relative convergence or divergence. Since, pre-lesion, each animal had a different 'baseline' phoria at the particular viewing distance at which it was measured, there must be a mechanism that sets this phoria value for individual subjects (Henson and Dharamshi, 1982). The cerebellum might play a specific role in, or have access to the networks that perform this function. The underlying FOR (fastigial oculomotor region) receives the sole (inhibitory) outflow from the Purkinje cells of the dorsal vermis. Therefore, the finding of a relative esophoria after dorsal vermal lesions implies that the FOR must contribute vergence tone towards a relative esodeviation, and that if the FOR itself were lesioned, the animals would show a relative exophoria. This seems to be the case (Gamlin and Zhang, 1996; Scheuerer et al., 2001).

Parenthetically, for *M2*, the lesion diminished its pre-lesion exophoria to almost perfect alignment, yet after recovery the alignment returned to the pre-le-

sion exophoria. This phenomenon is reminiscent of phoria adaptation in humans in whom a similar phenomenon occurs in response to wearing of a prism that corrects for a baseline deviation (Henson and Dharamshi, 1982). With sustained wearing of the prism the phoria returns to its initial value (clinically, this is related to 'eating up the prism').

Another aspect about the changes in phoria following the vermal lesions relates to the idea that the cerebellum functions to 'linearize' eye alignment as a function of the position of the eye in the orbit, i.e., to assure concomitancy. In this scenario, a cerebellar lesion might lead to an increased dependency of the phoria on orbital position, i.e., the phoria would become relatively noncomitant. Indeed, the horizontal misalignment — usually an esodeviation — that develops in human patients with more global cerebellar degenerations is relatively noncomitant compared to the natural phoria in intact human subjects (Versino et al., 1996). The findings in our monkeys were in accord with this idea since post-lesion there was an increase in the variability of the values of the phoria across the range of eye positions tested.

One might also have predicted that such effects on misalignment would be larger for more eccentric eye positions, where the effects of nonlinearities in orbital mechanical properties become more prominent. In our lesioned monkeys, however, the ocular misalignment became relatively more noncomitant in the more eccentric positions in only two of the animals (*M1* and *M3*). We cannot exclude, however, that if we had looked at even more eccentric positions we might have found relatively greater effects on eye alignment. To epitomize, the cerebellar vermis normally functions in the setting of the baseline vergence tone towards a relative exodeviation, and probably has a secondary effect on assuring that eye alignment is consistent across the visual field, i.e., preserves concomitancy.

Changes in dynamic properties of disparity-induced vergence

We also asked if lesions in the dorsal vermis led to changes in the dynamic properties of the initial, 'open-loop' portion of disparity-induced vergence. We have already shown that the same animals showed defects in the 'open-loop' control of two other types of visually guided eye movements, saccades and pursuit. Both the velocity and accuracy of saccades and the acceleration of the eyes during the initial portion of pursuit are affected by dorsal vermis lesions (Takagi et al., 1998, 2000). In the case of vergence, however, only in *M1* — the animal with the most enduring ocular motor abnormalities — was there a change in disparity-induced vergence, primarily a decrease in the rate of rise and the peak value of the velocity of divergence during the 'open-loop' period. There also may have been some increase in the rate of rise of convergence velocity, post-lesion. One might ask if these findings are simply an epiphenomenon of the static change in alignment, the relative esodeviation. This seems unlikely since the other animals also showed a relative esodeviation yet no change in the dynamic properties of divergence. Unfortunately, in all animals we only examined the vergence response to small-amplitude disparities, and then relatively late after the lesion. The effects of the lesion on the dynamic properties of vergence might have been more obvious with larger-amplitude stimuli or if we had examined disparity vergence earlier after the lesion, but this remains to be proven. Nevertheless, based upon the findings in *M1* it is attractive to speculate that since the dorsal vermis has a role in the control of the open-loop performance of the other foveally driven, visually driven eye movements (pursuit and saccades), that it might be the same for the open-loop, initial portion of disparity-induced vergence. In support of this idea is the finding of Gamlin and Zhang (1996) that inactivation of the FOR leads to a change in the dynamic properties of convergence.

Changes in saccade yoking

The most conspicuous changes in horizontal saccade conjugacy were noted in *M1*, in which the changes in static phoria were also most prominent. This animal, too, had the most striking changes in the control of the accuracy of conjugate saccades (Takagi et al., 1998). In the other two animals the changes were less prominent, though for each animal, in at least one direction, there was a clear change in saccade yoking following the lesion. Only *M2* showed a change in vertical saccade conjugacy; perhaps this was related to his lesion being more anterior, involving lobule VI to a greater degree than the other animals.

There is other evidence that the cerebellum might be involved in controlling saccade conjugacy. In humans, disconjugate dysmetria is a prominent finding (Versino et al., 1996). Cooling of the deep cerebellar nuclei, too, elicits alterations in saccade yoking (Vilis et al., 1983). Thus, we conclude that the dorsal vermis plays some role in assuring that saccades are conjugate.

Changes in phoria and disconjugate prism adaptation

The role for the cerebellum in phoria adaptation has been controversial. Judge (1987) studied monkeys after they had undergone removal of the flocculus and paraflocculus and found a normal range of phoria adaptation to a displacing prism. No pre-lesion data were available, however. Milder and Reinecke (1983) and Hain and Luebke (1990) studied human patients with cerebellar lesions and came to opposite conclusions about whether or not the cerebellum was involved in phoria adaptation. Hain and Luebke (1990) recorded adaptation to base-out prisms only; they found abnormalities in patients only when they had additional evidence for lesions outside the cerebellum. Milder and Reinecke (1983) studied responses to both base-in and base-out prisms in a smaller group of patients and found some abnormality in each patient but they also may have had lesions outside the cerebellum. Recently, Kono et al. (2002), studying patients with both acute and chronic dif-

Fig. 6. Disconjugate phoria adaptation, pre- and post-lesion. Values of phoria at each horizontal (left and middle columns) or vertical (right column) *relative* to pre-adaptation values are plotted on the ordinates. Panels are for *M1*, *M2* and *M3* from the top: in each panel the upper graph shows pre-lesion and the lower post-lesion data. Columns from the left are for 0–2Δ exo-prism, 0–2Δ eso-prism, 0–2Δ hyper-prism. Results from 1st, 2nd and 3rd day after wearing prism are plotted. Post-lesion, monkeys were tested with the 0–2 prisms between 26 and 57 days following surgery. Note the loss of precision in 'disconjugate' phoria adaptation for many of the prism combinations tested.

31

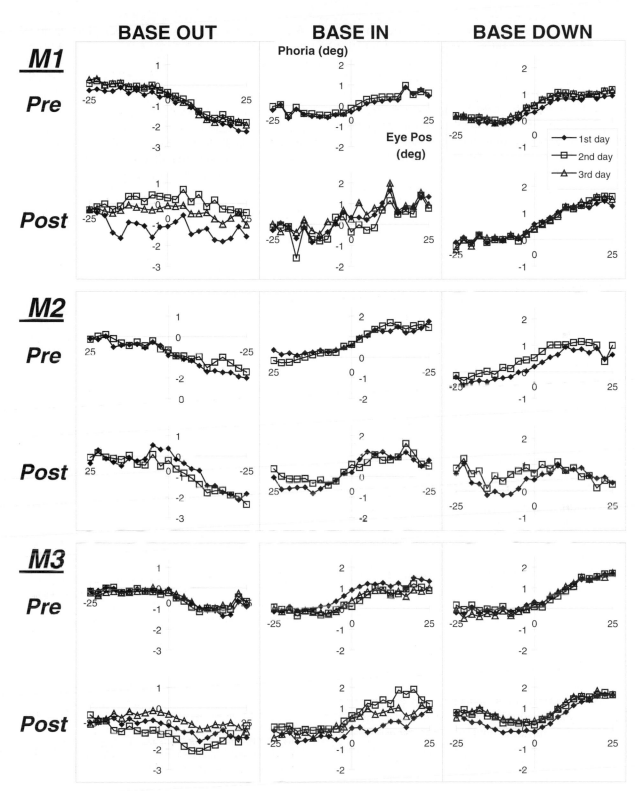

fuse cerebellar lesions, showed that vertical phoria adaptation was frequently impaired with cerebellar lesions, though the pattern of disturbance was somewhat idiosyncratic from patient to patient, and could even produce a change that overshot the desired effect. In the patients with transient cerebellar dysfunction there was recovery of phoria adaptation as their other cerebellar signs resolved

Our animals showed changes in phoria adaptation, though the pattern of change was idiosyncratic among animals. In response to wearing a prism that covered the entire field of one eye, which called for a constant change in eye alignment for all eye positions, there was a decreased adaptive response, especially for the larger prism calling for an esodeviation. One caveat is that since the animals had an esodeviation to begin with there could have been a relative limit or saturation value beyond which phoria adaptation could no longer operate.

Our animals also showed abnormalities in the disconjugate adaptation to a prism combination that called for orbital position-dependent adaptation. For static alignment some adaptation took place and usually in the right direction. The changes, however, were sometimes retarded and often not precisely tailored to the specific changes requested by the prism, implying perhaps some loss of ability to generate orbital-position dependent, adaptive responses.

In sum, our results point to a specific role for the oculomotor vermis in a variety of functions related to horizontal binocular eye movement control. Though the findings were idiosyncratic from animal to animal, there was a clear change in at least some aspect of binocular control in each animal. The most striking and enduring changes were in the animal (*M1*) that had the most profound changes in saccade and pursuit function. Many of the abnormalities of disconjugate eye movement control were similar to what has been reported in human patients with cerebellar disease. Disorders of static vertical alignment, however, which are also a feature of human cerebellar disease, were absent, with the exception of the one animal in which there was a change in dynamic vertical alignment during saccades. Taking into account all these findings, there must be areas of the cerebellar cortex apart from the vermal lobules lesioned here (predominantly VI and VII) that are involved with the control of both vertical and horizontal eye alignment. These remain to be discovered.

Acknowledgements

M. Takagi is supported by the Grants-in-Aid for Scientific Research 11671727 (the Japan Ministry of Education, Culture, Sports and Technology). D.S. Zee is supported by NIH grant R01-EY01849. Dr. R. John Leigh provided helpful suggestions.

References

Baker, R., Precht, W. and Llinas, R. (1972) Mossy and climbing fiber projections of extraocular muscle afferents to the cerebellum. *Brain Res.*, 38: 440–445.

Barash, S., Melikyan, A., Sivakov, A., Zhang, M., Glickstein, M. and Thier, P. (1999) Saccadic dysmetria and adaptation after lesions of the cerebellar vermis. *J. Neurosci.*, 19: 10931–10939.

Burde, R.M., Stroud, M.H., Roper Hall, G., Wirth, F.P. and O'Leary, J.L. (1975) Ocular motor dysfunction in total and hemi-cerebellectomized monkey. *Br. J. Ophthalmol.*, 59: 560–565.

Gamlin, P.D.R. and Clarke, R.J. (1995) Single-unit activity in the primate nucleus reticularis tegmenti pontis related to vergence and ocular accommodation. *J. Neurophysiol.*, 73: 2115–2119.

Gamlin, P.D.R. and Zhang, H.Y. (1996) Effects of muscimol blockade of the posterior fastigial nucleus on vergence and ocular accommodation in the primate. *Soc. Neurosci. Abstr.*, 22.

Gamlin, P.D.R., Yoon, K. and Zhang, H.Y. (1996) The role of cerebro-ponto-cerebellar pathways in the control of vergence eye movements. *Eye*, 10: 167–171.

Gulyás, B. and Roland, P.E. (1994) Binocularity disparity discrimination in human cerebral cortex: Functional anatomy by positron emission tomography. *Proc. Natl. Acad. Sci. USA*, 91: 1239–1243.

Hain, T.C. and Luebke, A. (1990) Phoria adaptation in patients with cerebellar lesions. *Invest. Ophthalmol. Vis. Sci.*, 31: 1394–1397.

Henson, D.B. and Dharamshi, B.G. (1982) Oculomotor adaptation to induced heterophoria and anisometropia. *Invest. Ophthalmol. Vis. Sci.*, 22: 234–240.

Holmes, G. (1922) Clinical symptoms of cerebellar disease and their interpretation (Croonian lectures III). *Lancet*, ii: 59–65.

Judge, S.J. (1987) Optically-induced changes in tonic vergence and AC/A ratios in normal monkeys and monkeys with lesions of the flocculus and the ventral paraflocculus. *Exp. Brain Res.*, 66: 1–9.

Kono, R., Hasebe, S., Ohtsuki, H., Kashihara, K. and Shiro, Y. (2002) Impaired vertical phoria adaptation in patients with cerebellar dysfunction. *Invest. Ophthalmol. Vis. Sci.*, 43: 673–678.

May, P.J., Porter, J.D. and Gamlin, P.D.R. (1992) Interconnections between the cerebellum and midbrain near response regions. *J. Comp. Neurol.*, 315: 98–116.

Milder, D.G. and Reinecke, R.D. (1983) Phoria adaptation to prisms. *Arch. Neurol.*, 49: 339–342.

Mossman, S. and Halmagyi, G.M. (1997) Partial ocular tilt reaction due to unilateral cerebellar lesion. *Neurology*, 49: 491–493.

Ohtsuka, K. and Noda, H. (1992) Burst discharges of mossy fibers in the oculomotor vermis of macaque monkeys during saccadic eye movements. *Neurosci. Res.*, 15: 102–114.

Oohira, A. and Zee, D.S. (1992) Disconjugate ocular motor adaptation in rhesus monkey. *Vis. Res.*, 32: 489–497.

Pélisson, D., Goffart, L., Guillaume, A. (2003) Control of saccadic eye movements and combined eye/head gaze shifts by the medio-posterior cerebellum. In: C. Prablanc, D. Pélisson and Y. Rossetti (Eds.), *Neural Control of Space Coding and Action Production. Progress in Brain Research*, Vol. 142. Elsevier, Amsterdam, pp. 69–89 (this volume).

Robinson, F.R. and Fuchs, A.F. (2001) The role of the cerebellum in voluntary eye movements. *Annu. Rev. Neurosci.*, 24: 981–1004.

Scheuerer, W., Petz, T., Eggert, T. and Straube, A. (2001) Static alignment after unilateral and bilateral pharmacological inactivation of the caudal fastigial nucleus in the monkey. *Soc. Neurosci. Abstr.*, 27: 2001.

Takagi, M., Zee, D.S. and Tamargo, R. (1998) Effects of lesions of the oculomotor vermis on eye movements in primate: saccades. *J. Neurophysiol.*, 80: 1911–1930.

Takagi, M., Zee, D.S. and Tamargo, R. (2000) Effects of lesions of the oculomotor cerebellar vermis on eye movements in primate: smooth pursuit. *J. Neurophysiol.*, 83: 247–262.

Takagi, M., Trillenberg, P. and Zee, D.S. (2001) Adaptive control of eye movements in humans: control of smooth pursuit, vergence and eye torsion. *Vis. Res.*, 41: 3329–3342.

Versino, M., Hurko, O. and Zee, D.S. (1996) Disorders of binocular control of eye movements in patients with cerebellar dysfunction. *Brain*, 119: 1933–1950.

Vilis, T., Snow, R. and Hore, J. (1983) Cerebellar saccadic dysmetria is not equal in the two eyes. *Exp. Brain Res.*, 51: 343–350.

Westheimer, G. and Blair, S. (1973) Oculomotor defects in cerebellectomized monkeys. *Invest. Ophthalmol.*, 12: 618–621.

Yamada, J. and Noda, H. (1987) Afferent and efferent connections of the oculomotor cerebellar vermis in the macaque monkey. *J. Comp. Neurol.*, 265: 224–241.

Zhang, H.Y. and Gamlin, P.D.R. (1996) Single-unit activity within the posterior fastigial nucleus during vergence and accommodation in the alert primate. *Soc. Neurosci. Abstr.*, 22.

Zhang, H.Y. and Gamlin, P.D.R. (1997) The dorsolateral pontine nucleus of the primate: neurons related to vergence and accommodation. *Soc. Neurosci. Abstr.*, 23.

C. Prablanc, D. Pélisson and Y. Rossetti (Eds.)
Progress in Brain Research, Vol. 142
© 2003 Published by Elsevier Science B.V.

CHAPTER 3

Single cell signals: an oculomotor perspective

David L. Sparks * and Neeraj J. Gandhi

Division of Neuroscience, Baylor College of Medicine, Houston, TX 77030, USA

Abstract: We examine the activity of individual neurons in three different brain areas where firing rate, number of spikes (the integral of discharge rate), and the location of the active cell within a motor map are used as coding schemes. The correlations between single cell activity and the parameters of a movement range from extremely tight (motoneurons) to non-existent (superior colliculus). We argue that the relationship between the activity of single cell activity and global aspects of behavior are best described as coarse coding for all three types of neuron. We also present evidence, in some cases in a preliminary and suggestive form, that the distribution of spikes in time, rather than average firing rate, may be important for all three neuron types, including those using a place code. Finally, we describe difficulties encountered in obtaining an estimate of the motor command when more than one oculomotor system is active.

Introduction

Many investigators have approached the problem of sensorimotor integration by asking how the activity of single sensory neurons in various subcortical and cortical regions contribute to neural representations of the environment. Complementary studies have addressed the question of how the activity of individual neurons residing at various locations in motor pathways contribute to the planning and execution of sensory initiated movements. Recently there has been renewed interest in the questions of what the activity of a single cell represents and which features of cellular activity are important (see, for example, Britten et al., 1992; Britten and Newsome, 1998; Shadlen and Newsome, 1998; Borst and Theunissen, 1999; Deneve et al., 1999; DeCharms and Zador, 2000; Kara et al., 2000; Movshon, 2000; Reinagel and Reid, 2000). Are perceptual and motor decisions based on the activity of a small number of neurons (sparse coding) or is it necessary to compile

* Corresponding author. Division of Neuroscience, Baylor College of Medicine, One Baylor Plaza, Houston, TX 77030, USA. Tel.: +1-713-798-4013; Fax: +1-713-798-3946; E-mail: sparks@cns.bcm.tmc.edu

inputs from a large population of neurons in order to make accurate perceptual and/or motor decisions (coarse coding)? Are sensory and motor signals conveyed by the average rate of firing over some short time period sufficient (rate coding), or is the precise placement of the spikes in time (temporal or interval coding) critical? Is knowing the location of the active neurons within a sensory or motor map (place coding) sufficient or does the rate of discharge of neurons in the active population provide additional information? Recent discussions of these and related questions have focused on the activity of cortical neurons. In this chapter we consider the same issues from the perspective of single cell activity observed in the oculomotor brainstem. The activity of motoneurons in the abducens nucleus, short-lead burst neurons in the paramedian pontine reticular formation, and saccade-related burst neurons in the superior colliculus will be examined in the context of coding schemes (rate, interval and place codes) and the relative importance of the activity of individual neurons (coarse vs. sparse coding). We will also explore the conditions in which the activity of a single neuron is a valid measure of motor performance by examining cellular activity from measurement and statistical perspectives. Reflecting on the properties of subcortical neurons involved in the control of movement could provide a different perspective on the significance of single cell signals in other sensory and motor systems.

Abducens neurons

Fig. 1A illustrates recordings from a single neuron in the right abducens nucleus. The top two traces plot horizontal and vertical eye position as a function of time. The next trace is a plot of instantaneous spike frequency, the reciprocal of interspike interval. The steady rate of action potentials observed while the eye is stationary near the center of the orbit is followed by a vigorous burst of activity before and during the rightward saccade. The burst of activity of motoneurons provides the innervation required to overcome the viscous resistance of the muscles and other orbital tissue and move the eye at a high speed. At the end of the saccade, there is a new, higher,

rate of firing that helps to overcome the elastic properties of the orbital tissue and hold the eye in the new position. As illustrated for two motoneurons in panel B, the relationship between tonic discharge rate and orbital position is linear. Motoneurons differ in the slope of the linear relationship and the orbital position at which they are recruited into action. Neurons that are recruited early have lower slopes than those that are recruited later (e.g., Robinson, 1970; Mays and Porter, 1984; Fuchs et al., 1988).

A measurement perspective

Table 1, modified from Stevens (1951), lists the different types of measurement scales, major defining features of each scale, and some of the types of statistical operations that are permissible with each type of measurement scale. For example, in *nominal scales*, numerals are merely used to label or classify numbers; words or letters would have been equally

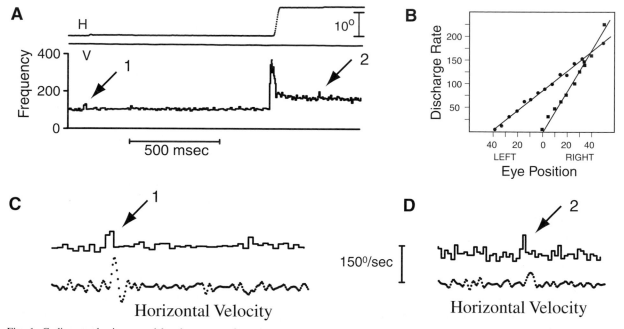

Fig. 1. Coding mechanisms used by the extraocular motoneurons. Horizontal and vertical eye position traces and the corresponding instantaneous spike rate of a motoneuron in the right abducens nucleus are plotted as a function of time (A). The motoneuron discharges at a constant rate during fixation, generates a burst to produce a rightward (on-direction) saccade and stabilizes at a higher, tonic rate during the post-saccadic fixation. The discharge rate recorded during fixation is a function of eye position, as illustrated for two motoneurons (B). While this result is suggestive of a rate-coding mechanism, a closer examination of the traces in (A) suggests that interval or temporal coding scheme is also prevalent. The instantaneous spike rate around arrows marked 1 and 2 in (A) are plotted with the corresponding horizontal eye velocity in (C) and (D), respectively. Note that the extra spike(s) above the tonic rate results in a momentary rightward deflection of the eye.

TABLE 1

Scales of measurement (modified from Stevens, 1951)

Scale	Empirical operations	Permissible statistics	Examples
Nominal	Determination of equality	Number of cases Mode Contingency correlation	'Numbering' of football players Assignment of type or model numbers to classes
Ordinal	Determination of greater or less	Median Percentiles Order correlation	Hardness of minerals Pleasantness of odors
Interval	Determination of equality of intervals or differences	Mean Standard deviation Order correlation Product–moment correlation	Temperature (Fahrenheit and Celsius) Energy Calendar dates
Ratio	Determination of equality of ratios	Geometric mean Coefficient of variation Decibel transformations	Length, weight, density resistance, etc. Loudness scale (sones)

effective. If classes containing several members have been formed it is possible to determine the mode or most numerous class. A number in an *ordinal scale* indicates the ranking of an item based upon some criterion, but the difference between rankings of 1 and 2 is usually not the same as the difference between rankings of 2 and 3. Review group ratings of grant applications are an example. An application assigned the score of 100 has a greater probability of being funded than an application assigned a score of 150. However, the difference between scores of 100 and 150 signify quite different things than the difference between scores of 300 and 350. The zero point on an *interval scale* is a matter of convention; the classic examples are the Fahrenheit and centigrade scales of temperature. Equal intervals of temperature are determined by measuring equal volumes of expansion, but lacking an absolute zero, it would be meaningless to state that 20°C is twice as hot as 10°C. Physical measurements of height, weight, and length are examples of measurements that meet the criteria for a *ratio scale* of measurement. It is meaningful to say that 10 m is twice as long as 5 m.

We examine the activity of brainstem neurons from this 'scales of measurement perspective' because only certain mathematical and statistical operations can be performed on each scale of measurement. For example, product moment correlations are permitted for data meeting the criteria of an interval scale, but not for data only meeting the criteria of an

ordinal scale. Why are these scales of measurement relevant to the activity of neurons? As will become apparent when the activity of neurons in the superior colliculus is discussed, measures of the activity of neurons residing in a motor map may not meet the criteria for any useful scale of measurement of the various attributes of a movement. Consequently, conventional statistical procedures may not be useful when trying to determine which aspect of a movement is coded by the activity of a cell.

For motoneurons, the tonic eye-position-related activity meets the criteria for an interval scale of measurement of horizontal eye position, at least under the experimental conditions used to obtain the slope and intercept of the linear regression line of best fit. The change in number of spikes/s when eye position changes from 10 to 20° is the same as when eye position changes from 20 to 30°. Because, the activity of these cells is a valid measure of a particular motor parameter, descriptive and inferential statistics such as mean, standard deviation and product moment correlations can be employed in additional analyses of the properties of these neurons.

Place, rate or interval coding?

In terms of the candidate coding schemes being considered, motoneurons appear to be coding eye position using a rate code. Periods of regular discharge rate are associated with stable eye positions and rapid changes in the rate of firing are associated with rapid changes in eye position (e.g., Fuchs et al., 1988). However, during slow movements of the eye, an additional increase or decrease in the instantaneous discharge rate is observed as the eye passes through a particular orbital position (Keller, 1981). A linear relationship is obtained when plotting instantaneous discharge rates as the eye passes through a fixed point at different velocities and the value of the slope, r, of the rate–velocity relationship has been used to construct a first-order differential equation relating each motoneuron's instantaneous firing rate to eye position and velocity (Keller, 1981). In a recent quantitative analysis of abducens neuron discharge dynamics during saccades and slow eye movements, Sylvestre and Cullen (1999) found that a single set of parameters could not be used to describe neuronal firing rates during both slow and rapid eye movements. The coefficients for eye velocity and position parameters consistently decreased as a function of the eye velocity that was generated.

DeCharms and Zador (2000) argue that the apparent distinction between the rate-coding hypothesis and the temporal-coding hypothesis is just one of time scale rather than of category. They note that the difference between rate coding and temporal coding for an individual spike train is based upon the interval chosen for counting the spikes and that the choice of interval is often based upon time scales believed to be relevant to a particular circumstance. According to this hypothesis, small variations in the exact timing of each spike could be important if we consider motoneuron activity during 5–10 ms periods rather than 200–400 ms intervals. Studies measuring motoneuron discharge with high temporal precision found the standard deviation of the interspike interval variability to be typically only about 6% of the mean discharge rate (Robinson, 1970; Keller and Robinson, 1972). However, in these experiments no attempt was made to relate small variations in the exact timing of each spike with minute changes in eye velocity or position. In our data archive we found recordings from several motoneurons in which small, brief deviations from the average firing rate were often *associated with* small, but observable, eye movements. As shown in Fig. 1C, the brief increment in the firing rate produced by two additional spikes was associated with a small eye movement having a

peak velocity of about $100°/s$. In Fig. 1D, a small increment in discharge rate produced by one additional spike was associated with a small movement having a peak velocity of $60°/s$. The prevalence of such correlations is unknown.

Coarse or sparse coding?

The coding scheme(s) employed (place, rate, or interval) need not determine whether the activity of a small number of neurons (sparse coding) or a large population of neurons (coarse coding) is used to make accurate perceptual decisions or to control accurate movements. The high correlations observed between the firing rate of individual motoneurons and eye position could be interpreted as evidence that the activity of a small number of motoneurons controls the position of the eye. However, consideration of a number of factors indicates that the contribution of each abducens motoneuron to the control of the orbital position of the eye is relatively small. The abducens nucleus contains approximately 1100 motoneurons (Steiger and Buttner-Ennever, 1978; Baker and Spencer, 1981). In terms of the steady firing rates observed during stable fixation intervals, most motoneurons have already been recruited into action when the eyes are in the center of the orbit (Robinson, 1970; Keller, 1977; Dean, 1996) and, accordingly, many motor units contribute to the muscle tension generated by the agonist muscle when the eye is in this position. It is likely that all the motoneurons have been recruited and all motor units participate in the generation of the tension required to hold the eye at a $25°$ eccentric position (in the pulling direction of the muscle). Furthermore, during the normal range of eye positions, motoneurons in the antagonist muscle motoneuron pool are also active and produce an innervation signal of opposite sign. Thus, as illustrated in Fig. 2A, horizontal eye position is controlled primarily by the ratio of motoneuron activity in the agonist and antagonist motoneuron pools. In theory, an infinite number of patterns of agonist and antagonist activity can maintain the eye in the same position. Three hypothetical examples are shown. In all three, the ratio of agonist and antagonist activity is the same and the eye is deviated $15°$ to the right. For the two cases shown on the left, the total output from the agonist and antago-

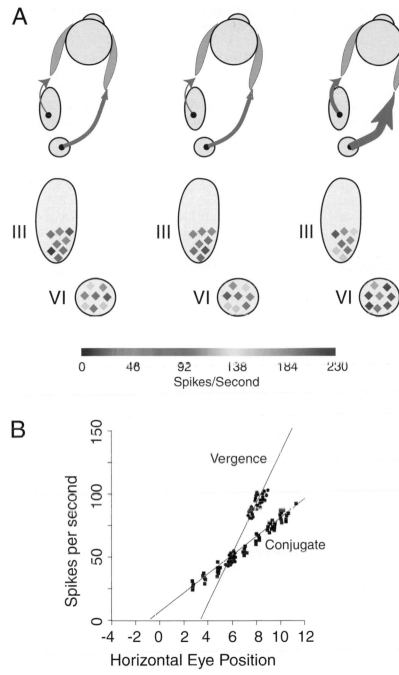

Fig. 2. Eye position is controlled by the ratio of activity in agonist and antagonist motoneuron pools. (A) The panel shows three schematics of the right globe connected to the lateral and medial recti muscles, their innervations from the abducens and oculomotor nuclei, respectively, and the level of activity in the representative motoneurons. The firing rates of the individual motoneurons in the three scenarios are different, as represented by the color scale, but the ratio of activity in the agonist and antagonist motoneuron pools is critical to maintain the eye in the same position. Thus, by recording the neural activity of any given neuron, we may not be able to determine the eye position. A perfect example is illustrated in the bottom panel (B), which demonstrates that the spike rate associated with the same eye position reached after a conjugate, saccadic eye movement and a disconjugate, vergence movement can be significantly different.

nist motoneuron pools is the same but the contribution of each of the neurons is different. In the third panel, the overall innervation level of both motoneuron pools is higher, but the same agonist/antagonist ratio is maintained. These patterns of activity constitute a motor equivalence class or 'motomere' (after the term 'metamere' used in color vision to describe two stimuli that are physically different but exactly matched perceptually).

What is the evidence that the eye may, in fact, be maintained in the same position by different patterns of motoneuron activity? Panel B of Fig. 2 illustrates one well-documented case (Mays and Porter, 1984). The firing rate of an abducens motoneuron is plotted as a function of horizontal eye position for eye positions reached by yoked movements of the two eyes during saccades and for the same positions reached by a convergence movement in which the two eyes move in opposite directions. Note that the same motoneuron fires at quite different rates, even though the eye is in the same orbital position. Henn and colleagues (Henn et al., 1984a) reported that the patterns of motoneuron activity associated with the same orbital eye position are different during alert waking behavior and light sleep.

To summarize, when the line of sight is shifted from one location to another at a fixed depth plane, the discharge rate of individual motoneurons is highly correlated with the steady position of the eye in the orbit. Under these specific conditions it is possible to accurately predict orbital eye position knowing only the firing rate of a single neuron. These correlations could be misinterpreted to suggest that the activity of a few neurons controls the orbital position of the eye when, as illustrated above, the sustained steady eye positions observed during fixation intervals are maintained by a large population of cells distributed throughout the motoneuron pools innervating the agonist and antagonist muscles. The same orbital position can be achieved by an infinite number of patterns of motoneuron activity. The relationship between firing rate and eye position obtained during fixation intervals in one depth plane cannot be used to accurately predict eye position during fixations in a different depth plane or to accurately predict when a particular eye position is reached during slow eye movements.

Short-lead burst neurons in paramedian pontine reticular formation

Accumulated evidence obtained from clinical, microstimulation, lesion, anatomical, and chronic single unit recording data indicates that neurons in the paramedian zone of the pontine reticular formation (PPRF) generate motor command signals responsible for the changes in the horizontal positions of the eyes during saccades and the quick phases of nystagmus (for reviews see Raphan and Cohen, 1978; Henn et al., 1984b; Fuchs et al., 1985; Hepp et al., 1989; Moschovakis and Highstein, 1994; Moschovakis et al., 1996). Fig. 3 illustrates the activity of a short-lead burst neuron (SLBN) in the PPRF. These neurons display extremely low rates of spontaneous activity and generate a vigorous burst of activity shortly before the onset of ipsilateral saccades. A series of horizontal saccades of different amplitudes and instantaneous frequency records of the associated bursts of activity are illustrated in panel A. For SLBNs burst duration is approximately the same as the saccade duration and, as illustrated in panel B, the number of spikes in the burst is highly correlated with the amplitude of the horizontal component of the saccade (Luschei and Fuchs, 1972; Keller, 1974; King and Fuchs, 1979; Van Gisbergen et al., 1981; Scudder et al., 1988). Also (not illustrated), the peak firing rates of SLBNs is highly correlated with peak saccadic velocity (Keller, 1974; Van Gisbergen et al., 1981). A subset of pontine SLBN, the excitatory burst neurons (EBNs) have monosynaptic connections with motoneurons in abducens nucleus and the timing and intensity of the discharge of EBNs are appropriate for producing the saccadic modulation in the motoneurons (Strassman et al., 1986).

Scales of measurement

From a measurement point of view, the number of spikes in the burst of a SLBN meets the criteria for an interval scale of measurement of the change in horizontal eye position, for the conditions under which the data were obtained. For the horizontal component of ipsilateral saccade, the difference in the number of spikes generated for 4° and 8° saccades, for example, is the same as the difference observed when saccades of 10° and 14° are observed. Thus, the statistical

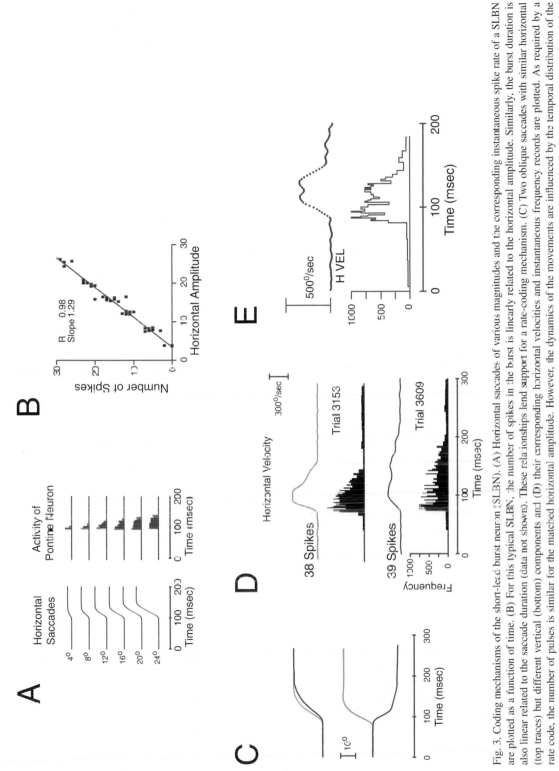

Fig. 3. Coding mechanisms of the short-lead burst neuron (SLBN). (A) Horizontal saccades of various magnitudes and the corresponding instantaneous spike rate of a SLBN are plotted as a function of time. (B) For this typical SLBN, the number of spikes in the burst is linearly related to the horizontal amplitude. Similarly, the burst duration is also linear related to the saccade duration (data not shown). These relationships lend support for a rate-coding mechanism. (C) Two oblique saccades with similar horizontal (top traces) but different vertical (bottom) components and (D) their corresponding horizontal velocities and instantaneous frequency records are plotted. As required by a rate code, the number of pulses is similar for the matched horizontal amplitude. However, the dynamics of the movements are influenced by the temporal distribution of the spike discharge, suggestive of a temporal code. (E) This observation is further illustrated for another neuron that dropped a spike during its burst and, consequently, resulted in a drop in the eye velocity. Therefore, like the motoneurons, the SLBNs may exhibit both rate and interval coding features.

analyses researchers have used to characterize these cells (see above) are appropriate.

Rate, interval, or place coding?

The time integral of firing rate, number of spikes, is highly correlated with the horizontal amplitude of saccades. Moreover, the distribution of spikes in time is also important, as indicated by the high correlation between the frequency of firing during the saccade-related burst and the velocity of the associated eye movement (Keller, 1974; King and Fuchs, 1979; Van Gisbergen et al., 1981; Cullen and Guitton, 1997a). Another example of the importance of the distribution of spikes in time is illustrated in panels C–E of Fig. 3. Panel D plots horizontal and vertical change in eye position as a function of time for the two oblique movements illustrated in panel C. Note that the horizontal amplitude of the two movements is the same but the movements have different durations because of variations in the amplitude of the vertical component of the movement. Beneath each velocity trace in panel D is a plot of the instantaneous discharge rate of the cell before and during that movement. Note that the cell generates 38 and 39 spikes in association with the top and bottom movements, respectively. The 38 spikes are distributed over about 80 ms and peak horizontal velocity is about 300°/s. The 39 spikes are distributed over about 150 ms; the peak velocity is much reduced and the movement duration is greater.

If, as suggested by DeCharms and Zador (2000), we examine the distribution of spikes over a shorter time period, does the exact placement of individual spikes become critical? We found no pertinent published data but were able to locate in our data archive recordings from cells in the medial vestibular nucleus indicating that this issue needs to be examined more carefully in future experiments. These neurons generate saccade-related bursts of activity and the number of spikes in the burst is highly correlated with the amplitude of the horizontal component of the saccade. For a few cells in our sample, the exact distribution of spikes in the burst was related to the velocity profile on a trial-by-trial basis. An example is shown in Fig. 3E. The close correspondence between the temporal pattern of activity of individual neurons and the profile of saccadic velocity on

a millisecond time scale suggests that either a few neurons have special effects upon the execution of saccades or, perhaps more likely, that the activity of some burst neurons can be synchronized.

Coarse or sparse coding?

Little is known about the relative contribution of individual EBNs to the generation of a saccade. Plots of number of spikes vs. saccade amplitude suggest that most EBNs are active before and during saccades larger than 5°. However, some SLBNs do not discharge before small (2–3° or smaller) saccades (see Fig. 3B). Based upon the information available, we conclude that a large population of pontine burst cells contributes to the generation of each saccade and that, despite the tight relationships between measures of spike activity and the parameters of the saccade, the contribution of each neuron to the movement is small. Other observations support this general conclusion. Strassman et al. (1986) found that the axonal terminals of individual EBNs were distributed in discrete patches in the abducens nucleus, covering a relatively small area of the nucleus. Local microstimulation at the site of putative EBNs rarely produces movements with saccadic velocity (Cohen and Komatsuzaki, 1972), suggesting that activation of a small number of EBNs does not recruit sufficient motoneurons to generate the innervation signal needed for a movement with saccadic velocity. Reversible inactivation of a small region of the pontine reticular formation produces reductions in saccadic velocity but does not prevent the occurrence of visually guided eye movements (Sparks et al., 2002). Collectively, these observations suggest that a large population of EBNs, spread over several millimeters, is active before and during each saccade and that the contribution of individual EBNs to the movement is small.

Saccade-related burst neurons in the superior colliculus

Fig. 4 illustrates properties of saccade-related burst neurons (SRBN) in the superior colliculus (SC). These cells generate a burst of action potentials before saccadic eye movements. The high frequency burst may reach instantaneous rates of 1000 or more

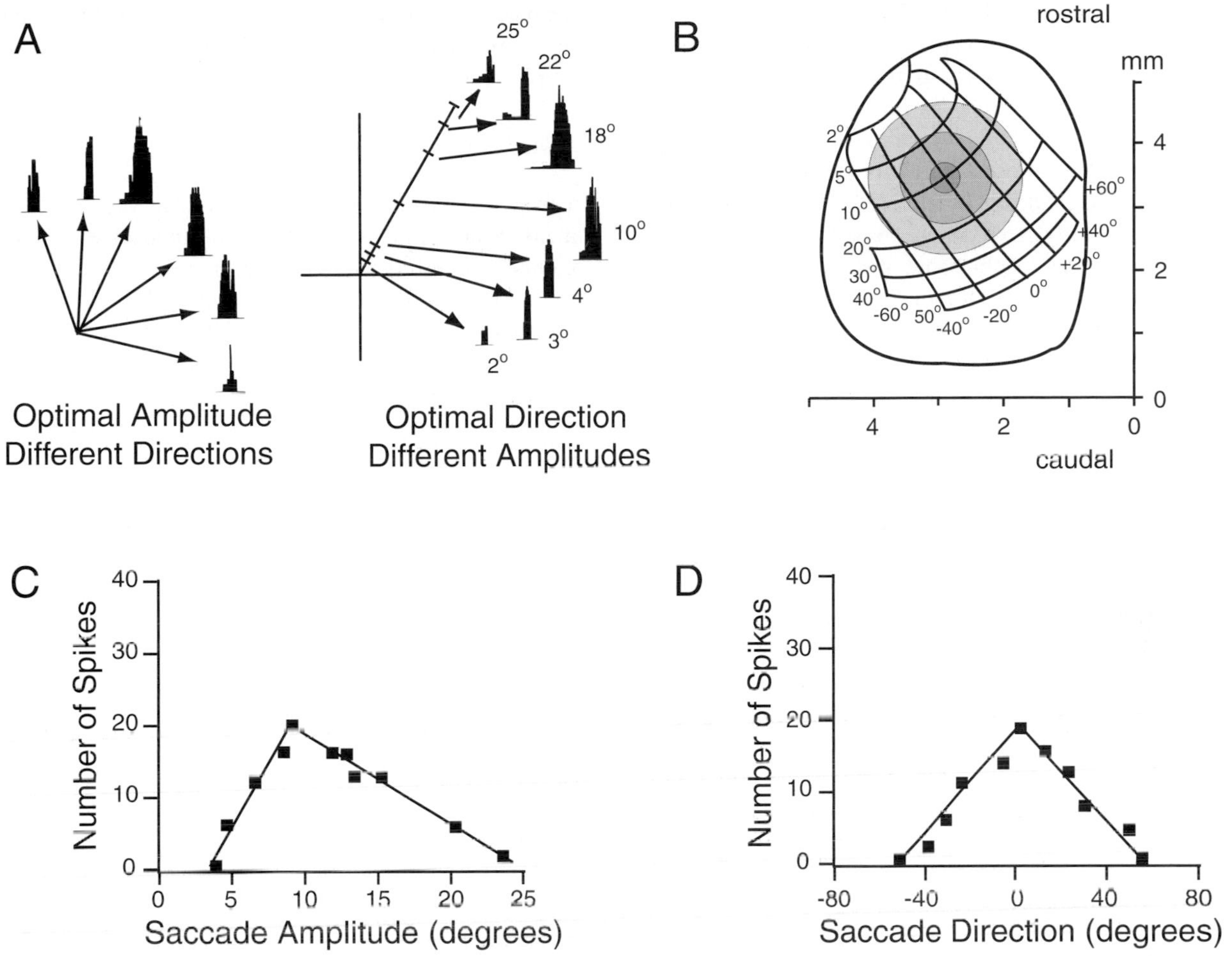

Fig. 4. Coding mechanisms and organization of the saccade-related burst neurons (SRBNs) in the superior colliculus. (A) The presaccadic discharge of a typical SRBN is plotted for eye movements of various amplitudes and directions to illustrate the properties of the movement field. The SRBN discharges a high frequency burst prior to onset of a saccade of optimal amplitude and direction. For movements of optimal amplitude but different directions and of variable amplitudes but in the optimal direction, the SRBN activity is later and weaker. (B) The motor map for saccadic eye movements, as constructed by Robinson (1972) is shown in the schematic. Neurons with small, optimal amplitudes reside in the rostral portion of the SC whereas cells discharging vigorously for large amplitudes are found in the caudal region. Similarly, neurons preferring saccades with upward (downward) components are localized within the medial (lateral) areas of the SC. The distribution is logarithmic along the rostral–caudal dimension (amplitude axis) but approximately linear along the medial–lateral extent (direction axis). A corollary of the observation that SRBNs are active for a large range of movements is that a large region of the superior colliculus is active during any given saccade. The shaded region depicts the spatial extent of activity for a horizontal 10° saccade. The gray scale indicates that neurons in the darkest region (center) discharge most vigorously while increasingly distant neurons (lighter shades) emit a later and weaker burst. This organization of neurons to form a motor map is a prime example of a place code. However, similar to the motoneurons and SLBNs, variability in the discharge rate for any given saccade often alters the dynamics of the movement (data not shown). In this sense, temporal coding features can also superimpose on a place code organization. (C,D) The plots quantify the qualitative assessment gathered from the format presented in (A). The data are from another SRBN. The number of spikes is plotted against amplitude for saccades in the optimal direction (C) and against direction for saccades of optimal amplitude (D). Neurons organized in a place code exhibit non-monotonic relationships between their spike count and saccade metrics, unlike the linear relationships observed for neurons (SLBNs and motoneurons) operating based on rate code. Thus, any given spike count of neurons in the SC does not reveal the amplitude of the executed saccade because each neural measure is associated with at least two saccade vectors. This trait of SRBNs does not meet the criteria for any useful scale of measurement, thereby preventing meaningful statistical measures on their activity (see text for details).

spikes per second. Each of these cells discharges maximally before movements of a particular direction and amplitude, but also discharges in association with a large range of eye movements. The activity of a typical SRBN is illustrated in panel A. This cell discharged most vigorously before upward and rightward saccades that were 14–18° in amplitude. Less vigorous activity was observed in association with movements of the same amplitude, but different directions. Similarly, for movements in the optimal direction, a weaker burst occurred for movements smaller or larger than the optimal amplitude.

Neurons of this type are organized according to the optimal amplitude and direction, and form a map of motor space. Fig. 4B illustrates the map of saccadic eye movement developed by Robinson (1972) (see figure legend for details). Because each cell discharges in association with a large number of saccades of different amplitudes and directions, a large population of cells is active before and during each saccade. The gray circles represents the hypothetical region of cellular activity associated with a 10° horizontal saccade. The population activity is characterized by a spatial and temporal gradient of activity: cells in the center of the active population (dark gray) discharge earliest and most vigorously whereas cells on the fringe of the active population (light gray) discharge later and less vigorously (Sparks and Mays, 1980).

The plots in panels C and D are sections through the movement field of a collicular cell. In panel C the number of spikes in the saccade-related burst is plotted as a function of the amplitude of the saccade for movements in the optimal direction. In panel D, the number of spikes in the burst is plotted as a function of saccade direction, for movement of the optimal amplitude. Note that the number of spikes, or peak frequency of the burst, or average frequency of the burst, or any other measure that we have considered is not linearly related to the amplitude — horizontal, vertical or vectorial component — or the direction of a saccade.

Thus, we observe a fundamental change in the relationship between spike activity and the metrics of movements when we move from motoneurons and pontine reticular formation to neurons in the SC. This change occurs because at the level of the SC, neurons are organized in a motor map and it is primarily the location of the cells in the map, not their rate of firing, that codes saccade direction and amplitude.

Scales of measurement

The non-monotonic relationships observed between measures of spike activity and the metrics of movements for neurons in superior colliculus is fundamentally different from the linear relationships observed for motoneurons and cells in PPRF. We postulated that the contribution of a single motoneuron or a single pontine EBN cell to the amplitude of a saccade or to the maintained position of the eye in the orbit is small. Nevertheless, because of the linear relationships between spike activity and measures of eye position and velocity, it is possible to make accurate predictions about the position of the eye in the orbit or changes in orbital position based upon the activity of a single neuron. In contrast, the activity of a single collicular neuron cannot be used to make accurate judgments about the direction or amplitude of a saccade. Referring to panel D, what could be concluded if it were known that two saccades occurred and the cell generated 5 spikes before the first saccade and 15 spikes before the second saccade? It is likely that 1 of 4 sequences of movements occurred: (a) a 5° saccade followed by a 7° saccade; (b) a 5° saccade and a 14° saccade; (c) a 20° saccade and a 7° saccade; or (d) a 20° saccade and a 14° saccade. Conclusions are limited because the activity of collicular neurons is ambiguous with respect to saccade direction and amplitude. As noted earlier, the same number of spikes is generated in association with a large range of movements having quite different directions and amplitude.

The activity of collicular neurons does not meet the criteria for any useful scale of measurement when used as a measure of the metrics of a saccade. Cell activity does not meet the criteria for an interval scale; equal changes in number of spikes do not indicate that equal changes in saccade amplitude have occurred. Measures of spike activity do not meet the criteria for an ordinal scale of measurement. A larger number of spikes does not mean that a movement with a larger (or smaller) amplitude has occurred. The practical consequences of this observation are that no useful statistics are permitted when using

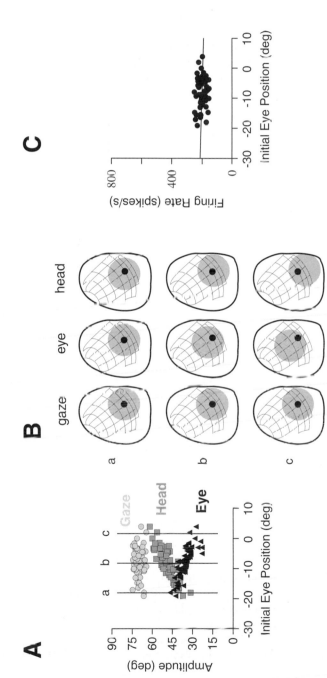

Fig. 5. Determining the role of superior colliculus neurons in the control of coordinated eye and head movements. Based on traditional head-restrained experiments in primates, the SRBNs are considered to encode saccadic eye movements. Recent studies have demonstrated that SRBNs also discharge during head-unrestrained gaze shifts. Is the activity of neurons that discharge before saccades in the head-restrained monkey coding for eye displacement or for a gaze displacement that is accomplished by an eye movement? If the head were free, would the activity correlate better with the ocular component, the head movement or the coordinated eye–head change in gaze? Constraints placed by scales of measurements principles prevent the use of statistical tests, such as multiple linear regression analysis, to address these questions. To circumvent these limitations, Freedman and Sparks (1997) analyzed activity of SC neurons recorded during gaze shifts of similar amplitude but starting from different initial eye position in the head (IEP). (A) Behavioral data: gaze amplitude (circles), eye contribution (triangles) and head contribution (squares) are plotted as a function of IEP. Note that for a group of amplitude-matched gaze shifts, the eye and head contributions vary inversely as the IEP changes. The eye (head) contributions increase (decrease) as the IEPs are increasingly more contralateral (negative values) to the direction of the gaze shifts. (The initial head position in space was not controlled in the study.) (B) Predictions regarding the spatial locus of activity in the SC (gray shade) depend on whether the SC encodes gaze (left column), eye (middle column) or head (right column). The three rows refer to the three vertical lines from panel (A) and indicate the active population of SC neurons during similar amplitude gaze shifts starting from three different IEPs. The black, filled circle corresponds to the site on the motor map encoding the executed gaze shift (see Fig. 4B). If SC neurons encode gaze shifts (left column) without regard to the individual eye and head contributions, the spatial distribution of active SC neurons (gray shade) remains the same across all initial eye positions. Furthermore, the black and gray circles remain concentric. If SC neurons encode only the ocular component (middle column), the population of active neurons will not correspond with the black circle. If SC neurons encode the head contribution (right column), the ensemble of active neurons will shift from rostral to caudal sites as the IEP becomes increasingly ipsilateral (top to bottom, sequentially). Also, the locus of the most intense activity will shift from rostral to caudal sites as the IEP becomes increasingly ipsilateral (top to bottom, sequentially). (C) Firing rate, averaged over the duration of each movement, from one SRBN is plotted against IEP for a set of similar-amplitude gaze shifts. The observation, that the firing rate is independent of IEP, supports the hypothesis that SC neurons encode gaze shifts.

the activity of a collicular SRBN as measure of movement parameters. Consequently, in their study of collicular activity in head-unrestrained animals generating coordinated movements of the eyes and head, Freedman and Sparks (1997) were not able to use statistical methods such as multiple regression techniques to determine if the activity of the cell was more related to eye, head, or gaze. As illustrated in Fig. 5, they were forced to use a more laborious experimental strategy to determine if the activity of a cell was specifying a movement of the eye, a movement of the head, or a change in gaze.

Rate, interval, or place coding?

As summarized above, although the vigor of discharge of a particular saccade-related burst cell varies for different movements within the movement field, information concerning saccade direction and amplitude is not contained within the discharge of a single cell. Unlike the primary vestibular afferents, for example, that encode head velocity by firing rate, the SC does not generate specific rates of firing to specify the direction or amplitude of a saccade. Saccade direction and amplitude are specified by the location of active neurons within the topographical map of movement fields, not their frequency of firing. Nonetheless, the level and temporal pattern of collicular activity does influence the velocity, duration, and amplitude of a saccade. A small number of stimulation pulses delivered to the SC during an on-going movement produces transient increases in the gaze velocity of cats (Munoz et al., 1991). Stanford et al. (1996) noted that stimulation trains must be continued until the site-specific maximal amplitude was obtained, otherwise the stimulation-evoked movement was truncated. They also observed, as previously reported in other animals (Du Lac and Knudsen, 1990; Pare et al., 1994) systematic effects of varying the frequency of stimulation upon the velocity of the evoked movements, indicating that the level of collicular activity is a determinant of saccade velocity. Results of experiments activating or inactivating the SC are consistent with this conclusion. The velocity of visually guided saccades is greatly reduced following inactivation of collicular neurons by local injections of muscimol or lidocaine (Hikosaka and Wurtz, 1985, 1986; Lee et al., 1988).

Manipulations in brain areas projecting to SC that indirectly affect the level or duration of collicular activity affect the speed and duration of saccades. Visually guided saccades are slowed or halted following electrical or pharmacological activation of areas that directly, or indirectly, inhibit saccade-related collicular activity (Munoz and Wurtz, 1993; Keller and Edelman, 1994). Inactivation of some of these same brain areas produces increases in saccade velocity (Munoz and Wurtz, 1993).

In summary, existing data are compatible with the hypothesis (Stanford et al., 1996) that a signal of desired displacement (amplitude and direction) is derived from the spatial location of collicular activity (a place code), the level of collicular activity influences movement velocity (a rate code), and ongoing collicular activity sustains the movement until the desired displacement is accomplished.

Sparse or coarse coding?

The case for coarse coding in the superior colliculus is strong. A large population of cells is active before and during each saccade and experiments in which a small subset of the active population was reversibly inactivated support the hypothesis that each member of the active population contributes to the movement (Lee et al., 1988). Saccadic accuracy results from the averaging of the movement tendencies produced by the entire active population (Lee et al., 1988; Sparks et al., 1990; Hanes and Wurtz, 2001). Small changes in the direction or amplitude of saccades are produced by slight shifts in the location of the large population of active cells. Interestingly, the large movement fields of collicular neurons may contribute to, rather than detract from, the accuracy of saccadic eye movements. The simulations of Baldi and Heiligenberg (1988) produced the apparently paradoxical result that, over a fairly large range, the wider the tuning curve of individual elements, i.e., the less precise they are, the more robust and precise the overall computation.

Single cell signals as estimates of commands being issued

According to traditional views of PPRF function, the excitatory burst neurons (EBNs) issue a saccadic eye movement command that is delivered, monosynaptically, to the extraocular motoneurons. More specifically, the number of spikes in the saccade-related burst generated by the EBNs is tightly correlated with saccade amplitude. However, during coordinated eye–head movements, the spike count of EBNs is better correlated with gaze amplitude than with the amplitude of the eye component (Ling et al., 1999). This observation also holds for the inhibitory burst neurons (Cullen et al., 1993; Cullen and Guitton, 1997b), which are thought to reflect the activity of EBNs. There is disagreement about the interpretation of these findings, but some investigators find these data consistent with models (e.g., Galiana and Guitton, 1992) in which a reference signal of desired gaze displacement, derived from the superior colliculus (SC), serves as the input to a single gaze motor error comparator that controls both eye and head movements (see Guitton et al., 2003, this volume).

To distinguish between the traditional and recently suggested roles of the EBNs in the control of gaze, we exploited the antagonistic relationship of EBN and omnipause neurons (OPNs). Located within nucleus raphe interpositus, OPNs form a discrete collection of cells that discharge tonically during fixation and are silent during saccades. They gate the output of EBNs through a monosynaptic inhibitory connection (Curthoys et al., 1984). Microstimulation can be used to selectively activate OPNs and interrupt ongoing saccades or delay their onset (Keller, 1977, 1977; King and Fuchs, 1977). If EBNs encode eye movements only, then stimulation of the OPNs during a gaze shift will perturb only the eye component; the head movement will be unattenuated. If, on the other hand, the EBN output is relayed to both eye and neck motoneurons, stimulation of the OPNs should attenuate both eye and head movements.

We found that OPN microstimulation triggered on the onset of a gaze shift halted the change in gaze, typically until the end of stimulation, but had little, if any, effect on the head movement (Gandhi and Sparks, 2001). The interruption in gaze was mediated via a perturbation in the eye movement: the ocular component of the gaze shift stopped in mid-flight and the eyes immediately began to counter-rotate to stabilize gaze (the gain of the vestibulo-ocular reflex was approximately 1). Stimulation

prior to the onset of the gaze shift delayed the onset of gaze, but not the onset of the head movement. Head movements were typically initiated during the microstimulation and, therefore, led gaze onset. The direction of gaze was stable during the stimulation because the eyes counter-rotated compensating for the ongoing head movement. At the end of the microstimulation train, the gaze shift was initiated by a saccadic eye movement in the same direction as the ongoing head movement (Gandhi and Sparks, 2001; Sparks et al., 2002). These results provide strong support for the hypothesis that the EBNs participate in the eye pathway and that commands to motoneurons innervating the neck muscles originate from structures upstream of the EBNs. This raises the question of why, in head unrestrained animals the number of spikes generated by pontine burst neurons is more highly correlated with the amplitude of the gaze shift than it is with the amplitude of the eye movement.

One possibility that has been suggested (Sparks, 1999; Sparks et al., 2002) is illustrated in Fig. 6. Panels B and C represent the output of a Simulink (Mathworks, Inc.; Natick, MA) model that simulates the commands illustrated in panel A. The model utilizes local gaze feedback (Laurutis and Robinson, 1986; Guitton and Volle, 1987; Pelisson et al., 1988; Galiana and Guitton, 1992) and assumes that EBNs generate commands for eye movements whereas commands for moving the head originate in an independent, parallel pathway, as illustrated in panel A. Movements of the head can influence the command signals reaching extraocular muscles via the vestibulo-ocular reflex (VOR) which, in the simulations shown, has a gain of 1. In panel B, gaze (bold, solid lines), eye (dashed lines), and head (thin, solid lines) position are plotted as a function of time for 9 gaze shifts. Three sets of movements are shown. In each set, independent commands to move the eye and head were issued. Eye movement commands were either 25, 30, or 35°. Associated head movement commands were 20% smaller than the eye movement command (20, 24, or 28°). Variations in the amplitude of the head contribution to gaze were introduced by having the head movement begin 50 ms before the eye movement or 10 or 50 ms after the eye movement. Note the accuracy of the gaze shifts. Despite differences in the commands sent to

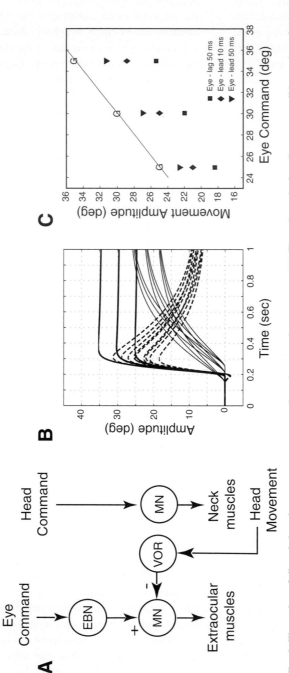

Fig. 6. Illustration of dissociations between motor commands and executed movements. (A) The schematic describes one possible version of the neural circuit that can implement coordinated movements of the eyes and head. The eye and head pathways receive separate inputs for desired eye and head movements, respectively. Furthermore, the gain of the vestibulo-ocular reflex is assumed to equal 1 during all gaze shifts and, therefore, the activity of the extraocular muscle motoneurons is reduced by an amount proportional to the amplitude of the head movement. This model was simulated on Simulink (Mathworks, Inc.). (B) The panel plots gaze (thick, solid lines), eye-in-head (dashed traces) and head (thin, solid curves) amplitudes as a function of time for a total of 9 simulations based on changing two variables: eye command and relative latency of eye with respect to head onset. Eye command was 25, 30 or 35°. Eye onset lagged head by 50 ms, led head onset by 10 ms or led head onset by 50 ms. The head command was always 80% of the eye command. (C) A quantification of the movements showed that gaze amplitude (G) always equaled the eye command. The slope of the best-fit line was one. Similarly, the total head amplitude equaled the head command (data not shown). In contrast, the eye component of the gaze shift was significantly less than the requested eye movement. Moreover, the perfect correlation between the eye command and the gaze amplitude wrongly leads to the suggestion that the EBNs encode gaze shifts (i.e., both eye and head movements), even though the EBNs encode the eye component only. See text for a discussion of the consequences of reducing the gain of the VOR during active gaze shifts.

the eye and head, changes in the relative timing of eye and head movements, and variations in the eye and head contributions to gaze, the change in gaze was exactly the displacement requested by the eye movement command. This occurred in the absence of an explicit gaze command. The changes in eye position were not those requested by the EBN signal. In this model, gaze, not eye, obeys the eye command. These observations are illustrated graphically in panel C. The amplitude of the gaze shift (G) and the eye movement (filled symbols) observed during the movements illustrated in panel B are plotted as a function of the command issued to the EYE. The thin solid line represents the unity gain slope. The points representing the amplitude of the gaze shift fall on the line representing unity gain for the eye movement command. The points representing the amplitude of the eye movement fall short of the unity gain line, depending upon the amplitude of the head movement occurring during the time period when the EBNs are active. Thus, if we were recording the activity of EBNs during these simulations, we would observe that the correlation between number of spikes in the burst and gaze amplitude was higher than the correlation between number of spikes and the amplitude of the eye movement. But, as demonstrated by examples, it would be incorrect to conclude that the output of the EBNs were relayed to motoneurons innervating neck muscles.

Motor physiologists would like to know how the activity of cortical and subcortical neurons is related to the motor command being issued. How do we know which motor command is being issued? In the absence of a head movement, measures of executed eye movements provide accurate estimates of the saccadic commands transmitted to the extraocular motoneurons. The estimates of the motor command are accurate because the motoneurons receive no additional inputs from other oculomotor subsystems (e.g., vergence, pursuit, vestibular) during the time when the saccade command is being implemented. Under these conditions, the amplitude of the movement is tightly correlated with the number of spikes in the saccade-related burst of pontine EBNs, and the peak velocity of the movement is tightly coupled to the peak frequency of the burst. However, when the motoneurons are receiving inputs from parallel oculomotor subsystems while a saccade is being generated, measures of the amplitude, direction or velocity of the executed saccade provide unreliable and potentially misleading estimates of the saccadic command issued to the motoneurons. Correlations of activity of premotor neurons with the amplitude, velocity, and duration of the executed eye movement cannot be used to make solid inferences about the motor signals being generated by the cells because of the dissociation between the command that is issued and the movement that is executed. This dissociation is illustrated by the simulated eye movements shown with dashed lines (Fig. 6B). The EBNs generated commands for a 25, 30, or 35° movement. Because the head was moving and the vestibulo-ocular reflex (VOR) was active with a gain of 1, the executed eye movements had amplitudes smaller than the movements that would have occurred if the head had not been moving. Because of the dissociation between the issued command and the executed movement, relationships between movement parameters and the activity of any neuron issuing an oculomotor command above the level of the motoneurons are misleading *in the absence of accurate information about other influences on motoneuron activity*. When more than one oculomotor subsystem is active (e.g., during combined eye–head gaze shifts or during static changes in the orientation of the head relative to gravity; Scherberger et al., 2001), the data obtained by correlating the activity of neurons above the level of motoneurons with various movement parameters must be interpreted cautiously.

The simulations illustrated in Fig. 6 were based upon the assumption that the gain of the vestibulo-ocular reflex was 1 during the executed movements. Numerous studies have shown that the gain of the VOR is reduced during gaze shifts and that the amount of the attenuation increases as the amplitude of the gaze shift increases (for references, see Roy and Cullen, 1998). However, large individual differences in the VOR attenuation observed during perturbations in head position occurring during large combined eye–head gaze shifts have been reported (Huterer and Cullen, 2001) and there is disagreement about the exact time course of the changes in VOR gain during the gaze shift (for references, see Roy and Cullen, 1998). Nevertheless, because the gain of the VOR is reduced during large gaze shifts, the actual differences between executed eye movements and the commands to move the eye will be smaller than those illustrated in Fig. 6C. Nonetheless, when there is a significant head contribution to the gaze shift, the executed eye movement will be an unreliable estimate of the command signal sent to the motoneuron because the VOR gain is not reduced to 0 during the entire time course of the gaze shift. Interpretation of the data correlating the activity of EBNs or other pre-motoneuron signals with changes in eye, head, and gaze position is difficult because, at this time, methods of measuring the instantaneous state of VOR gain during a single gaze shift or of estimating trial-to-trial variability in VOR gain are not readily available.

Summary and conclusions

Contemporary conceptual considerations of the role of the activity of individual neurons in the representation of sensory and perceptual phenomena and in the control of movements is largely restricted to data obtained from cortical neurons. In this chapter we have made an initial attempt to include data obtained from the oculomotor brainstem in our thinking about the significance of single cell activity. Our major conclusions and conjectures are summarized below.

For oculomotor motoneurons, a tight linear relationship (correlation coefficients in the 0.9 to 0.99 range) is observed between firing rate during fixation intervals and the orbital position of the eye. It would be possible to make extremely accurate estimates of eye position based upon the rate–position curves of a small number of motoneurons selected to cover the normal oculomotor range of eye position (see Fig. 1B). The ability to make accurate predictions of global behavior on the basis of a small number of cells does not constitute strong evidence for sparse coding. The number of neurons required to generate accurate predictions about motor outcomes is not necessarily an accurate estimate of the number of neurons required to implement the action. Indeed, in terms of the relative importance of individual neurons (coarse or sparse coding), we argue that the motoneuron control of orbital position is a coarse code. Each motoneuron innervates a small number of muscle fibers. The twitch and tetanic tension of each motor unit is small compared to total tension required to hold the eye in eccentric positions (see,

for example, Goldberg et al., 1998; Goldberg and Shall, 1999). Moreover, it is the ratio of the activity of neurons in the agonist and antagonist motoneuron pools that controls eye position. Finally, the question of coarse or sparse coding depends upon the level of analysis. The tension generated by individual extraocular muscle fibers is sparsely coded but, at a more global level, the position of the eye in the orbit is coarsely coded.

The relationship between motoneuron activity and eye position is not static. The firing rate associated with a given orbital position depends upon how that position was obtained (conjugate or disjunctive movements) and upon whether the eye is stationary or slowly moving through that position. We also presented preliminary data suggesting that rate and interval coding may coexist, depending upon the time scale being considered. In a few cells, small variations in the exact distribution of spikes were associated with minute changes in eye position. The prevalence of this phenomenon is unknown and if it occurs frequently, it will be important to determine if the relationship is due to synchronous activity in a subset of the neurons in the motoneuron pool.

The activity of SLBNs in PPRF also constitutes a rate code. The integral of spike rate (number of spikes) is correlated with saccade amplitude and it would be possible to make accurate predictions about the horizontal amplitude of a movement based upon a small number of pontine neurons. We speculate, however, that the representation of saccade amplitude by the activity of pontine neurons should be labeled coarse coding, not sparse coding. This speculation is based upon the large number of these cells located in a widespread region of pontine reticular formation, and upon the restricted effects of local microstimulation and reversible inactivation of a small subset of pontine cells. We also reported preliminary data suggesting that the exact distribution of spikes in the saccade-related burst of premotor neurons is associated with fine changes in the details of the velocity profile of a saccade. This result seems to contradict the coarse coding argument presented above, but that is not a necessary conclusion. Should further investigations indicate that small variations in the exact timing of each spike in the saccade-related burst are tightly coupled to measurable changes in saccadic velocity, the possibility that subgroups of pontine burst neurons have a tendency to discharge synchronously would need to be examined.

In the superior colliculus information about saccade direction and amplitude is represented as a place code, the location of the active population within the motor map. Yet, the duration and level of activity are important determinants of saccade duration and velocity. This indicates that the spatial and temporal pattern of activity within the collicular motor map is 'read out' by more than one mechanism, as previously suggested (Stanford et al., 1996).

Acknowledgements

This project was supported by NIH grants EY-01189 (DLS), EY-02520 and EY-07009 (NJG).

References

Baker, R. and Spencer, R. (1981) Synthesis of horizontal conjugate eye movement signals in the abducens nucleus. *Jap. J. EEG EMG Suppl.*, 31: 49–59.

Baldi, P. and Heiligenberg, W. (1988) How sensory maps could enhance resolution through ordered arrangements of broadly tuned receivers. *Biol. Cybern.*, 59: 313–318.

Borst, A. and Theunissen, F.E. (1999) Information theory and neural coding. *Nat. Neurosci.*, 2: 947–957.

Britten, K.H. and Newsome, W.T. (1998) Tuning bandwidths for near-threshold stimuli in area MT. *J. Neurophysiol.*, 80: 762–770.

Britten, K.H., Shadlen, M.N., Newsome, W.T. and Movshon, J.A. (1992) The analysis of visual motion: a comparison of neuronal and psychophysical performance. *J. Neurosci.*, 12: 4745–4765.

Cohen, B. and Komatsuzaki, A. (1972) Eye movements induced by stimulation of the pontine reticular formation: evidence for integration in oculomotor pathways. *Exp. Neurol.*, 36: 101–117.

Cullen, K.E. and Guitton, D. (1997a) Analysis of primate IBN spike trains using system identification techniques. I. Relationship to eye movement dynamics during head-fixed saccades. *J. Neurophysiol.*, 78: 3259–3282.

Cullen, K.E. and Guitton, D. (1997b) Analysis of primate IBN spike trains using system identification techniques. II. Gaze versus eye movement based models during combined eye–head gaze shifts. *J. Neurophysiol.*, 78: 3283–3306.

Cullen, K.E., Guitton, D., Rey, C.G. and Jiang, W. (1993) Gaze-related activity of putative inhibitory burst neurons in the head-free cat. *J. Neurophysiol.*, 70: 2678–2683.

Curthoys, I.S., Markham, C.H. and Furuya, N. (1984) Direct projection of pause neurons to nystagmus-related excitatory burst neurons in the cat pontine reticular formation. *Exp. Neurol.*, 83: 414–422.

Dean, P. (1996) Motor unit recruitment in a distributed model of extraocular muscle. *J. Neurophysiol.*, 76: 727–742.

DeCharms, R.C. and Zador, A. (2000) Neural representation and the cortical code. *Annu. Rev. Neurosci.*, 23: 613–647.

Deneve, S., Latham, P.E. and Pouget, A. (1999) Reading population codes: a neural implementation of ideal observers. *Nat. Neurosci.*, 2: 740–745.

Du Lac, S. and Knudsen, E.I. (1990) Neural maps of head movement vector and speed in the optic tectum of the barn owl. *J. Neurophysiol.*, 63: 131–1460.

Freedman, E.G. and Sparks, D.L. (1997) Activity of cells in the deeper layers of the superior colliculus of rhesus monkey: Evidence for a gaze displacement command. *J. Neurophysiol.*, 78: 1669–1690.

Fuchs, A.F., Kaneko, C.R.S. and Scudder, C.A. (1985) Brainstem control of saccadic eye movements. *Annu. Rev. Neurosci.*, 8: 307–337.

Fuchs, A.F., Scudder, C.A. and Kaneko, C.R.S. (1988) Discharge patterns and recruitment order of identified motoneurons and internuclear neurons in the monkey abducens nucleus. *J. Neurophysiol.*, 60: 1874–1895.

Galiana, H.L. and Guitton, D. (1992) Central organization and modeling of eye–head coordination during orienting gaze shifts. *Ann. NY Acad. Sci.*, 656: 452–471.

Gandhi, N.J. and Sparks, D.L. (2001) Accuracy of head-unrestrained gaze shifts interrupted by stimulation of the omnipause neurons in monkey *Soc. Neurosci. Abstr.*, 784.3.

Goldberg, S.J. and Shall, M.S. (1999) Motor units of extraocular muscles: recent findings. *Prog. Brain Res.*, 123: 221–232.

Goldberg, S.J., Meredith, M.A. and Shall, M.S. (1998) Extraocular motor unit and whole-muscle responses in the lateral rectus muscle of the squirrel monkey. *J. Neurosci.*, 18: 10629–10639.

Guitton, D. and Volle, M. (1987) Gaze control in humans: eye–head coordination during orienting movements to targets within and beyond the oculomotor range. *J. Neurophysiol.*, 58: 427–459.

Guitton, D., Bergeron, A., Choi, W.Y. and Matsuo, S. (2003) On the feedback control of orienting gaze shifts made with eye and head movements. In: C. Prablanc, D. Pélisson and Y. Rossetti (Eds.), *Neural Control of Space Coding and Action Production. Progress in Brain Research*, Vol. 142. Elsevier, Amsterdam, pp. 55–68 (this volume).

Hanes, D.P. and Wurtz, R.H. (2001) Interaction of the frontal eye field and superior colliculus for saccade generation. *J. Neurophysiol.*, 85: 804–815.

Henn, V., Lang, W., Hepp, K. and Reisine, H. (1984a) The sleep–wake transition in the oculomotor system. *Exp. Brain Res.*, 54: 166–176.

Henn, V., Lang, W., Hepp, K. and Reisine, H. (1984b) Experimental gaze palsies in monkeys and their relation to human pathology. *Brain*, 107: 619–636.

Hepp, K., Henn, V., Vilis, T. and Cohen, B. (1989) Brainstem regions related to saccade generation. In: R.H. Wurtz and M.E. Goldberg (Eds.), *The Neurobiology of Oculomotor Research*. Elsevier, Amsterdam, pp. 105–212.

Hikosaka, O. and Wurtz, R.H. (1985) Modification of saccadic eye movements by GABA-related substances. I: Effect of muscimol and bicuculline in monkey superior colliculus. *J. Neurophysiol.*, 53: 266–291.

Hikosaka, O. and Wurtz, R.H. (1986) Saccadic eye movements following injections of lidocaine into the superior colliculus. *Exp. Brain Res.*, 61: 531–539.

Huterer, M. and Cullen, K.E. (2001) Time course of vestibulo-ocular reflex suppression during gaze shifts. *Soc. Neurosci. Abstr.*, 403.23.

Kara, P., Reinagel, P. and Reid, R.C. (2000) Low response variability in simultaneously recorded retinal, thalamic, and cortical neurons. *Neuron*, 27: 635–646.

Keller, E.L. (1974) Participation of medial pontine reticular formation in eye movement generation in monkey. *J. Neurophysiol.*, 37: 316–332.

Keller, E.L. (1977) Control of saccadic eye movements by midline brain stem neurons. In: R. Baker and A. Berthoz (Eds.), *Control of Gaze by Brain Stem Neurons*. Elsevier/North-Holland, Amsterdam, pp. 327–336.

Keller, E.L. (1981) Oculomotor neuron behavior. In: B.L. Zuber (Ed.), *Models of Oculomotor Behavior*. CRC Press, Boca Raton, FL, pp. 1–19.

Keller, E.L. and Edelman, J.A. (1994) Use of interrupted saccade paradigm to study spatial and temporal dynamics of saccadic burst cells in superior colliculus in monkey. *J. Neurophysiol.*, 72: 2754–2770.

Keller, E.L. and Robinson, D.A. (1972) Abducens unit behavior in the monkey during vergence movements. *Vis. Res.*, 12: 369–382.

King, W.M. and Fuchs, A.F. (1977) Neuronal activity in the mesencephalon related to vertical eye movements. In: R. Baker and A. Berthoz (Eds.), *Control of Gaze by Brain Stem Neurons*. Elsevier/North-Holland, Amsterdam, pp. 319–326.

King, W.M. and Fuchs, A.F. (1979) Reticular control of vertical saccadic eye movements by mesencephalic burst neurons. *J. Neurophysiol.*, 42: 861–876.

Laurutis, V.P. and Robinson, D.A. (1986) The vestibulo-ocular reflex during human saccadic eye movements. *J. Physiol.*, 373: 209–233.

Lee, C., Rohrer, W. and Sparks, D. (1988) Population coding of saccadic eye movements by neurons in the superior colliculus. *Nature*, 332: 357–360.

Ling, L., Fuchs, A.F., Phillips, J.O. and Freedman, E.G. (1999) Apparent dissociation between saccadic eye movements and the firing patterns of premotor neurons and motoneurons. *J. Neurophysiol.*, 82: 2808–2811.

Luschei, E.S. and Fuchs, A.F. (1972) Activity of brain stem neurons during eye movements of alert monkeys. *J. Neurophysiol.*, 35: 445–461.

Mays, L.E. and Porter, J.S. (1984) Neural control of vergence eye movements: Activity of abducens and oculomotor neurons. *J. Neurophysiol.*, 52: 743–761.

Moschovakis, A.K. and Highstein, S.M. (1994) The anatomy and physiology of primate neurons that control rapid eye movements. *Annu. Rev. Neurosci.*, 17: 465–488.

Moschovakis, A.K., Scudder, C.A. and Highstein, S.M. (1996) The microscopic anatomy and physiology of the mammalian saccadic system. *Prog. Neurobiol.*, 50: 133–254.

Movshon, J.A. (2000) Reliability of neuronal responses. *Neuron*, 27: 412–414.

Munoz, D.P. and Wurtz, R.H. (1993) Fixation cells in monkey superior colliculus. II. Reversible activation and deactivation. *J. Neurophysiol.*, 70: 1–14.

Munoz, D.P., Guitton, D. and Pélisson, D. (1991) Control of orienting gaze shifts be tectoreticulospinal system in the head-free cat. III. Spatiotemporal characteristics of phasic motor discharges. *J. Neurophysiol.*, 66: 1642–1666.

Pare, M., Crommelinck, M. and Guitton, D. (1994) Gaze shifts evoked by stimulation of the superior colliculus in the head-free cat conform to the motor map but also depend on stimulus strength and fixation activity. *Exp. Brain Res.*, 101: 123–139.

Pelisson, D., Prablanc, C. and Urquizar, C. (1988) Vestibuloocular reflex inhibition and gaze saccade control characteristics during eye–head orientation in humans. *J. Neurophysiol.*, 59: 997–1013.

Raphan, T. and Cohen, B. (1978) Brainstem mechanisms for rapid and slow eye movements. *Annu. Rev. Physiol.*, 40: 527–552.

Reinagel, P. and Reid, R.C. (2000) Temporal coding of visual information in the thalamus. *J. Neurosci.*, 20: 5392–5400.

Robinson, D.A. (1970) Oculomotor unit behavior in the monkey. *J. Neurophysiol.*, 33: 393–404.

Robinson, D.A. (1972) Eye movements evoked by collicular stimulation in the alert monkey. *Vis. Res.*, 12: 1795–1808.

Roy, J.E. and Cullen, K.E. (1998) A neural correlate for vestibulo-ocular reflex suppression during voluntary eye–head gaze shifts. *Nat. Neurosci.*, 1: 404–410.

Scherberger, H., Cabungcal, J.H., Hepp, K., Suzuki, Y., Straumann, D. and Henn, V. (2001) Ocular counterroll modulates the preferred direction of saccade-related pontine burst neurons in the monkey. *J. Neurophysiol.*, 86: 935–949.

Scudder, C.A., Fuchs, A.F. and Langer, T.P. (1988) Characteristics and functional identification of saccadic inhibitory burst neurons in the alert monkey. *J. Neurophysiol.*, 59: 1430–1454.

Shadlen, M.N. and Newsome, W.T. (1998) The variable discharge of cortical neurons: implications for connectivity, computation, and information coding. *J. Neurosci.*, 18: 3870–3896.

Sparks, D.L. (1999) Conceptual issues related to the role of the superior colliculus in the control of gaze. *Curr. Opin. Neurobiol.*, 9: 698–707.

Sparks, D. and Mays, L. (1980) Movement fields of saccade-related burst neurons in the monkey superior colliculus. *Brain Res.*, 190: 39–50.

Sparks, D.L., Lee, C. and Rohrer, W.H. (1990) Population coding of the direction, amplitude, and velocity of saccadic eye movements by neurons in the superior colliculus. *Cold Spring Harb. Symp. Quant. Biol.*, 55: 805–811.

Sparks, D.L., Barton, E.J., Gandhi, N.J. and Nelson, J. (2002) Studies of the role of the paramedian pontine reticular formation (PPRF) in the control of head-restrained and head-unrestrained gaze shifts. *Ann. NY Acad. Sci.*, 956: 85–98.

Stanford, T.R., Freedman, E.G. and Sparks, D.L. (1996) The site and parameters of microstimulation determine the properties of eye movements evoked from the primate superior colliculus: Evidence for independent collicular signals of saccade displacement and velocity. *J. Neurophysiol.*, 76: 3360–3381.

Steiger, H.J. and Buttner-Ennever, J. (1978) Relationship between motoneurons and internuclear neurons in the abducens nucleus: a double retrograde tracer study in the cat. *Brain Res.*, 148: 181–188.

Stevens, S.S. (1951) Mathematics, measurement, and psychophysics. In: S.S. Stevens (Ed.), *Handbook of Experimental Psychology*. Wiley, New York, pp. 1–49.

Strassman, A., Highstein, S.M. and McCrea, R.A. (1986) Anatomy and physiology of saccadic burst neurons in the alert squirrel monkey. I. Excitatory burst neurons. *J. Comp. Neurol.*, 249: 337–357.

Sylvestre, P.A. and Cullen, K.E. (1999) Quantitative analysis of abducens neuron discharge dynamics during saccadic and slow eye movements. *J. Neurophysiol.*, 82: 2612–2632.

Van Gisbergen, J.A.M., Robinson, D.A. and Gielen, S. (1981) A quantitative analysis of generation of saccadic eye movements by burst neurons. *J. Neurophysiol.*, 45: 417–442.

C. Prablanc, D. Pélisson and Y. Rossetti (Eds.)
Progress in Brain Research, Vol. 142
© 2003 Published by Elsevier Science B.V.

CHAPTER 4

On the feedback control of orienting gaze shifts made with eye and head movements

Daniel Guitton *, Andre Bergeron, Woo Young Choi and Satoshi Matsuo

Montreal Neurological Institute, McGill University, 3801 University Street, Montreal, QC H3A 2B4, Canada

Abstract: Combined eye–head movements are routinely used to orient the visual axis (gaze) rapidly in space. The gaze control system can be modeled using a feedback system in which an internally created instantaneous gaze position error signal equivalent to the distance between the target and the current gaze position is used to drive brainstem eye and head motor circuits. The visual axis is driven until this gaze position error (GPE) is zero. The neural structure of the feedback system is discussed here. The midbrain's superior colliculus (SC) is implicated in gaze control but its 'location' in the feedback circuitry is debated. Our moving hill hypothesis proposed that the SC is within the feedback loop and that GPE is encoded topographically by a moving locus of activity on the motor map. In cat, fixation neurons of the superior colliculus encode GPE, which supports this model. Our preliminary evidence in both monkey and cat shows that neurons on the motor map respond to and encode, at very short latency, gaze shift perturbations. This further supports the hypothesis that the SC is within the gaze feedback loop.

Introduction

In current models of the saccadic eye movement system, derived from experiments in which the head of the animal under study is mechanically *fixed*, the eye saccade is driven by a burst generator that responds to a signal proportional to eye error (also called here eye-position-error), which equals the desired change of eye position in the head minus the actual change in eye position (Fig. 1A; reviewed in Scudder et al., 2002). Here we consider the control of the eyes' movement through space (gaze) during coordinated eye–head orienting gaze shifts. In our discussion of this subject we define gaze (G) = eye-in-space = eye-in-head (E/H) + head-in-space (H/S).

It has been proposed that the conceptual model of Fig. 1A can be extended to gaze control when the head is unrestrained (Roucoux et al., 1980; Fuller et al., 1983; Guitton et al., 1984, 1990; Laurutis and Robinson, 1986; Guitton and Volle, 1987; Pélisson et al., 1988; Tomlinson, 1990; reviewed in Guitton, 1992). A conceptual model of a gaze control system similar in structure to that shown in Fig. 1A but now incorporating the head motor system is shown in Fig. 1B. In this model, brainstem, eye and head motor circuits are driven by a signal encoding gaze error (hereafter called gaze-position-error, GPE). We have proposed a model, using this structure, that permits compensation for gaze trajectory perturbations and which also predicts non-intuitive properties of the gaze motor system such as eye position saturation (Galiana and Guitton, 1992).

In the schema of Fig. 1B, an estimate of the actual change in gaze position is obtained by integrating the sum of eye and head velocities. The signal for 'head velocity relative to space' ($\dot{H}^*/S$) is assumed to be derived from the output of the semicircular canals (see section below). The head and eye motor systems are driven to nullify GPE, i.e. until the

* Correspondence to: D. Guitton, Montreal Neurological Institute, 3801 University Street, Montreal, QC H3A 2B4, Canada. Tel.: +1-514-398-1954; Fax: +1-514-398-8106; E-mail: dguitt@mni.mcgill.ca

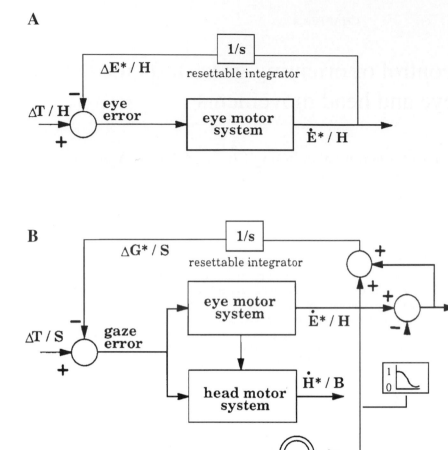

Fig. 1. Simplified feedback circuits for controlling saccades. (A) Classic scheme that controls eye saccades in the head-fixed condition. Input to system is desired angular change in eye position, equivalent to target offset angle ($\Delta T/S$). A signal proportional to eye position error (eye error) drives the saccade generator and is constructed by subtracting an internal signal encoding the actual change in eye position ($\Delta E^*/H$) from $\Delta T/S$. $\Delta E^*/H$ is obtained by integrating eye velocity in the box labeled '1/s' (the Laplacian symbol for integration). Eye velocity is provided by brainstem burst neurons. After the saccade the integrator is reset to zero. (B) Analogous scheme for controlling gaze saccades made head-unrestrained. The signal driving the eye and head motor circuits is gaze error (or gaze position error). Actual change in gaze position is obtained by integrating the sum of eye velocity relative to head and head velocity relative to space. The signal encoding head velocity is provided by the semicircular canals (SCC). The actual eye velocity depends on the influence of the SCC on the eye; i.e. on the interaction between the VOR and saccade signals. Before being added to the eye motor system's output, the VOR signal is attenuated in relation to gaze error, by the function in the box whose horizontal axis is gaze error and vertical axis is the canal signal impinging on the eye circuitry. Asterisk indicates that the designated parameter is an internal signal. Dots overlying letter indicate velocity.

desired change in gaze position ($\Delta T/S$) minus the actual change in gaze position ($\Delta G^*/S$) equals zero. At that point the saccadic gaze-generating system of Fig. 1B is disengaged and the compensatory phase of eye rotation, driven by the vestibulo-ocular reflex (VOR), commences. The gaze stabilization system is not shown in Fig. 1B. In this paper we will not consider in detail either the boxes labeled eye and head motor systems, or the influence of the VOR on the eye system. We will focus mainly on the question of feedback control and the generation of a GPE signal.

Experimental verification of gaze feedback

The diagram in Fig. 1B suggests that excellent gaze accuracy can be obtained, independent of the characteristics of the gaze trajectory and of whether head motion is normal, or perturbed. The system attempts to nullify the GPE no matter what the trajectories of eye and head are. I will now summarize different lines of evidence obtained in humans, monkeys and cats that support such a gaze feedback scheme.

Behavioral observations

Fig. 2 shows different eye, head and gaze trajectories that result when a human subject in the light makes three very large gaze shifts of the same amplitude (120°) but with different head velocities (Guitton and Volle, 1987). Initial gaze position was on a fixation point 60° to the left of the body midline, and when it was extinguished the subject oriented to the remembered location of a peripheral target at

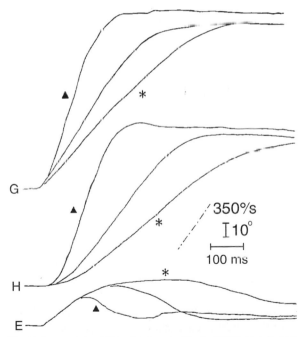

Fig. 2. Large gaze shifts of same amplitude (120°) in a human subject instructed to move head at different velocities. Associated eye (E) head (H) and gaze (G) traces are marked by same symbol. Initial eye trajectories are the same irrespective of head trajectory, indicating absence of vestibulo-ocular reflex (VOR) on eye motion.

60° to the right. The traces have been aligned on the onset of the gaze shifts. Trajectories that correspond to the same movement are identified by the same symbol. Consider first the gaze trace resulting from the fastest head movement, marked by the black triangle. The early part of the gaze shift is driven by an ocular saccade. As the gaze shift progresses, the eye soon begins to slow down and turn around in the orbit, such that for the final 1/3 of the gaze trajectory the eye is moving in a direction opposite to head motion. The ocular counter-rotation, whose velocity is too low to counter head motion, may be the result of either a low-gain VOR, with no saccade signal, or of summing signals that drive respectively the eye saccade in one direction and the VOR in the other. The precise mechanisms underlying this are not the subject of this paper. Consider now the slowest head movement. In this case, the eye saccade reaches a position saturation and the eye remains immobile there until gaze is in the final 1/3 of its trajectory, after which the eye begins counter-rolling in the orbit. The saturation position (at about 35°) is not at the mechanical limits (about 52° in this subject) of eye motion (Guitton and Volle, 1987). In all three examples gaze gets on target within a few degrees, irrespective of the very different head and eye trajectories. In particular, for the slow head movements the eye hovers, immobile in the orbit, until gaze approaches target, at which point the counter rotation begins. This phenomenon, combined with the excellent gaze accuracy in these movements, suggests the action of a feedback loop. A method for testing more rigorously this hypothesis is to perturb a gaze trajectory, in-flight, and verify that the system compensates for this perturbation such that gaze accuracy remains intact. Such experiments have been done in cat, monkey and human subjects and will be reviewed in the next section.

Mechanical perturbations of head motion that perturb gaze motion

A simple method of perturbing a gaze trajectory is to mechanically interfere with head motion. This occurs naturally in real life, for example as animals bump on obstacles, or carry objects or food in their mouth as they orient their head to new positions. A strongly perturbed gaze shift, obtained in monkey, is shown in

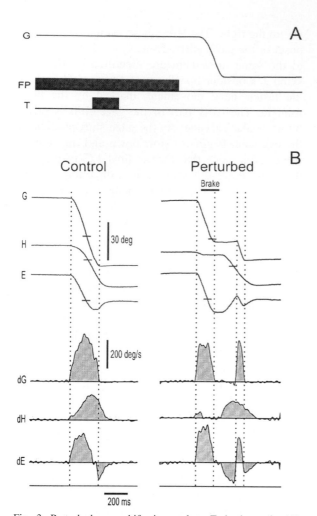

Fig. 3. Perturbed gaze shifts in monkey. Task shown in (A). Monkey with head-unrestrained starts by fixating fixation point, FP. During fixation, target (T) flashes. When FP off, monkey makes gaze shift in dark to remembered location of T. (B) Left panel, control gaze shift. Right panel, gaze shift perturbed by mechanically braking head rotation for about 150 ms. Brake occurs early in head motion. dG, dH, dE: gaze, head and eye velocities. Horizontal tic-marks on movement traces indicate central positions of gaze and head relative to body midline and eye relative to head. Other symbols as in Fig. 2. See text for details.

Fig. 3. In this laboratory task, the monkey looked at a central fixation point (FP) during which time a peripheral target (T) was briefly flashed (Fig. 3A). The extinction of FP signaled to the head-unrestrained monkey to look, in the dark, at the remembered location of T. The typical resulting pattern of eye–head coordination and the resulting gaze shift to a target at 50° is shown in the left panel of Fig. 3B. Gaze shift onset and the rapid initial movement of the gaze trajectory were determined by the eye saccade (see also Fig. 2). At the end of the latter, final eye position eventually saturated in the orbit, and the head carried gaze. When gaze arrived at the intended position, the eye counter-rotated to oppose head motion, thereby stabilizing the visual axis in space. The right panel of Fig. 3B shows a perturbed gaze shift, obtained by briefly halting head motion. (This was done by using a friction clutch, which immobilized a vertical shaft to which the monkey's head was attached via multiple universal joints.) The brake was applied just after the start of head movement and therefore prevented significant early head motion. Consequently, the initial gaze saccade was due essentially to the eye saccade. The latter reached its terminal position in the orbit, well under the mechanical limits of eye motion, and remained immobile there until head release. At that moment, the eye counter-rotated in the orbit to compensate for ongoing head rotation thereby stabilizing gaze in space, called here a gaze plateau. The plateau implies that the oculomotor system had come out of the saccade mode into the slow-phase mode. In all trials, the onset of the second eye saccade always followed, after a variable time, the moment at which head motion resumed after brake release. The mechanisms that determine the onset of the second eye saccade are unknown to us. We have hypothesized elsewhere (Guitton et al., 1984; Guitton and Volle, 1987) and reiterate here that the second eye saccade may be a quick-phase of vestibular nystagmus.

The sum of the second eye saccade plus head motion generated a second gaze saccade which compensated for the perturbation and brought final gaze position close to the target zone. This is shown in Fig. 4 for the same animal. In the control, unperturbed condition, this monkey overshot targets at <40°, and undershot targets at >40°. Notice that in the perturbed condition, the first gaze saccade undershot the target even when the target was well within the oculomotor range (e.g. at 40° and with initial eye position typically starting 10–15° off-center, on the side away from the target, Fig. 3B). However, the amplitude of the second gaze saccade was sufficient to compensate for the gaze perturbation and brought

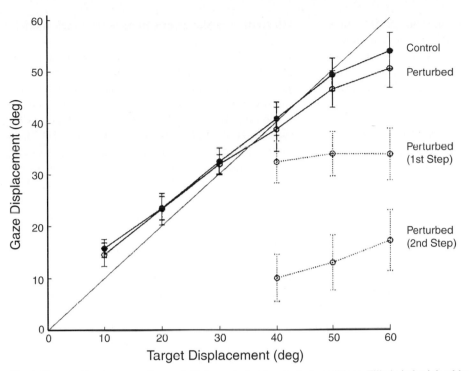

Fig. 4. Comparative accuracy of gaze shifts in control and perturbed conditions. Filled circles joined by full line show gaze displacement during control gaze shifts to targets ranging in offset from 10 to 60°. Unity line at 45° shows where points should lie for perfect accuracy. Open circles joined by filled line show final gaze position after second saccade (see Fig. 3B) in perturbed gaze shifts. Top light dotted line shows amplitude of first gaze saccade (see Fig. 3B) in perturbed trials. Lower light dotted line shows amplitude of second gaze saccade. Between gaze saccades, gaze is immobile. Therefore the overall gaze displacement, open circles, is the sum of 1st and 2nd saccades.

gaze close to the control value. These results support feedback control of gaze.

Similar experimental results have been reported previously in cat, monkey and humans. They will be briefly reviewed here. Laurutis and Robinson (1986) perturbed human head motion very briefly during large gaze saccades of about 180°, made between two visible targets in a dimly lit room. The perturbation did not halt head motion, nor cause a plateau in gaze position; the gaze velocity was however slowed by about 180°/s. In the perturbed gaze trajectories, the duration of the overall gaze shift was longer and final gaze position compensated for the perturbation: control gaze shifts were within about 3° of target compared to 4° for the perturbed trials, a nonsignificant difference.

Guitton and Volle (1987) studied gaze accuracy in two human subjects that made active eye–head gaze shifts *in the dark* to briefly flashed targets. In the control condition, on average for both subjects, the

gaze undershot targets in the offset range 30–50°, by about 4° and overshot targets in the 60–80° range by about 2°. By comparison, when the head movement was mechanically braked — sometimes halting gaze motion, sometimes slowing it as in Laurutis and Robinson (1986) — subjects undershot targets in the 30–50° range on average by only 0.5°, and undershot targets in the 60–80° range by 1°. Clearly, for each subject, gaze accuracy was not significantly dependent on whether the gaze shifts were performed with or without perturbed head motion.

Tomlinson (1990) perturbed 65° gaze saccades to visible targets in monkey, with a torque motor that could briefly either momentarily slow down or speed up head movements. Perturbations to the gaze trajectory amounted to about ±10% of the intended amplitude, and were compensated for within about 1°.

In cat, Matsuo et al. (2002) (see also Guitton et al., 1984) have found that gaze shifts in the dark to remembered targets at an eccentricity of 50° show excellent compensation for gaze trajectory perturbations that halt the gaze trajectory in mid-flight for periods ranging from 50 to 400 ms: control gaze shift $43.2 \pm 2.4°$, compared to perturbed gaze shifts, $43.0 \pm 2.6°$.

In summary, in all experiments that have tested compensation for gaze trajectory changes induced by mechanically perturbing head motion, there is unanimous agreement that compensation is excellent and accuracy is indistinguishable from control data.

Gaze shifts perturbed by electrical stimulation of superior colliculus

The hypothesis that ocular saccades in the head-fixed monkey are controlled by feedback was supported by the experiments of Sparks and Mays (1983). They perturbed the eye position by stimulating the superior colliculus (SC) just before a monkey was to make a saccade to the location of a briefly flashed visual target. In spite of the change in eye position, the monkey — in the dark — made a saccade to the location of the target. Using similar techniques, a test of the gaze feedback concept was made in head-unrestrained cats trained to orient in the dark to a target that had flashed but was extinguished when the gaze shift began (Pélisson et al., 1989). Despite a gaze position perturbation — involving changes to both eye and head positions — and the absence of visual feedback, a corrective saccadic gaze shift, using coordinated eye–head movement, terminated on target. In a subsequent and complementary study (Pélisson et al., 1995), goal-directed gaze shifts were perturbed 'in-flight' — rather than before onset, as in the previous experiment — by a brief stimulation of the SC. The movements were not halted. Following stimulation offset, the transient perturbations were compensated for, 'on-line', before gaze shifts terminated. It is important to note that at the end of a compensated gaze shift, the contributing eye and head amplitudes and positions were different than those contributing to the control unperturbed gaze shift. This is evidence against the separate comparator model described and discussed in the next section.

Alternative explanations to gaze feedback model

In early theories of eye–head coordination it was thought that the VOR acts throughout the entire eye saccade: head motion is first added to that of the eye because the head carries the eye, but then it is subtracted out by the VOR (Bizzi et al., 1971; Morasso et al., 1973; reviewed in Guitton, 1992). In this oculocentric view of the gaze control system, the head motion is irrelevant to target acquisition; it is the eye saccade that gets gaze on target. This hypothesis is incorrect for large gaze shifts. Indeed, many experiments have shown that the VOR is not transmitted to ocular motoneurons during large gaze shifts (e.g. Roy and Cullen, 1998). Furthermore, for the 120° gaze shifts in Fig. 2, it is unrealistic to postulate that the brain programs 120° eye saccades.

Sparks (1999) has argued that the finding that subjects compensate for perturbations to gaze trajectories does not unequivocally support the gaze feedback control scheme of Fig. 1B, i.e. a single GPE comparator that drives the eye and head motor circuits (see Sparks and Gandhi, 2003, this volume). He argues that compensation can also be explained by so-called 'separate comparator' models (Phillips et al., 1995) which assume that the gaze displacement command is decomposed into separate eye and head displacement commands that drive separate generators, each controlled by its individual feedback circuit. Sparks is incorrect in this assertion. Although the latter scheme may be true in specific experimental conditions, it is inadequate for controlling perturbed gaze movements. Consider the perturbed trajectory in Fig. 3B. When head motion is halted the eye completes its displacement and therefore, in the separate comparator model, *eye* position error becomes zero. (The observation that brainstem 'omnipause' neurons are on during a brake-induced gaze plateau (Paré and Guitton, 1998) supports this aspect of the model's prediction.) However, since gaze is only about half-way to the target, the Phillips et al. (1995) model would have the VOR fully or partly turned *off*, in line with the results of Roy and Cullen (1998) cited above. This part of the model is not compatible with the experimental observations: in Fig. 3B, when the head is released, the VOR moves the eye in a direction opposite to head motion and gaze is stabilized in space. A further and critical drawback of the separate comparator model is its failure to predict the new eye saccade that is generated when the head is released. Put another way, in the separate comparator model the question arises as to how the new eye position error in the independent eye loop is calculated if remaining gaze position error is unknown to the eye system. Reestablishing the same value as before is clearly inadequate because after the gaze plateau, eye and head starting positions relative to the target are now different and a new amplitude is required (Fig. 4). These points have been discussed in the previous section in relation to electrically perturbed gaze shifts in cat (Pélisson et al., 1995).

Evidence that semicircular canals provide gaze feedback loop with information on head motion

Pélisson et al. (1988) studied the accuracy of gaze saccades made when human subjects made eye saccades to follow a target that stepped from one location to another (ΔT) whilst their head was being passively rotated about a vertical axis, relative to a fixed trunk. In the control condition, when the subject was not rotated and the head was fixed, the saccadic eye movements undershot the target by $0.06\Delta T$ on average for five subjects. By comparison, when the head was passively driven there was a large increase in variability but the mean error was not significantly affected when the target jumped in a direction either 'with' or 'against' head motion. These observations suggest that signals from the semicircular canals and/or neck proprioceptors provide the feedback information in the model (Fig. 1B). Support for the hypothesis that feedback information originates in the semicircular canals comes from the experiments of Bloomberg et al. (1988). They asked human subjects to match the amplitude of a preceding head angular displacement with a voluntary saccade of equal but opposing amplitude. They found that subjects correctly made saccades back to the position of a previously seen earth-fixed target one second after a passive whole-body rotation in the dark with eyes centered in the head. A further line of evidence is that cats with bilateral semicircular canal plugs, make large gaze overshoots in the dark to the location of a remembered target (Fakhri et al., 1994).

Neural implementation of the gaze feedback model: role of superior colliculus

Deficits in gaze shift accuracy due to subcortical lesions in the head-unrestrained cat have been reported to result from inactivation of the fastigial nucleus (Goffart and Pélisson, 1997, 1998; Goffart et al., 1998a,b; Pélisson et al., 1998), semicircular canals (Fakhri et al., 1994) and mesencephalic reticular formation (Waitzman et al., 2002). With regard to feedback control, Goffart et al. (1998a) have studied whether the caudal fastigial nucleus is implicated in compensating for gaze shift perturbations generated by stimulating the SC. They showed that following lesions of the caudal fastigial nucleus the amplitude of the compensatory gaze shift to a given target was inaccurate but nevertheless comparable with the amplitude of control, unperturbed, gaze shifts starting from similar positions. Therefore, irrespective of the deficit caused by a caudal fastigial nucleus lesion, a perturbation is still compensated for and therefore neither the feedback loop pathway nor the summing junction resides in the fastigial nucleus (see Klier et al., 2003, this volume, for a further discussion of the neural encoding of gaze). In this paper we focus on the role of the SC.

It has been known for some time that the cat SC encodes *gaze* displacements, but it is only recently that the monkey SC has been accorded this property, having traditionally been thought of as an oculomotor structure (Roucoux et al., 1980; Munoz et al., 1991; Freedman et al., 1996; Freedman and Sparks, 1997a,b; Paré and Guitton, 1998). Traditional models of how the SC controls eye and/or gaze shifts postulate that the SC provides the brainstem with a signal encoding the initial desired displacement vector; e.g. target offset angle and direction (e.g. Scudder, 1988). In such a model the neural circuits downstream of the SC implement the feedback control loop. The SC has also been considered as the source of the error signal. The SC's involvement in feedback control has been well reviewed recently by Scudder et al. (2002) (see also Quaia et al., 1999).

Regarding gaze control, we have proposed that the gaze position error signal is continuously encoded on the motor map of the SC. Specifically, in Munoz and Guitton (1991) and Munoz et al. (1991) we argued that: (1) an ensemble of discharging neurons, whose locus of activity moves on the topographically organized map, instructs brainstem eye and head circuits as to the current GPE (the 'moving hill' hypothesis), (2) activity begins at the site appropriate for encoding the desired gaze saccade vector, (3) when activity invades the rostral SC, collicular 'fixation' neurons are activated which activate omnipause neurons that in turn suppress cat gaze saccades (Paré and Guitton, 1998).

This hypothesis places the SC within the gaze feedback loop, a mechanism that has been vigorously debated, particularly as to whether it applies to the head-fixed monkey. We will briefly overview some key points in this debate. Munoz and Wurtz (1995a,b) have described, for the head-fixed monkey, two cell types in the SC related to saccade generation; buildup neurons (BUNs) and burst neurons (BNs). Buildup neurons were reported to have a prelude of activity at a frequency > 30 spikes/s, that preceded by about 100 ms, eye saccades of the optimal amplitude and direction in the delayed saccade paradigm. Buildup neurons also have 'open-ended' movement fields; i.e. the cell discharged for all saccades larger than the amplitude of the 'optimal' vector encoded by the cell's position on the motor map. They described a moving front of activity that, during a saccade, spreads across the BUN layer towards the SC's rostral pole as the saccade progresses. As in Munoz et al. (1991), the saccade is hypothesized to stop when the front activates fixation neurons. By comparison, collicular BNs showed a burst of activity that precedes a saccade, but negligible buildup activity. These neurons have a 'closed' movement field: they discharge only during saccades that have a vector close to the 'optimum'. According to Munoz and Wurtz (1995b) in the BN layer, activity remains topographically immobile during a saccade.

Further experiments, involving recording simultaneously the activity of two buildup neurons in the head-fixed monkey, have supported rostrally moving activity during saccades (Port et al., 2000): during a saccade activity in the rostral SC occurs later than in the caudal SC. However, Soetedjo et al. (2002b) argue that the time difference between the respective activations of rostral and caudal neurons is too small compared to that calculated from motor error. Put another way, they argue that the rostrally moving

activity in the Port et al. (2000) experiments goes faster than the movement itself and arrives in the rostral zone too early to stop the saccade.

A further argument advanced against the moving hill hypothesis is that the prediction, by Munoz et al. (1991) and Munoz and Wurtz (1995b), that saccades would be hypermetric if the rostral SC is deactivated is not borne out experimentally (Aizawa and Wurtz, 1998; see also Quaia et al., 1999).

Four other reports have looked specifically for moving activity in the *head-fixed* monkey and cat and all report no significant rostral movement of the locus of activity during eye saccades (imaging SC in monkey: Moschovakis et al., 2001; single-cell recording in monkey: Anderson et al., 1998; Soetedjo et al., 2002b; single-cell recording in cat: Kang and Lee, 2000). One can criticize certain deficiencies in methods and analysis techniques in each study, but we will not overview these here. Suffice it to say that if moving activity exists in the SC of head-fixed monkey it is not a robust phenomenon. Nevertheless, evidence does exist for the head-fixed monkey that the SC is in some type of feedback loop whose role in controlling saccades in unclear (Goossens and Van Opstal, 2000; Soetedjo et al., 2002a).

In recent experiments we have reexamined the moving hill hypothesis. First, we have exploited a specific behavior of the cat, which is to orient to targets using multiple-step gaze shifts. Second, we have perturbed gaze trajectories, as discussed above, while recording on the collicular motor map. We will now briefly review some key observations.

Collicular fixation neurons in cat encode gaze position error

Superior colliculus fixation neurons (SCFNs; reviewed in Bergeron and Guitton, 2000) are located in the rostral pole of the SC. They discharge tonically during steady fixation of a behaviorally significant target, irrespective of whether it is visible or not. The example in Fig. 5A shows that when the cat fixated the food target in the light, SCFNs discharged tonically. When ambient illumination was extinguished, and the animal was suddenly in complete darkness, but gaze was still aligned on the now invisible food target, tonic discharge continued for at least 400 ms. In some cells the rate in the dark during this protocol

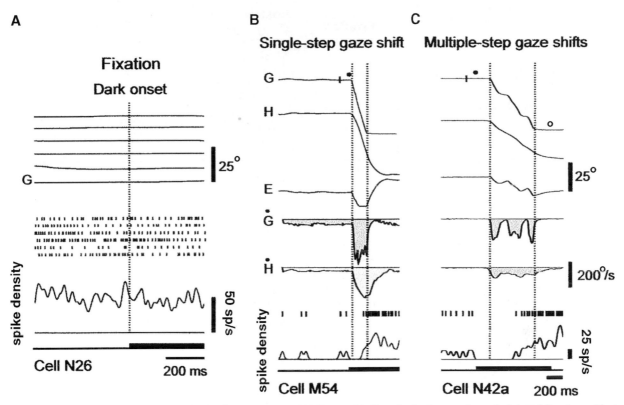

Fig. 5. Typical discharges of superior colliculus fixation neurons. (A) Cat steadily fixated a food target. At vertical dotted line the ambient lighting was extinguished and the cat was in total darkness, as also indicated by thick horizontal dark bar at bottom. This procedure was repeated six times. From top to bottom: six gaze (G) traces showing steady fixation; the associated six discharges of SCFN, cell N26 in right SC. Each tic-mark represents an action potential and each line of action potentials corresponds to the equivalently placed gaze trace above. Below the action potential traces is the averaged discharge, the spike density histogram, in spikes/s. (B) A 45° single-step gaze shift and associated discharge of another SCFN, cell M54. Associated action potentials shown as tic-marks below head velocity trace. Vertical mark on G trace indicates when target shown to cat. Gaze in the dark is at the remembered target location at the right vertical dotted line. (C) A 45° multiple-step gaze shift and associated discharges of another SCFN, cell N42a in right superior colliculus. Dark circle indicates when ambient lighting was extinguished; open circle when it was re-illuminated. Letters $\dot{G}$ and $\dot{H}$ indicate gaze and head velocity.

was similar to that in the light, in other cells less but never below 25 spikes/s.

Fig. 5B shows SCFN activity during a large single-step gaze shift made by a cat in our protocol and in a direction contralateral to the recording site. Note that this gaze shift is qualitatively similar to that in humans Fig. 2 and monkey (Fig. 3B). Before a gaze shift, the cat faced an opaque barrier on which there was no target of significance and the SCFN had a characteristically low tonic discharge, lower than during attentive fixation in the dark. During this contralateral gaze shift in the dark, the cell was silent until near the end of the gaze trajectory. We focus now on what determines when SCFN firing

intensifies after the initial low-frequency discharge, by studying multiple-step gaze shifts in the dark, a typical example being shown in Fig. 5C. In this example, the target at about 50° from initial gaze position, was attained using a sequence of three gaze saccades separated by short periods (gaze position plateaus) during which gaze was either immobile or moving much slower than at saccade velocity. An important feature of multiple-step gaze shifts is that, for a given overall amplitude, they are very variable in structure in terms of the number of saccades, their amplitude and the duration of the gaze plateaus. Fig. 6 shows a series of leftward multiple-step gaze shifts made by a cat as it oriented, in the dark, to

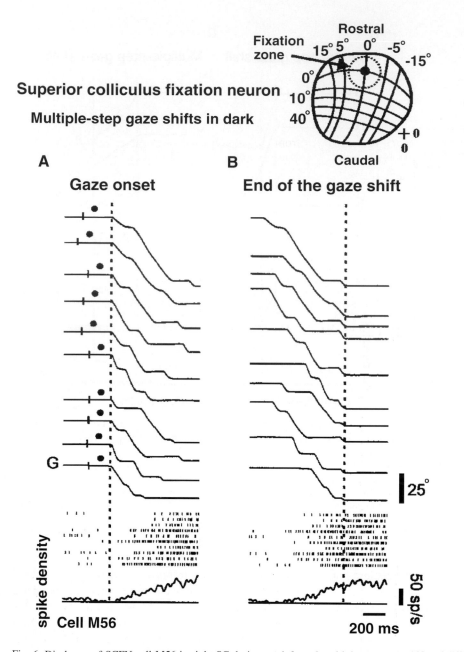

Superior colliculus fixation neuron

Multiple-step gaze shifts in dark

A
Gaze onset

B
End of the gaze shift

G

spike density

Cell M56

25°

50 sp/s

200 ms

Fixation zone

Rostral
15° 5° 0° -5°
-15°
0°
10°
40°
+0
0

Caudal

Fig. 6. Discharge of SCFN cell M56 in right SC during ten leftward multiple-step gaze shifts of different amplitudes. Cat initiated gaze shifts from different initial positions to a fixed remembered target location. (A) Traces aligned on onset of multiple-step sequences, indicated by vertical dotted line. (B) Traces aligned on end of multiple-step sequences. Spike density histogram shown below action potential traces. Same symbols and conventions as in Fig. 5. Inset at top right shows dorsal view of superior colliculus' motor map. Recording made in rostral fixation zone.

a target at distances varying from about 50° (top trace) to 25° (bottom trace) from different initial fixation positions. In Fig. 6A,B the same movements

are aligned on the beginning and end of the gaze shifts, respectively. The bottom trace in each panel shows that this cell, in the right SC, was silent at the onset of the first gaze saccade and discharged at peak frequency at the end of the last gaze saccade. Between start and end, there was a gradual increase in firing frequency.

We showed in Bergeron and Guitton (2000) that the first spike after the pause in activity at gaze start, occurred when the visual axis arrived at a particular distance from the target; i.e. at a particular GPE. The GPE at which the first spike occurs is called the cell's 'preferred' GPE and its value varies from cell to cell. The value for cell M56 was 16° and the average for all cells was 13°. After the fist spike, as the gaze shift evolved, the firing frequency increased as GPE decreased (Bergeron and Guitton, 2000, 2002). Fig. 7A shows one of the multiple-step gaze shifts of Fig. 6, now plotted as GPE versus time. The associated cell discharge is shown below the gaze trace and clearly increases as GPE → 0. This is shown quantitatively in Fig. 7B where each numbered point

corresponds to a plateau in Fig. 7A. An analysis of many multiple-step gaze shifts produces the group of points in Fig. 7B through which it is possible to fit a Gaussian function. All SCFNs that we recorded had a frequency of discharge that increased as GPE → 0, similar to that shown in Fig. 7B. All Gaussian fits peaked at GPE = 0, but the width of the curve varied from cell to cell. The width, defined as 1.6 × standard deviation, equaled the preferred GPE calculated as the time of onset of the first spike.

The observations just reviewed support the hypothesis that there is feedback to the cat's SC, at least to the fixation zone, and that this feedback generates a GPE signal. Furthermore, the rising frequency in SCFNs, of the rostral SC, as the multiple-step gaze shift approaches the target is compatible with the moving hill hypothesis. Note that in yet unpublished results, we have found by recording at different locations on the motor map in cat, that for large

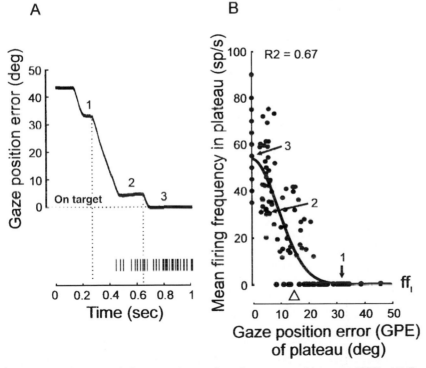

Fig. 7. Firing frequency during gaze plateaus depends on gaze position error (GPE). (A) Example of one multiple-step gaze shift (part of the ten shown in Fig. 6) and the associated action potential trace of cell M56, shown by short vertical lines below. (B) Mean firing frequency during gaze plateaus increases as GPE → 0. Points numbered 1–3 correspond to firing frequency during equivalently numbered plateaus in (A). Other points are from plateaus in other multiple-step gaze traces. Solid line through points is a Gaussian fit giving a variance-accounted-for (R2) of 0.67. ff$_i$ is firing frequency at start, GPE = 0. Open triangle at bottom indicates when discharge rises significantly above zero.

multiple-step gaze shifts of overall amplitude of, say 60°, a hill of activity begins at the 60° location and moves forward on the map, sequentially activating caudo-rostral sites with each step, until it reaches the SC's fixation zone. *Thus we continue to observe phenomena in the SC of the head-unrestrained cat that are compatible with the moving hill hypothesis.* Furthermore, if gaze shift trajectories are mechanically halted (as in Fig. 3B) during the pause in fixation neuron activity, the pause is prolonged in relation to the increased duration to the end of the compensatory gaze saccade (Fig. 8) (Matsuo et al., 2002). Furthermore, neurons on the SC's motor map, at the appropriate location for encoding the remaining GPE, stay tonically active until the gaze trajectory is allowed to complete its trajectory (Matsuo et al., 2002).

Our recent observations in *head-unrestrained* monkey (Choi and Guitton, 2002) also support gaze feedback to the primate SC. Indeed, as in cat, when *large* gaze shifts are mechanically perturbed (Fig. 3B) activity in fixation cells remains low until the end of the 2nd saccade that corrects for the perturbation (see Fig. 8). Furthermore, during the perturbation-induced gaze plateau, the saccade-related firing frequency of buildup neurons in the rostral motor map, remains at its value at the time of the gaze perturbation, 'on-hold' until the end of the 2nd saccade. We still do not know how this gaze feedback relates to the moving hill phenomenon, but contrary to that suggested by Soetedjo et al. (2002b), we believe it is premature to lay to rest the moving hill hypothesis, particularly for monkey whose head is unrestrained. When the causes of possible differences between experimental conditions and between cat and monkey are discovered they should provide valuable insight into the gaze motor circuitry.

Acknowledgements

Supported by the Canadian Institutes of Health Research (CIHR). A. Bergeron and W.Y. Choi were supported by studentships from the CIHR and le Fonds de Recherche en Santé du Québec (FRSQ). S. Matsuo was supported by a Grant-in-Aid for Scientific Research from the Japanese Ministry of Education, Science and Culture.

References

Aizawa, H. and Wurtz, R.H. (1998) Reversible inactivation of monkey superior colliculus. I. Curvature of saccadic trajectory. *J. Neurophysiol.*, 79: 2082–2096.

Anderson, R.W., Keller, E.L., Gandhi, N.J. and Das, S. (1998) Two-dimensional saccade-related population activity in superior colliculus in monkey. *J. Neurophysiol.*, 80: 798–817.

Bergeron, A. and Guitton, D. (2000) Fixation neurons in the superior colliculus encode distance between current and desired gaze positions. *Nat. Neurosci.*, 3: 932–939.

Bergeron, A. and Guitton, D. (2001) The superior colliculus and its control of fixation behavior via projections to brainstem omnipause neurons. *Prog. Brain Res.*, 134: 97–107.

Bergeron, A. and Guitton, D. (2002) Discharge of superior colliculus fixation neurons (SCFNs) and brain stem omnipause neurons (OPNs) during multiple-step gaze shifts in cat: OPNs, not SCFNs, gate saccades; both cells encode gaze position error. *J. Neurophysiol.*, 88: 1726–1742.

Bizzi, E., Kalil, R.E. and Tagliasco, V. (1971) Eye–head coordination in monkeys: evidence for centrally patterned organization. *Science*, 173: 452–454.

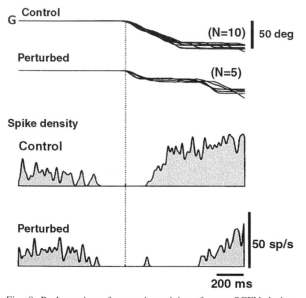

Fig. 8. Prolongation of pause in activity of a cat SCFN during perturbed gaze shifts. Top trace shows ten superimposed control single-step gaze traces, no perturbation. Below are five superimposed gaze shifts perturbed by mechanically stopping head motion, as in Fig. 3B. All gaze traces aligned on start of gaze displacement. Below the gaze traces are the associated spike density histograms giving average firing frequency of cell. Note that control discharge show typical pause in activity at start of gaze shift and reactivation near end to higher frequency than at start. Note that in perturbed gaze shifts the pause in firing frequency is prolonged.

Bloomberg, J., Jones, G.M., Segal, B., McFarlane, S. and Soul, J. (1988) Vestibular-contingent voluntary saccades based on cognitive estimates of remembered vestibular information. *Adv. Otorhinolaryngol.*, 41: 71–75.

Choi, W.Y. and Guitton, D. (2002) Discharge characteristics of saccade-related neurons in primate superior colliculus during head-perturbed gaze shifts. *32nd Annual Meeting, Society for Neuroscience*, abstract.

Fakhri, S., Pélisson, D. and Guitton, D. (1994) Compensation for perturbations of gaze and role of vestibular signals in gaze control. In: J.M. Delgado-Garcia, E. Godaux and P.P. Vidal (Eds.), *Information Processing Underlying Gaze Control*. Pergamon Studies in Neuroscience No. 12. Elsevier Science Inc., New York, pp. 53–63.

Freedman, E.G. and Sparks, D.L. (1997a) Activity of cells in the deeper layers of the superior colliculus of the rhesus monkey: evidence for a gaze displacement command. *J. Neurophysiol.*, 78: 1669–1690.

Freedman, E.G. and Sparks, D.L. (1997b) Eye–head coordination during head-unrestrained gaze shifts in rhesus monkeys. *J. Neurophysiol.*, 77: 2328–2348.

Freedman, E.G., Stanford, T.R. and Sparks, D.L. (1996) Combined eye–head gaze shifts produced by electrical stimulation of the superior colliculus in rhesus monkeys. *J. Neurophysiol.*, 76: 927 952.

Fuller, J.H., Maldonado, H. and Schlag, J. (1983) Vestibular–oculomotor interaction in cat eye–head movements. *Brain Res.*, 271: 241–250.

Galiana, H.L. and Guitton, D. (1992) Central organization and modeling of eye–head coordination during orienting gaze shifts. In: B. Cohen, D.L. Tomko and F. Guedry (Eds.), *Sensing and Controlling Motion. Vestibular and Sensorimotor Function.* Annals of the New York Academy of Sciences, Vol. 656, New York Academy of Sciences, New York, pp. 452–471.

Goffart, L. and Pélisson, D. (1997) Changes in initiation of orienting gaze shifts after muscimol inactivation of the caudal fastigial nucleus in the cat. *J. Physiol.*, 503: 657–671.

Goffart, L. and Pélisson, D. (1998) Orienting gaze shifts during muscimol inactivation of caudal fastigial nucleus in the cat. I. Gaze dysmetria. *J. Neurophysiol.*, 79: 1942–1958.

Goffart, L., Guillaume, A. and Pélisson, D. (1998a) Compensation for gaze perturbation during inactivation of the caudal fastigial nucleus in the head-unrestrained cat. *J. Neurophysiol.*, 80: 1552–1557.

Goffart, L., Pélisson, D. and Guillaume, A. (1998b) Orienting gaze shifts during muscimol inactivation of caudal fastigial nucleus in the cat. II. Dynamics and eye–head coupling. *J. Neurophysiol.*, 79: 1959–1976.

Goossens, H.H.L.M. and Van Opstal, A.J. (2000) Blink-perturbed saccades in monkey. II. Superior colliculus activity. *J. Neurophysiol.*, 83: 3430–3452.

Guitton, D. (1992) Control of eye–head coordination during orienting gaze shifts. *Trends Neurosci.*, 15: 174–179.

Guitton, D. and Choi, W.Y. (2002) Discharge characteristics of fixation neurons in primate superior colliculus during head-perturbed gaze shifts. *32nd Annual Meeting, Society for Neuroscience*, abstract.

Guitton, D. and Volle, M. (1987) Gaze control in head-free humans: eye–head coordination during orienting movements to targets within and beyond the oculomotor range. *J. Neurophysiol.*, 58: 427–459.

Guitton, D., Douglas, R.M. and Volle, M. (1984) Coordinated eye–head movements in the cat. *J. Neurophysiol.*, 52: 1030–1050.

Guitton, D., Munoz, D.P. and Galiana, H.L. (1990) Gaze control in the cat: Studies and modelling of the coupling between orienting eye and head movements in different behavioral tasks. *J. Neurophysiol.*, 64: 509–531.

Kang, I. and Lee, C. (2000) Properties of saccade-related neurons in the cat superior colliculus: patterns of movement fields and discharge timing. *Exp. Brain Res.*, 131: 149–164.

Klier, E.M., Martinez-Trujillo, J.C., Medendorp, W.P., Smith, M.A. and Crawford, J.D. (2003) Neural control of 3-D gaze shifts in the primate. In: C. Prablanc, D. Pélisson and Y. Rossetti (Eds.), *Neural Control of Space Coding and Action Production. Progress in Brain Research*, Vol. 142. Elsevier, Amsterdam, pp. 109–124 (this volume).

Laurutis, V.P. and Robinson, D.A. (1986) The vestibulo-ocular reflex during human saccadic eye movements. *J. Physiol.*, 373: 209–233.

Matsuo, S., Bergeron, A. and Guitton, D. (2002) Activity of superior colliculus neurons during gaze trajectory perturbations in head-unrestrained cat. *32nd Annual Meeting, Society for Neuroscience*, abstract.

Morasso, P., Bizzi, E. and Dichgans, J. (1973) Adjustment of saccade characteristics during head movements. *Exp. Brain Res.*, 16: 492–500.

Moschovakis, A.K., Gregoriou, G.G. and Savaki, H.E. (2001) Functional imaging of the primate superior colliculus during saccades to visual targets. *Nat. Neurosci.*, 4: 1026–1031.

Munoz, D.P. and Guitton, D. (1991) Control of orienting gaze shifts by the tecto-reticulo-spinal system in the head-free cat. II. Sustained discharges related to motor preparation and fixation. *J. Neurophysiol.*, 66: 1624–1641.

Munoz, D.P. and Wurtz, R.H. (1995a) Saccade-related activity in monkey superior colliculus. I. Characteristics of burst and buildup cells. *J. Neurophysiol.*, 73: 2313–2333.

Munoz, D.P. and Wurtz, R.H. (1995b) Saccade-related activity in monkey superior colliculus. II. Spread of activity during saccades. *J. Neurophysiol.*, 73: 2334–2348.

Munoz, D.P., Pélisson, D. and Guitton, D. (1991) Movement of neural activity on the superior colliculus motor map during gaze shifts. *Science*, 251: 1358–1360.

Paré, M. and Guitton, D. (1998) Brainstem omnipause neurons and the control of combined eye–head gaze saccades in the alert cat. *J. Neurophysiol.*, 79: 3060–3076.

Paré, M., Crommelinck, M. and Guitton, D. (1994) Gaze shifts evoked by stimulation of the superior colliculus in the head-free cat conform to the motor map but also depend on stimulus strength and fixation activity. *Exp. Brain Res.*, 101: 123–139.

Pélisson, D., Prablanc, C. and Urquizar, C. (1988) Vestibuloocular reflex inhibition and gaze saccade control characteristics during eye–head orientation in humans. *J. Neurophysiol.*, 59: 997–1013.

Pélisson, D., Guitton, D. and Munoz, D.P. (1989) Compensatory eye and head movements generated by the cat following stimulation-induced perturbations in gaze position. *Exp. Brain Res.*, 78: 654–658.

Pélisson, D., Guitton, D. and Goffart, L. (1995) On-line compensation of gaze shifts perturbed by micro-stimulation of the superior colliculus in the head-free cat. *Exp. Brain Res.*, 106: 196–204.

Pélisson, D., Goffart, L. and Guillaume, A. (1998) Contribution of the rostral fastigial nucleus to the control of orienting gaze shifts in the head-unrestrained cat. *J. Neurophysiol.*, 80: 1180–1196.

Phillips, J.O., Ling, L., Fuchs, A.F., Siebold, C. and Plorde, J.J. (1995) Rapid horizontal gaze movement in the monkey. *J. Neurophysiol.*, 73: 1632–1652.

Port, N.L., Sommer, M.A. and Wurtz, R.H. (2000) Multielectrode evidence for spreading activity across the superior colliculus movement map. *J. Neurophysiol.*, 84: 344–357.

Quaia, C., Lefevre, P. and Optican, L.M. (1999) Model of the control of saccades by superior colliculus and cerebellum. *J. Neurophysiol.*, 82: 999–1018.

Roucoux, A., Guitton, D. and Crommelinck, M. (1980) Stimulation of the superior colliculus in the alert cat. II. Eye and head movements evoked when the head is unrestrained. *Exp. Brain Res.*, 39: 75–85.

Roy, J.E. and Cullen, K.E. (1998) A neural correlate for vestibulo-ocular reflex suppression during voluntary eye–head gaze shifts. *Nat. Neurosci.*, 1: 404–410.

Scudder, C.A. (1988) A new local feedback model of the saccadic burst generator. *J. Neurophysiol.*, 59: 1455–1475.

Scudder, C.A., Kaneko, C.S. and Fuchs, A.F. (2002) The brainstem burst generator for saccadic eye movements: a modern synthesis. *Exp. Brain Res.*, 142: 439–462.

Soetedjo, R., Kaneko, C.R. and Fuchs, A.F. (2002a) Evidence that the superior colliculus participates in the feedback control of saccadic eye movements. *J. Neurophysiol.*, 87: 679–695.

Soetedjo, R., Kaneko, C.R. and Fuchs, A.F. (2002b) Evidence against a moving hill in the superior colliculus during saccadic eye movements in the monkey. *J. Neurophysiol.*, 87: 2278–2789.

Sparks, D.L. (1999) Conceptual issues related to the role of the superior colliculus in the control of gaze. *Curr. Opin. Neurobiol.*, 9: 698–707.

Sparks, D.L. and Gandhi, N.J. (2003) Single cell signals: an oculomotor perspective. In: C. Prablanc, D. Pélisson and Y. Rossetti (Eds.), *Neural Control of Space Coding and Action Production. Progress in Brain Research*, Vol. 142. Elsevier, Amsterdam, pp. 35–53 (this volume).

Sparks, D.L. and Mays, L.E. (1983) Spatial localization of saccade targets. I. Compensation for stimulation-induced perturbations in eye position. *J. Neurophysiol.*, 49: 45–63.

Tomlinson, R.D. (1990) Combined eye–head gaze shifts in the primate. III. Contributions to the accuracy of gaze saccades. *J. Neurophysiol.*, 64: 1873–1891.

Waitzman, D.M., Pathmanathan, J., Presnell, R., Ayers, A. and DePalma, S. (2002) Contribution of the superior colliculus and the mesencephalic reticular formation to gaze control. *Ann. N.Y. Acad. Sci.*, 956: 111–129.

C. Prablanc, D. Pélisson and Y. Rossetti (Eds.)
Progress in Brain Research, Vol. 142
© 2003 Elsevier Science B.V. All rights reserved

CHAPTER 5

Control of saccadic eye movements and combined eye/head gaze shifts by the medio-posterior cerebellum

Denis Pélisson *, Laurent Goffart and Alain Guillaume [1]

Espace et Action, INSERM Unité 534, 16 avenue Doyen Lépine, 69500 Bron, France

Abstract: The cerebellar areas involved in the control of saccades have recently been identified in the medio-posterior cerebellum (MPC). Unit activity recordings, experimental lesions and electrical microstimulation of this region in cats and monkeys have provided a considerable amount of data and allowed the development of new computational models. In this paper, we review these data and concepts about cerebellar function, discuss their importance and limitations and suggest future directions for research. The anatomical data indicate that the MPC has more than one site of action in the visuo-oculomotor system. In contrast, most models emphasize the role of cerebellar connections with immediate pre-oculomotor circuits in the reticular formation, and only one recent model also incorporates the ascending projections of the MPC to the superior colliculus. A major challenge for future studies, in continuation with this initial attempt, is to determine whether the various cerebellar output pathways correspond to distinct contributions to the control of saccadic eye movements. Also, a series of recent studies in the cat have indicated a more general role of the MPC in the control of orienting movements in space, calling for an increasing effort to the study of the MPC in the production of head-unrestrained saccadic gaze shifts.

Introduction

There has been a long-standing tradition of studying the role of the cerebellum in motor functions. This interest originates in the 19th century with the first detailed description of the cerebellar syndrome (Flourens, 1824) and with the pioneering anatomical description of the cerebellar architecture (Cajal, 1888) and was later renewed by the use of computers to simulate the processing performed by the cerebellar cortex (Marr, 1969; Albus, 1971). More recently,

the use of neurophysiological and functional imaging techniques has contributed to the establishment of several cerebellar theories in motor control and in other cognitive functions (see reviews in: Ito, 1984; Thach et al., 1992; Schmamann, 1996). The present paper focuses on motor aspects and specifically reviews the recently emerging effort allocated to the study of the cerebellar role in the production of quick orienting movements (saccades) of the line of sight.

Saccadic shifts of the line of sight (gaze) towards a visual target represent a good model for studying the role of the cerebellum in the control of goal-directed action (Robinson and Fuchs, 2001). Indeed, saccadic eye movements are relatively simple motor responses and our knowledge about their dynamical and metrical properties as well as their underlying neural control is much more advanced than for any other motor response involving the squeletomotor system (see Guitton et al., 2003, this volume; Lünenburger et al., 2003, this volume; Sparks and Gandhi,

* Corresponding author: D. Pélisson, Espace et Action, INSERM U 534, 16 avenue Doyen Lépine, 69500 Bron, France. Tel: +33-472-913417; Fax: +33-472-913401; E-mail: pelisson@lyon.inserm.fr
[1] Present address: UMR Mouvement et Perception, Univ. de la Méditerranée, CP 910, 163 av. de Luminy, 13288 Marseille, France.

2003, this volume). In addition, the understanding of the physiopathological bases of saccade dysmetria will help in alleviating the disastrous consequences of cerebellar damage in patients.

In this paper, we review experimental data and theoretical studies addressing the role of the cerebellum in the control of orienting gaze shifts. We will first review anatomical and functional data and then confront these data to the predictions of recent models of saccadic control that incorporate the cerebellum. The cerebellar adaptive control will be treated in this paper only when providing complementary information as to the neural processes and pathways underlying the control of saccades. Neurophysiological data have been provided mostly by studies performed in the monkey, and in the cat especially in relation to head-unrestrained gaze shifts.

Cerebellar territories involved in saccadic control

According to the functional organization of the cerebellum into parasagittal zones, the vermis and underlying fastigial nucleus are involved in the control of eye movements, reflexive postural adjustments and autonomic function. Early studies led to the notion that the cerebellar vermis of the posterior lobe is specifically involved in oculomotor control. In particular, stimulation studies (Cohen et al., 1965; Ron and Robinson, 1973; Llinas and Wolfe, 1977; Gauthier and Stark, 1979) disclosed a widespread territory from which saccadic eye movements can be elicited with a preferential locus at the level of the posterior vermis. Lesion studies (Optican and Robinson, 1980; Optican et al., 1986) revealed that two distinct cerebellar territories are involved in the control of saccade: the vermis participates in generating the pulse of activity required to overcome the visco-elastic forces of the oculomotor plant and the flocculus contributes to the sustained activity required for holding the eye against passive elastic forces.

Using anatomical, electrophysiological and pharmacological approaches, Noda and colleagues (Noda, 1991) delineated within the medio-posterior cerebellum (MPC) the cerebellar territories involved in the control of saccade metrics (amplitude and direction). This 'oculomotor cerebellum' comprises the lobules VIc and VII of the cerebellar vermis and their output target neurons in the caudal portion

of the fastigial nucleus (cat: Courville and Diakiw, 1976; Hirai et al., 1982; monkey: Noda et al., 1990). This caudal part of the fastigial nucleus (cFN) thus constitutes the exclusive output of the MPC and has been named fastigial oculomotor region (FOR) by Noda. Together with the flocculus, the MPC is also involved in the control of smooth pursuit eye movements (Suzuki and Keller, 1988a,b; Pierrot-Deseilligny et al., 1990; Büttner et al., 1991; Kurzan et al., 1993; Fuchs et al., 1994; Robinson et al., 1997; Krauzlis and Miles, 1998; Takagi et al., 2000). Another functional zone of the fastigial nucleus, rostrally located (rFN), responds to optokinetic or vestibular stimulation (Büttner et al., 1991, 1999; Gruart and Delgado-Garcia, 1994; Siebold et al., 1997) and would be involved in the control of the somatic musculature (Büttner et al., 1991). The rFN will be discussed for comparison with the cFN in the light of its recently demonstrated involvement in the control of head-unrestrained gaze shifts.

Other cerebellar zones have saccade-related activity and project to oculomotor centers but there are no data showing a direct involvement in saccadic control (Takikawa et al., 1998; Robinson, 2000). More recently, the ventral zone of the interposed nucleus was proposed to be involved in the control of the vertical component of saccadic eye movements (Robinson, 2000).

Input/ouput relationship of the MPC

Anatomical data show a wide network with the cerebellum situated in parallel with respect to major motor and sensory pathways (Fig. 1). Afferent projections to the MPC contact both the vermis and the cFN, and many vermal projecting neurons produce a collateral to the cFN (Noda et al., 1990). MPC input, like other cerebellar afferents, can be segregated into mossy fiber input and climbing fiber input.

Afferent projections to the MPC

According to the anatomical data in the monkey, the following structures provide the MPC with mossy fibers input, through mainly bilateral projections (Hoddevik et al., 1977; Batini et al., 1978; Gould, 1980; ; Carpenter and Batton, 1982; Dietrichs and Walberg, 1987; Gerrits and Voogd, 1987; Yamada

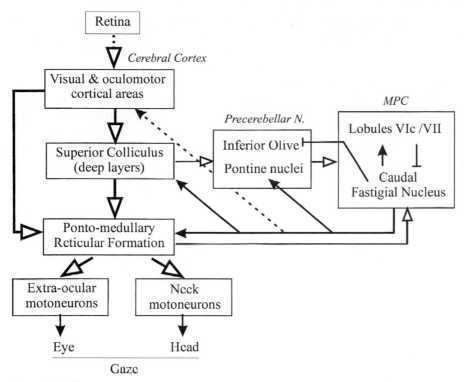

Fig. 1. This diagram shows the main anatomical connections of the medio-posterior cerebellum (MPC) with the centers involved in the production of orienting gaze shifts toward a visual target. Inputs and outputs of the MPC are shown by open and filled arrows, respectively, indirect projections by dotted arrows, and inhibitory connections by a dash-terminated arrow.

and Noda, 1987; Blanks, 1988; Noda et al., 1990; Thielert and Thier, 1993). Dorsolateral pontine nuclei (DLPN) and nucleus reticularis tegmenti pontis (NRTP) provide the most numerous synaptic inputs, followed by the pontine paramedian reticular formation (PPRF), pontis raphe nucleus and the medullary reticular formation (MRF). The MPC also gets bilateral input, although less intense, from the vestibular complex (MVN, IVN, SVN) and NPH and directly from the vestibular apparatus (Kotchabhakdi and Walberg, 1978). Concerning the climbing fibers input, the exclusively crossed projections originate in the caudal portion of the medial accessory olive (MAO) (Hoddevik et al., 1977; Groenewegen and Voogd, 1977; Dietrichs and Walberg, 1985; Yamada and Noda, 1987; Noda et al., 1990).

Efferent projections of the MPC

The cFN constitutes the exclusive output of the MPC. It sends feedback projections to all struc-

tures afferenting it. Thus, the cFN projects to the brainstem reticular formation (Carpenter and Batton, 1982; McCrea and Baker, 1985; Noda et al., 1990; Homma et al., 1995), including the PPRF and the MRF where saccade-related premotor neurons have been found, and vestibular complex (mostly MVN), the NRTP and DLPN nuclei, and the controlateral MAO (Dietrichs and Walberg, 1985). Whereas the NPH receives projections from the rFN (McCrea and Baker, 1985), it is debated whether this nucleus also gets input from the cFN (McCrea and Baker, 1985; Ohtsuka, 1988). The cFN is also contacting premotor neurons involved in the control of head movements, either through the vestibular complex and the reticulo-spinal neurons or directly by projections to the spinal cord cervical segments (Eccles et al., 1975; Matsushita and Hosoya, 1978). Other cerebellar influences over eye and head movements contributing to the saccadic shift of gaze in space also involve ascending projection of the cFN to the deep layers of the superior colliculus (SC). However, whether and how the fastigial terminals in the SC motor map show a topographical organization is still a controversial issue, since the different studies suggest a preferential termination of fastigial fibers either in the rostral SC (Batton et al., 1977; May et al., 1990; Hirai et al., 1982), in the caudal SC (Roldan and Reinoso-Suarez, 1981) or do not show any clear topographical arrangement along the rostro-caudal axis of the SC (Kawamura et al., 1982; Sugimoto et al., 1982). Ascending projections towards the ventro-median thalamus (Nakano et al., 1980; Sugimoto et al., 1982; Jimenez-Castellanos and Reinoso-Suarez, 1985; Katoh and Deura, 1993) suggest a cerebellar influence upon areas of cerebral cortex (frontal and parietal lobe in the monkey: Sasaki et al., 1976; and in the cat: Kyuhou and Kawaguchi, 1987; Steriade, 1995). The contribution of these projections to the translation of sensory input into oculomotor commands is not known. Notably, these thalamic and collicular ascending projections originate exclusively from the caudal part of the FN, and not from its rostral portion.

In general, efferent neurons from the deep cerebellar nuclei are thought to exert an excitatory drive onto target neurons (see for example Ito et al., 1970, and Ohtsuka, 1988), the only known exception are inhibitory fastigial neurons projecting to the MAO (De Zeeuw et al., 1989; Ruigrok and Voogd, 1995). However, deep cerebellar nuclei neurons may contact different neuronal elements in the target structure, as demonstrated for cerebellar projections to the superior colliculus (Warton et al., 1983) and for fastigial projections to the thalamic nuclei (Kultas-Ilinsky et al., 1980a,b). Thus, the fastigial projections may directly drive the output neurons of the targeted structure or the local interneurons.

Closed anatomical loops through the MPC

In agreement with the closed loop general organization of the cerebellum input/output channels (Allen and Tsukuhara, 1974; Middleton and Strick, 1998), the MPC can be involved in closed anatomical loops with most neural circuits of the brainstem involved in the control of saccadic eye movements and/or saccadic gaze shifts. This postulated closed loop arrangement may not be restricted to short brainstem–cerebellar interactions (MPC–reticular formation–

MPC and MPC–vestibular complex–MPC loops) but could extend to longer loops including the superior colliculus (SC) (MPC–SC–NRTP–MPC), the spinal cord (MPC–spinal cord–lateral reticular nucleus–MPC) and the cerebral cortex (MPC–thalamus–FEF–DLPN–MPC loop in cat and monkey, MPC–thalamus–parietal lobe–DLPN–MPC loop in the cat). Thus, the MPC is ideally situated to influence the various sensorimotor transformation stages involved in the production of saccadic gaze shifts, including attentional mechanisms related to target selection and localization, specification of saccade metrics, movement initiation, trajectory control and eye–head coordination. We address now the neurophysiological data that highlight which of these roles are achieved by the MPC, starting from the simplified situation where saccadic eye movements are performed without head movement.

Role of the MPC in saccadic control: head-restrained condition

Neuronal activity

The presence of saccade-related activity in the MPC has been reported by several studies (Llinas and Wolfe, 1977; Kase et al., 1980; Waterhouse and McElligott, 1980; McElligott and Keller, 1982; Suzuki and Keller, 1988a,b; Ohtsuka and Noda, 1990, 1991a,b; Gruart and Delgado-Garcia, 1994; Helmchen et al., 1994; Helmchen and Büttner, 1995; Ohtsuka and Noda, 1995; Thier et al., 2000), in the vermal lobules VI/VII, in the caudal part of the fastigial nucleus, but not in its rostral part.

To understand the functional significance of these saccade-related activities, several studies have tried to determine their specificity relative to the type of saccades (Ohtsuka and Noda, 1992; Helmchen et al., 1994; Helmchen and Büttner, 1995), their dependency relative to orbital eye position (McElligott and Keller, 1982; Ohtsuka and Noda, 1991a; Fuchs et al., 1993; Helmchen et al., 1994; Ohtsuka et al., 1994; Thier et al., 2000) and their tuning relative to the saccade direction (Hepp et al., 1982; Ohtsuka and Noda, 1991a; Fuchs et al., 1993; Ohtsuka et al., 1994; Ohtsuka and Noda, 1995; Thier et al., 2000). As a general cerebellar feature (see Mushiake and Strick, 1993), the motor discharges of MPC saccadic neurons are in general stronger for visually triggered saccades than for spontaneous or internally triggered saccades (Ohtsuka and Noda, 1992; see also Mano et al., 1996 for saccadic neurons recorded from the cerebellar hemisphere). In addition, the burst discharge during spontaneous saccades is indistinguishable from the burst observed during quick phases of vestibular and optokinetic nystagmus, and is stronger when these fast eye movements are produced in the light than in darkness (Helmchen et al., 1994; Helmchen and Büttner, 1995). Concerning the initial eye position dependency, a few studies have directly investigated this influence and failed to reveal any consistent effect (Ohtsuka and Noda, 1991; Helmchen et al., 1994; Ohtsuka et al., 1994; Haas et al., 1999) or found a rather weak effect (Fuchs et al., 1993; but see McElligott and Keller, 1982). This tuning of MPC neurons discharge by eye position is rather weak and contrasts with the activity found in structures supplying a strong input to it such as the NRTP (Crandall and Keller, 1985). It also contrasts with the gain field modulation found in extracerebellar structures like the deep superior colliculus (Van Opstal et al., 1995) and the posterior parietal cortex (Andersen et al., 1990). At the level of the oculomotor vermis, Ohtsuka and Noda (1995) reported three types of saccade-related Purkinje cells according to their discharge pattern: phasic, pause and phasic–tonic. The phasic neurons were further classified as bi- and uni-directional, the majority of uni-directional neurons discharging for ipsiversive saccades (but see Helmchen and Büttner, 1995). At the level of the cFN, all studies have found that neurons generate a burst during the saccade irrespective of its direction and amplitude. For contraversive saccades, the burst duration generally increases with saccade duration (Ohtsuka and Noda, 1990, 1991a; Fuchs et al., 1993; Helmchen et al., 1994). Thus, for a given saccade amplitude, neither the frequency nor the duration of the burst can be used to extract any relevant information about saccade direction. Many fastigial neurons also show a pause in activity either before or after the burst, especially for large saccades. The clearest distinctive feature of the burst activity of cFN neurons in the context of directional coding appears to be the timing of the burst of activity relative to saccade onset. Indeed, the burst of cFN neurons tends to be timed to the onset of contraversive saccades with an average lead time of 20 ms ('early burst'), while the burst of the same neurons occurs later during the course of ipsiversive movements ('late burst'). From these observations and from lesion data, it was suggested that the cFN helps to accelerate contraversive saccades and to decelerate ipsiversive saccades. Given the inhibition exerted by the cerebellar vermis onto the deep nuclei, the fast decline and the fast rise of the burst activity produced by omnidirectional Purkinje cells in relation to ipsiversive and contraversive saccades, respectively, would contribute to the cessation of the cFN early burst and to the sudden onset of cFN late burst (Ohtsuka and Noda, 1992).

Although much less investigated, a strong sustained activity is also typical of neurons in the deep cerebellar nuclei and is classically reported also for neurons in the cerebellar vermis. This tonic activity is found for both saccade-related and non-saccade-related neurons. A weak relationship with eye position has been reported only for a minority of cFN tonic neurons in the cat (type I eye position: Gruart and Delgado-Garcia, 1994) and in the monkey (Fuchs et al., 1993). Although they do not report any spontaneous or gaze-evoked nystagmus, the lesion studies suggest a possible function of MPC tonic activity in maintaining tonic gaze direction (see below). Proprioceptive inputs from the extraocular and neck muscles (Fuchs and Kornhuber, 1969; Batini et al., 1974; Berthoz and Llinas, 1974; Schwartz and Tomlinson, 1977) could account for this activity. Responses related to slow eye movements (during vestibular or optokinetic stimulation or during smooth pursuit) have also been reported in the cerebellar vermis (Precht et al., 1977; Suzuki and Keller, 1988a,b) and in the fastigial nucleus (Furuya et al., 1975; Fuchs et al., 1994; Gruart and Delgado-Garcia, 1994). Finally, old studies have reported a number of non-motor activities in the MPC, including responses to visual (Koella, 1959; Freeman, 1970; Buchtel et al., 1972; Donaldson and Hawthorne, 1979; Kawamura et al., 1990) and auditory stimuli (Wolfe, 1972; Altman et al., 1976).

Electrical microstimulation

Several authors have found that saccadic eye movements can be evoked in the head-restrained animal by electrical microstimulation of the cerebellar posterior lobe and of the underlying fastigial nucleus (Cohen et al., 1965; Ron and Robinson, 1973; Llinas and Wolfe, 1977; Gauthier and Stark, 1979; Keller et al., 1983; McElligott and Keller, 1984; ; Fujikado and Noda, 1987; Noda and Fujikado, 1987a,b; Ohtsuka et al., 1987; Noda et al., 1988, 1991; Murakami et al., 1991; Sato and Noda, 1992; Godschalk et al., 1994; Goffart et al., 1998c). The use of low-intensity (<10 μA) high-frequency electrical stimulation in the monkey led to delineate the so-called 'oculomotor vermis' in the lobules VIc and VII and the fastigial oculomotor region (FOR) in the caudal part of the fastigial nucleus (Noda and Fujikado, 1987a,b; Noda et al., 1988). The metrics of the evoked saccades depend both on the stimulation locus and the stimulation parameters. Saccades evoked from the oculomotor vermis are directed toward the stimulation side and their vertical component varies in a topographically ordered manner. These saccades likely result from the activation of Purkinje cells since their occurrence is suppressed when Purkinje cells are lesioned by local injection of kainic acid or when Purkinje cells connections to cFN neurons are blocked by local injection of bicuculline (Noda and Fujikado, 1987a,b; Noda et al., 1988; Sato and Noda, 1992). When the electrical stimulation is applied to the fastigial nucleus, both ipsiversive and contraversive saccades can be elicited depending on the stimulated site and on the stimulation parameters. Ipsiversive saccades are produced by stimulation of the dorso-caudal part of the fastigial nucleus and disappear after local injection of bicuculline, suggesting that these saccades result from the recruitment of the Purkinje cells axons (Noda et al., 1988). Contraversive saccades are evoked from the rostro-ventral portion of the fastigial nucleus, seemingly by recruiting the axons of FOR neurons (Noda et al., 1988). In a more recent study, using electrical microstimulation with lower-frequency and longer-duration stimulation trains, contraversive saccades could also be evoked from the dorso-caudal part of the fastigial nucleus (Goffart et al., 1998c, 1999). Interestingly, these saccades are triggered by the offset of the stimulation train, suggesting that they resulted from a microstimulation-induced postinhibitory rebound in the firing of FOR neurons (Aizenman and Linden, 1999). Finally, electrical microstimulation

of the fastigial nucleus in the head-unrestrained cat evokes a rapid head movement in addition to the saccadic eye movement, and the metrics of both eye and head movements vary as a function of microstimulation parameters (Goffart et al., 2001; Pélisson et al., 2002).

In sum, the short latency of saccades evoked from stimulating the MPC (15–20 ms), the low current threshold (about 10 μA) and the effect of stimulation temporal parameters on the duration and velocity of evoked saccades are consistent with the anatomical projections from the FN to the brainstem regions where the premotor saccade-related neurons are located. This conclusion is further supported by experiments where the electrical stimulation interferes with the production of a visually triggered saccade, as described in the following.

A first series of experiments used very brief stimulation trains during the on-going saccade to investigate how this would perturb the saccade. Such intra-saccadic stimulations have been applied in the monkey lobules V–VI (Keller et al., 1983), or over the oculomotor vermis through trans-cranial magnetic stimulation in human subjects (Hashimoto and Ohtsuka, 1995). A common observation of these two studies is the hypometria of contraversive saccades during the perturbed trials, with a perturbation latency estimated at 12 ms by Keller et al. (1983). However, whereas the local electrical stimulation failed to modify ipsiversive saccades, the trans-cranial magnetic stimulation increased the amplitude of ipsiversive saccades. This difference may be accounted for by the type of stimulation (electrical versus magnetic) or by the amount of tissue that was stimulated. Note that another study indicated that supra-threshold electrical stimulation of the cFN leads to similar perturbation of all on-going saccades, irrespective of their direction relative to the stimulated side (Noda et al., 1991). This study further demonstrated that monkeys did not compensate for the stimulation-evoked saccade, since no secondary saccade was subsequently generated to bring the eyes back to the remembered location of the flashed target.

A second class of studies applied the short stimulation train prior to the onset of a visually triggered saccade to investigate how the electrically and visually elicited signals interact. Noda et al. (1991)

have applied a supra-threshold stimulation in the monkey fastigial nucleus in a paradigm similar to that originally designed by Mays and Sparks (1980). They reported that the stimulation-induced perturbation was not compensated during the subsequent saccade toward the remembered target location, i.e. the direction and amplitude of the saccade were the same as unperturbed saccades. This finding is reminiscent of the absence of compensation reported for some stimulated sites in the PPRF (Sparks et al., 1987) but contrasts with the compensation which is observed when supra-reticular structures like the deep SC (Schiller and Sandell, 1983; Sparks and Mays, 1983; Pélisson et al., 1989; Schlag-Rey et al., 1989), the thalamic IML (Schlag and Schlag-Rey, 1987) and the FEF (Schiller and Sandell, 1983; Schlag and Schlag-Rey, 1987) are stimulated. However, another study from the same group (Ohtsuka and Noda, 1991b) suggests that correction saccades can be observed even in the case of a cerebellar microstimulation. This was observed when a sub-threshold stimulation, applied to the oculomotor vermis prior to saccade onset, reduces the amplitude of contraversive saccades. Recordings from cFN neurons further showed that the hypometria is associated with a truncation of the cFN presaccadic burst (Ohtsuka and Noda, 1991b). A tentative conclusion would be that a compensation is observed when a sub-threshold electrical microstimulation is applied to the oculomotor vermis level but not when a supra-threshold microstimulation is applied at the cFN level. However, given the recent observations reported by Goffart et al. (1999, see above), it is possible that the secondary saccades observed in the first case are not corrective but are simply due to a poststimulation rebound of FOR activity. Thus, further experiments are necessary to resolve the issue of the functional role of the oculomotor vermis and the cFN in the feedback control of saccade amplitude (Robinson, 1975). The other main outcome of these microstimulation studies provides a substrate for the MPC control of contraversive saccades and emphasizes the role of the cFN early burst. Indeed, they show that the amplitude of the contraversive saccade is correlated with the duration of the early cFN burst which is in turn controlled by the oculomotor vermis.

Lesion/inactivation

Several clinical studies and experimental studies in animals have contributed to the description of the oculomotor deficits induced by permanent or reversible lesions of the cerebellum (Aschoff and Cohen, 1971; Ritchie, 1976; Selhorst et al., 1976; Zee et al., 1976; Optican and Robinson, 1980; Vilis and Hore, 1981; Sato and Noda, 1992; Kurzan et al., 1993; Goldberg et al., 1993; Robinson et al., 1993; Ohtsuka et al., 1994; Vahedi et al., 1995; Goffart and Sparks, 1997; Takagi et al., 1998; Barash et al., 1999). When restricted to the MPC, the deficits concern the saccadic eye movements, eye fixation and spontaneous eye position. The vestibulo-ocular reflex remains normal when the cFN is inactivated (Kurzan et al., 1993) and the absence of spontaneous nystagmus indicates a normal vestibular balance and gaze holding (Goffart and Pélisson, 1998).

The most severe and consistent deficit of goal-directed saccades is the dysmetria, namely a disruption of the relationship between target eccentricity and saccade amplitude. Lesions restricted to the cerebellar vermis lead to hypometric horizontal saccades and asymmetric lesions or unilateral pharmacological decortications decrease the amplitude of ipsiversive saccade (Sato and Noda, 1992; Vahedi et al., 1995; Takagi et al., 1998; Barash et al., 1999). Conversely, lesions or inactivations restricted to the cFN lead to an opposite pattern. Following unilateral lesion, ipsiversive saccades become hypermetric and contraversive saccades hypometric, whereas following bilateral lesions a general saccade hypermetria is observed (Vilis and Hore, 1981; Goldberg et al., 1993; Kurzan et al., 1993; Robinson et al., 1993; Ohtsuka et al., 1994; Straube et al., 1995). The same pattern is observed after lesions involving both the vermis and cFN (Ritchie, 1976; Optican and Robinson, 1980). In general, lesions of the MPC alter the horizontal component of saccades performed in all directions, thereby modifying the amplitude of horizontal saccades, the amplitude and direction of oblique saccades and, in the case of unilateral lesions, the direction of vertical saccades (Robinson et al., 1993; Ohtsuka et al., 1994; Goffart et al., 1999). Although this pattern of errors corresponds to the ocular lateropulsion seen in different neurological patients (e.g. Straube et al., 1994), most experimental studies have focused on the dysmetria of horizontal saccades.

An important issue is related to the type of error made by cerebellar subjects. Classically, saccade dysmetria has been described as a change in gain, i.e. in the ratio of the eye displacement to the target displacement. This type of analysis led to the notion that the MPC adjusts the gain of the transformation of retinal signals into saccadic motor commands, with different suggestions regarding the neural implementation of the postulated gain change (target position signal: Optican, 1982; eye position feedback signal: Keller, 1989; feedback comparator: Dean, 1995). More recently, following studies performed in the head-unrestrained cat (see below), the dysmetria of head-unrestrained gaze shifts in the cFN-inactivated monkey was described by plotting the relationship between the horizontal amplitude of the actual gaze displacement and that of the required gaze displacement (or target eccentricity or retinal error). A linear regression analysis disclosed that the slope of this relationship was systematically increased or reduced for ipsi- or contra-versive gaze saccades, respectively, consistent with the gain modifications reported earlier. However, the analysis also systematically reported changes in the intercept of the relationship. Thus the horizontal dysmetria can be decomposed in two errors, a proportional error that increases with horizontal target eccentricity and a constant error that, in contrast, is not sensitive to horizontal target eccentricity (Goffart et al., in preparation).

Another important question which must be solved to better understand the cerebellar deficits is whether the saccade dysmetria depends on the triggering mode and on the nature of the visual stimulation. To address this question, some authors have recorded in cerebellar patients saccades elicited either toward a suddenly appearing visual stimulus (reactive mode), toward the remembered location of a visual stimulus (delayed mode), or toward permanently displayed visual targets (self-paced mode). On the one hand, two studies have compared the reactive and the delayed (memory) modes, in a single patient with an angioma of the dorsal vermis (Kanayama et al., 1994) or in a group of cerebellar patients (Kori et al., 1998). Both studies found that the saccade dysmetria was similar in the two tested triggering modes. On the other

hand, two other studies compared internally generated saccades to saccades elicited in other modes, in a group of patients (Gaymard et al., 1994) or in a patient with bilateral ablation of the fastigial nuclei (Straube et al., 1995). Both found that the dysmetria of saccades toward a permanent visual target was smaller than that of saccades toward a brief target flash or toward a remembered target. Altogether, these data suggest that the role of the MPC in saccadic control is more prominent for reactive visually elicited saccades than for internally generated ones, in agreement with the somewhat stronger activation of MPC neurons during the former than during the latter. Data describing the saccades towards auditory or somesthetic targets are lacking, so it is yet unclear whether the MPC contributes to the production of saccades induced by other sensory modalities.

A third important issue is whether the cerebellar saccade dysmetria depends on eye position. Many investigators observed in the head-restrained cerebellar patient (Vahedi et al., 1995) or monkey (Ritchie, 1976; Optican and Robinson, 1980; Vilis and Hore, 1981; Sato and Noda, 1992; Robinson et al., 1993; Takagi et al., 1998) that the dysmetria does vary with initial orbital eye position such that centripetal saccades are more hypermetric than centrifugal ones (L. Goffart et al., unpublished data) or that centrifugal saccades are more hypometric than centripetal ones. From these studies it was concluded that the MPC takes into account the mechanical properties of the oculomotor apparatus by adding an orbital-dependent signal to the saccadic command in order to compensate for these peripheral nonlinearities. However, a major limitation of this hypothesis concerns the paucity of orbital-dependent modulation of neuronal activity recorded in the MPC (see above). In addition, under natural circumstances, shifting gaze involves a head movement together with the saccadic eye movement, and the mechanisms that compensate for initial eye position may be overestimated by artificially restraining the head.

Although less studied than the dysmetria of saccades, other oculomotor deficits have been reported after the lesion of the MPC, such as changes in the dynamics and latency of saccades, in fixating a visual target and in the spontaneous exploration of a visual scene. Modifications in saccade dynamics have been reported by different groups (Robinson et al., 1993; Goffart et al., 2002), but not by others (see Selhorst et al., 1976; Zee et al., 1976; Ohtsuka et al., 1994). Takagi et al. (1998) reported that decortication could in some cases change the relationship between saccade amplitude and saccade duration or peak velocity (main sequence relationship) but further showed that the presence of a modification was not related to the size of the dysmetria. Similar observations were made in the head-unrestrained cat (Goffart et al., 1998a, see below). Concerning saccade latency, changes were not systematically examined. Modifications were found to various degrees between experimental subjects and studies (Robinson et al., 1993; Takagi et al., 1998). Systematic studies in the monkey revealed a slight but significant reduction in the latency of ipsiversive saccades in the head-restrained monkey (Goffart et al., 2002). In the head-unrestrained cat, an additional increase in latency for contraversive saccades was observed (Goffart and Pélisson, 1997). A peculiar observation made during unilateral MPC inactivation is the presence of an error in fixating a visual target. On average this fixation offset is about 1–2 degrees in the trained monkey (Robinson et al., 1993), but values up to 7 degrees can be reached in some trials (Goffart et al., 2002; see also Ohtsuka et al., 1994). In the head-unrestrained cat, the fixation offset is larger, 5 degrees on average (Goffart and Pélisson, 1998). This type of error indicates either a difficulty in generating saccades with small amplitude or a bias in the processing of target-related signals or in the specification of the desired saccade amplitude. In either case, the fixation offset could be related to an imbalance in neuronal tonic activity between the two cFN. This fixation offset is reminiscent of that observed after lesions of other oculomotor structures such as the SC (Keating and Gooley, 1988) and the FEF (Dias and Segraves, 1999).

A final clue regarding saccade deficits following cerebellar dysfunction concerns the type and the timing of cerebellar signals which are required for generating accurate saccades and for appropriate visual fixation. Indeed, the studies reviewed above used an inactivation or lesion method that suppressed cerebellar output signals for a period which is very long relative to the time scale of events contributing to the production of a single saccade. A first attempt to specifically suppress the phasic saccade-related cFN

activity was introduced by Noda and colleagues by electrical stimulation of the Purkinje cell afferents to the cFN (Ohtsuka and Noda, 1991b). By applying a sub-threshold electrical microstimulation prior to contraversive saccades, these authors could experimentally truncate the early burst of cFN neurons and then shorten the amplitude of the impending saccade. More recently, Goffart et al. (1999) used sub-threshold electrical microstimulation of the cFN afferents to study the various time windows during which the cerebellar control signals could influence the generation of saccades. The electrical microstimulation was too weak to evoke any immediate eye movement (instead, a delayed contraversive saccade timed with the offset of the stimulus was triggered, presumably reflecting a postinhibitory rebound phenomenon) but when applied in the period of a visually triggered saccade, saccades were strongly dysmetric in a way very similar to what is observed during local muscimol injection. The second major observation from this study is that the maximum dysmetria was obtained when the stimulation was applied during the on-going saccade, and not when restricted to the period prior to saccade onset. This result indicates that the critical time period for the influence of MPC output signals on saccade accuracy corresponds to the period when cFN neurons produce a saccade-related burst of action potential.

Role of the MPC in saccadic control: head-unrestrained condition

Neuronal activity, electrical microstimulation

Data describing the activity of MPC neurons in the head-unrestrained animal are not yet available. However, several studies have described neuronal responses to vestibular (Precht et al., 1977; Suzuki and Keller, 1982; Gruart and Delgado-Garcia, 1994) and neck-proprioceptive (Berthoz and Llinas, 1974) stimulation. During studies related to visual–vestibular interactions, neurons that respond in a synergistic manner to eye and head movements (gaze velocity neurons) and also to target retinal slip (target velocity neurons) were recorded in the vermal lobules VIc–VII (Suzuki and Keller, 1988b) and in the cFN (Büttner et al., 1991). These data together indicate that the role of the MPC is not restricted to the sole control of the eye displacement in the orbit, but extends to the control of head movements and gaze shifts.

Concerning electrical microstimulation, no study performed in the head-unrestrained condition has been published so far. We have recently explored the MPC in the cat to localize the areas from which saccades can be evoked at a low current intensity (threshold <30 μA). We then selected a few sites for a detailed analysis of head-restrained and head-unrestrained evoked responses. Although the histological verification is not yet available because the experiments are still going on, these sites are likely situated in the close vicinity of the cFN. All sites tested so far indicate the presence of a head movement that accompanies the evoked saccade. Depending on the stimulated site, the direction of the head movement can be similar or different from the direction of the concurrent gaze shift.

Lesion/inactivation

Very limited information about the role of the MPC in the control of gaze shifts in the head-unrestrained condition can be obtained from monkey studies (Ritchie, 1976) or clinical studies (Shimizu et al., 1981a,b). Using large lesions of the MPC in the monkey, Ritchie (1976) noted that the dysmetria of saccadic gaze shifts (eye in space) is largely independent of whether the animal can also move its head. This observation was also made in a first group of cerebellar patients by Shimizu et al. (1981b), but in a second group, only hypermetric patients and some hypometric patients showed the same tendency, whereas the gaze hypometria of the remaining subjects was reduced in the head-unrestrained condition as compared to the head-restrained condition. On the whole, these data are inconclusive because the data regarding head movements have not been systematically analyzed. Thus, it is not yet possible to determine whether the lesion affected the head movement and to which extent the head actually contributed to the dysmetria of gaze.

cFN inactivation and visually triggered gaze shifts

During the last decade we have used unilateral injections of muscimol to investigate in the head-un-restrained cat the role of the cFN in the control of visually triggered gaze shifts (Goffart and Pélisson, 1994, 1997, 1998; Goffart et al., 1998a,b). The main deficits found after cFN unilateral inactivation are spontaneous gaze deviation, fixation offset, dysmetria of the gaze displacements, marked modifications in the latency and moderate changes in the dynamics of gaze saccades. We present in the following these deficits and emphasize on the type of dysmetria and on the coordination between eye and head components.

Spontaneous gaze deviation and fixation offset

After unilateral cFN inactivations the spontaneous scanning of the lighted environment was mostly restricted to the ipsilesional visual hemifield. When a food target was presented to the animal, an offset ranging from 1 to 9.4 degrees toward the inactivated cFN (average value 4.9 degrees) was observed between the gaze and the target positions. The offset involved the head to a major extent, since the deviation of the eyes in the orbit was very small in these situations. When the head was restrained, the average deviation of the eyes in the orbit increased but with a smaller magnitude than the deviation of gaze observed in the head-unrestrained condition. These deviations of gaze in light with or without presentation of a visual target are reminiscent of the behavior of the head-restrained monkey, but in this last situation the reported ocular deviation was much smaller (1–2 degrees average fixation offset reported by Robinson et al., 1993, and Goffart et al., 2002; but see the 7-degrees fixation offset illustrated in the work of Ohtsuka et al., 1994). This quantitative difference of gaze deviation between the head-restrained and head-unrestrained studies could be due to the head mobility, to the constraints to make accurate fixation during both training and recording phases and/or to difference in visual system between the cat and the monkey. The deviation of the head is likely responsible for the gaze deviation since it is maintained when a food target is approached toward the animal's yaw and when the animal tries to bite the food. Finally, when the animal is walking on the floor toward a food target located about 2 m in front, the locomotion path of the body is systematically curved toward the inactivated cFN (Guillaume et al.,

2000). Such curved paths are predicted by a simple model assuming a systematic bias in the specification of the heading direction relative to the current target direction with a bias similar to the constant error of ipsiversive gaze shifts recorded before the locomotion tests (see below).

Gaze dysmetria

The amplitude of the primary saccadic gaze shift was strongly affected by inactivation of the cFN. Like the dysmetria observed in the head-restrained condition, gaze shifts were hypermetric or hypometric depending on their direction relative to the side of injection (ipsi- or contra-versive, respectively). Beyond this amplitude difference, a marked difference in the type of error emerged from our study: the contraversive hypometria could mainly be described by a slope decrease in the relationship between the horizontal amplitude of the gaze displacement response and the horizontal amplitude of the required gaze displacement (gain reduction), whereas the ipsiversive hypermetria was essentially related to an increase in the y-intercept. This relationship revealed the major contribution of a constant error (mean 10 degrees, ranging from 4 to 20 degrees) to the ipsilateral hypermetria with a rather limited change in gain. Several points which qualify the pattern of saccadic dysmetria are worth considering.

First, when the target was presented at the location of the actual gaze position, above or below it, the injected animals produced an inappropriate response bringing gaze away from the target toward the inactivated side, toward a position that corresponded approximately to the horizontal constant error value. Such responses reject the possibility that the change in y-intercept would be due to an erroneous extrapolation of the relationship between the horizontal gaze amplitude and the horizontal amplitude of the required gaze displacement. Also, when the target was presented in the contralesional visual hemifield with an eccentricity smaller than the bias, the animal produced an ipsiversive gaze shift bringing again gaze away from the target. The horizontal constant error that characterizes the hypermetria of ipsiversive gaze shifts was interpreted as reflecting an impairment in the localization of the target or in the specification of the movement metrics prior to

movement onset (Goffart and Pélisson, 1994, 1998). Qualitative observation of the straight trajectory of oblique ipsiversive gaze shifts toward a target presented on the horizontal azimuth and initiated from different vertical positions suggests that impairment is already acting at the gaze shift onset.

Second, for both the ipsiversive and contraversive gaze shifts, the dysmetria of gaze shifts is related to modifications in the amplitude of both eye and head components. These modifications of eye and head movements are such that their relative contributions to the amplitude of the gaze shift are barely changed relative to control gaze shifts with matched amplitudes. This result indicates that the injection of muscimol in the cFN does not interfere with mechanisms subtending the eye–head coordination and suggests an influence of cFN upon functional processes that are located centrally rather than peripherally along the visuomotor pathways involved in gaze shifts production.

Gaze latency

As suggested by the inappropriate gaze shifts, cFN inactivation also interfered in a consistent manner with mechanisms prior to gaze shift onset and more particularly with those involved in its initiation: the latency of ipsiversive movements of the eye and head decreased, whereas that of contraversive movements increased. Although the former effect was rather limited in amplitude because the latencies of control movements were already quite short in these food target paradigms, the maximum mean increase of contraversive responses latency reached 109% in these paradigms where both the direction and amplitude of the desired response were unpredictable. The modifications of latency were very similar in magnitude between the eye and the head movements such that the changes in eye/head delay were small (7.5 ms on average).

Gaze dynamics

The dynamics of dysmetric gaze shifts and of their eye and head components were first studied by plotting for each experiment the main sequence relationships. Qualitative examination of all these nonlinear relationships revealed a tendency for the velocity of ipsiversive gaze shifts to be reduced after musci- mol injection. The larger range of amplitudes after muscimol injection for ipsiversive gaze shifts facil- itated the detection of a main sequence change for these gaze shifts as compared to contraversive ones. The quantitative comparison of normal and postin- activation peak gaze velocity for matched amplitude gaze shifts within a common range of 30 degrees revealed a consistent reduction in gaze velocity for both movement directions ($55°/s$ on average). This slowing of gaze velocity resulted from combined modifications in the velocity of both eye and head components. In some experiments where the slowing of ipsiversive gaze shifts exceeded that of contraver- sive responses, the detailed analysis of the accel- eration and the deceleration durations disclosed a predominant increase in the duration of the decel- eration phase. Notably, in two experiments, a large reduction of gaze velocity has been observed dur- ing the postinactivation period without concomitant change in the size of gaze dysmetria, suggesting that modifications in the dynamics and metrics of gaze shifts following cFN inactivation are not related to each other but instead result from partly independent mechanisms.

Specificity of deficits: comparison between cFN and rFN inactivation

In another study we made similar muscimol injec- tions in the rostral part of the fastigial nucleus (rFN) and compared in the same animals the resulting deficits to those induced by injections in the caudal part (Pélisson et al., 1998). Since the cFN and rFN have both common and specific outputs, this compar- ison allowed to test the link between gaze dysmetria and the inactivated fastigial efferences. Some deficits induced by cFN inactivation could also be observed when the injection was made in the rFN. For ex- ample, ipsiversive gaze shifts were hypermetric and their latency reduced, whereas contraversive gaze shifts were hypometric and their latency increased during rFN and cFN inactivations. A moderate de- crease in gaze velocity was also observed in both conditions. Modifications of eye–head coordination were quite limited, and were significantly smaller after inactivation of the cFN than after inactivation of the rFN. Other deficits induced by rFN inactiva-

tion differed from those induced by cFN inactivation. Indeed, in the head-unrestrained condition, the eyes were severely deviated in the orbit in the former case and barely in the latter. After muscimol injection in the rFN, the dysmetria was characterized by a rather small change in *y*-intercept of the relationship between the horizontal target eccentricity and the horizontal amplitude of the subsequent gaze shift. Fi- nally, a strong postural deficit was found exclusively after muscimol injection in the rFN, but not when the cFN was inactivated. Three conclusions can be drawn from these data. First, a previously unknown contribution of the rFN to the control of head-un- restrained gaze shifts is demonstrated. Second, the modified pattern of deficits according to the inacti- vation locus in the fastigial nucleus underlines the specificity of our inactivation methods. Third, this pattern defining a functional distinction between rFN and cFN can be used to relate some deficits to differ- ent fastigial output pathways: the ipsiversive bias of gaze shifts and fixation offset could be related to as- cending fastigial projections to the thalamus and SC which arise specifically from the cFN, whereas the deviation of the eyes in the orbit could be due to the descending projections from the rFN to the nucleus prepositus hypoglossi (McCrea and Baker, 1985).

cFN inactivation and SC stimulation

To better understand the functional nature of gaze dysmetria during cFN inactivation and get further insight into the neural processes controlled by the MPC, we combined in the head-unrestrained cat unilateral inactivation of the cFN with electrical mi- crostimulation of the deep superior colliculus (dSC). Gaze shifts have been evoked by dSC microstim- ulation with two objectives: first, to modify the position of gaze prior to its launch toward a pre- viously presented visual target and to test whether cFN inactivation impaired the feedback mechanisms that compensate for such gaze perturbation (Mays and Sparks, 1980; Pélisson et al., 1995), and second, to elicit gaze shifts from various dSC loci and to test whether the SC motor map is impaired by cFN inactivation.

The first study was motivated by the hypothesis that the MPC would be part of the local feedback loop controlling the on-going trajectory of saccades

(Vilis and Hore, 1981; Keller, 1989). Assuming that the compensatory mechanisms are part of this local feedback loop, this hypothesis predicts that the animal's capability to compensate for an unexpected saccade perturbation should be altered during dysfunction of the MPC. Since the dynamic feedback concept has been extended to the control of head--unrestrained gaze shifts (Laurutis and Robinson, 1986; Pélisson et al., 1988; Munoz et al., 1991; Guitton, 1992; Lefèvre and Galiana, 1992; Pélisson et al., 1995; Phillips et al., 1995), we tested the involvement of the MPC in the feedback mechanisms controlling combined eye–head gaze shifts (Goffart et al., 1998a). A previous study has indicated that in a similar experimental situation with the head unrestrained, normal cats do produce an accurate compensation to a gaze perturbation induced by SC stimulation during the reaction time period (Pélisson et al., 1995). In cFN-inactivated animals, perturbations were again followed by compensations which brought gaze to the same location as gaze shifts during unperturbed trials. This is true for both ipsiversive and contraversive perturbations, indicating that irrespective of the dysmetria induced by cFN inactivation, the encoding of gaze (or separate eye and head) feedback signals are still operating normally in the cFN-inactivated animals. In agreement with the limited modification of gaze dynamics reported above, these results suggest that the dysmetria of gaze shifts are not related to an impaired feedback control.

The second study addressed the question of the state of the SC motor map during cFN inactivation (Guillaume and Pélisson, 2001). To this aim, we studied the effect of cFN inactivation on the properties of head unrestrained gaze shifts evoked by SC microstimulation. Focussing on near-horizontal gaze shifts, we varied the location of the stimulated sites along the SC rostro-caudal axis and for each site ($n = 18$ in two cats) we tested various stimulation currents. The analysis of the metrics and latency of evoked gaze shifts indicated that the cFN inactivation resulted in a strong distortion of the SC motor map coding for ipsiversive responses (SC contralateral to inactivated cFN) and for a moderate reduction of the amplitude coding in the opposite SC. Indeed, the amplitude of ipsiversive gaze shifts was modified — relative to responses elicited before cFN

inactivation — in a manner that depended on the position of the stimulated SC site: it increased for sites located in the rostral 2/3 of the SC, but decreased for the remaining caudal zone, with one site in the transition zone providing gaze shifts with an unchanged amplitude. In contrast, contraversive gaze shifts elicited from the opposite SC all had a moderately reduced amplitude, except for the most caudal site (no change). Based on these results, Guillaume and Pélisson (2001) proposed that the MPC influences both the SC and downstream centers through parallel fastigial output pathways.

Role of the MPC in saccadic control: models

Models of saccadic and gaze control systems that include the medio-posterior cerebellum and make predictions about saccade dysmetria can be distinguished into system theory models (Optican, 1982; Keller, 1989) based on the local feedback loop structure of the original model of Robinson (1975) and neurophysiologically oriented models which additionally attempt to incorporate detailed neurophysiological data (Dean, 1995; Quaia et al., 1999). In the former category, the models suggest that the medio-posterior cerebellum is located upstream from the feedback control of saccades (Optican, 1982) or is part of the feedback loop (Keller, 1989). These formal models do not simulate the actual neural activity and do not consider the connectivity of cerebellar neurons but provide formal predictions regarding the saccade metrics and dynamics following cerebellar dysfunction. Although they both predict saccade dysmetria, their predictions differ when one considers the dynamics of saccades, since only the feedback model predicts changes in saccade dynamics. Note that in this latter case, the predicted changes associated with hypometric and hypermetric saccades are opposite to each other. These predictions are not consistent with the lesion data since changes in the main sequence relationships, when they occur, always correspond to a reduction of saccade velocity. The second category of models (Dean, 1995; Quaia et al., 1999) has recently been developed to incorporate the accumulating neurophysiological data in the monkey. These models follow the concept, initially proposed by Noda (1991) and supported by data from Fuchs' laboratory (Fuchs et al., 1993), that the cFN helps accelerate contraversive saccades and decelerate ipsiversive saccades by sending to the pre-oculomotor burst neurons an early and a late burst of activity, respectively. Thus, contrary to the above formal models, the postulated influence of the cFN on the saccadic circuitry is non-linear, i.e. do not act as a simple gain control. Whereas the model published by Dean (1995) focuses on these fastigio-reticular projections (see also the models by Schweighofer et al., 1996, and Gancarz and Grossberg, 1999, regarding the adaptive control of saccades), the model proposed later by Optican and colleagues (Quaia et al., 1999) also attributes a role to fastigial efferences toward the SC. Dean proposed a way to combine neurophysiological data in a Robinson type model (Van Gisbergen et al., 1981) by suggesting that the cFN adds temporally coded signals at the level of the feedback comparator. Specifically, in the model, the early burst of the contralateral cFN and the late burst of the ipsilateral cFN ('braking signal') are respectively added and subtracted from the EBNs saccade-related activity at a postsynaptic level. This model accurately simulates the generalized hypermetria of saccades following bilateral cFN inactivation as well as the metrics of saccades following unilateral cFN inactivation in the head-unrestrained monkey. The limitation of this model rests on its structure which excludes any other MPC outputs, particularly ascending fastigial projections to the thalamus and SC. Besides a conceptual schema proposed by Houk et al. (1992), the model published by Optican's group (Quaia et al., 1999) is the first to present a synergic contribution of the cerebellar output pathways to the brainstem reticular formation and SC. It is suggested that (1) the SC provides the brainstem pulse generator with an initial directional drive, (2) the medio-posterior cerebellum, which is located inside the local feedback loop, monitors on-line saccadic motor error and is responsible for terminating the saccade by turning off ('choke signal') the motoneurons drive through a projection from the cFN to the contralateral IBNs, and (3) the cerebellum also modulates SC activity.

This model is a valuable effort to incorporate the contribution of many oculomotor structures (parietal and frontal cortices, SC, cerebellum, brainstem reticular formation) in a functionally tractable scheme compatible with the main features of SC and cerebellar contribution to saccade production. However, this model fails to predict the well established hypometria of saccades directed away from a lesioned cFN. Also, the hypothesized topographically coded wave of activity between the two cFN assumes a recruitment of cFN neurons that depends on the saccade size, which is not consistent with the evidence of cFN neurons discharging in relation to all saccades, regardless of their amplitude. In addition, predictions regarding electrically evoked saccades and compensatory responses to stimulation-induced perturbations have not been found experimentally, and instead, the electrical SC stimulation can still produce staircase saccades during cFN inactivation (Guillaume and Pélisson, 2001) and the capability to compensate for such collicular-evoked saccades is preserved (Goffart et al., 1998a). Finally, both Dean's and Quaia's models predict that the pre-oculomotor burst neurons (EBN, IBN) should demonstrate a late burst of activity during OFF-directed saccades, a possibility which is debated given the controversial empirical data (Van Gisbergen et al., 1981; Cullen and Guitton, 1997).

In summary, models of the MPC need to incorporate the results reviewed above. In addition, given the evidence that the role of the MPC is not restricted to the movement of the eyes in the orbit, future modelling studies should specify how the cerebellum controls saccadic gaze shifts and eye–head coordination processes when these two platforms are synergistically involved.

Concluding remarks and perspectives

Beyond the precise delineation of the various cerebellar zones involved in saccadic eye movements, the spectacular explosion of empirical data observed during the last decade in cerebellar saccadic neurophysiology has led to the elaboration of the first testable models incorporating both neurophysiological and functional information. An immense hope shared by researchers and clinicians is that, due to its relatively circumscribed structure and known neurophysiology, the saccadic system offers a valuable model to study the cerebellar role in sensorimotor transformations.

While current models focus on the production of horizontal saccadic eye movements (with the exception of the model of Quaia et al., 1999, which deals with both horizontal and vertical saccadic components), shifting gaze in space under natural conditions rarely corresponds to such a simplified case, but instead involves 3-D movements of the eyes in the orbit, the coupling between versional and vergence ocular responses as well as between eye, head and sometimes torso movements (see Takagi et al., 2003, this volume, and Klier et al., 2003, this volume). As recent data already suggest, addressing these various aspects in more detail will tell us that the role of the cerebellum in gaze shifts is more general than just controlling the motion of the eyes in the orbit. These new studies will also provide fruitful information on the neural signals influenced by cerebellar activity and will have to differentiate whether: (1) the cerebellum controls desired displacement signals, feedback signals or downstream motor commands; (2) signals related to eye, head and body axis are influenced by parallel cerebellar output pathways or a gaze- (or target-) related signal is directly under cerebellar control; (3) version and vergence signals are controlled separately or the desired displacement of gaze in space is directly modulated by cerebellar activity; (4) the cerebellum is involved in the computation necessary for the kinematic control of eye, head and gaze movements to account for the neural implementation of Donders' law and Listing's law.

Evidently, the answers to these functionally oriented questions will bring new information about the functional input–output relationships of the cerebellum with other oculomotor structures. For example, the demonstration of an involvement of the MPC in controlling desired gaze displacement will advocate for a significant involvement of fastigio-tectal reciprocal projections, given the strongly suggested involvement of the SC in the encoding of a gaze displacement command (Munoz et al., 1991; Freedman and Sparks, 1997; Guitton et al., 2003, this volume; Sparks and Gandhi, 2003, this volume). Given all these possible modes and levels of control, what then can we expect from these future studies? There are at least three reasons why we believe that the MPC influences the saccadic orienting gaze behavior through multiple levels of actions. The first is related to the cerebellar connectivity which is organized in closed loops with multiple neural centers situated at different levels along the sensorimotor pathways.

The second reason comes from our recent study of gaze shifts evoked electrically from the SC in the head-unrestrained cat. Indeed, the pattern of modifications of gaze amplitude and latency following cFN inactivation is consistent with a dual role of the MPC, through parallel fastigial projections toward the SC and toward downstream centers (Guillaume and Pélisson, 2001). The third reason is more indirect and is related to the neural substrate of saccadic adaptation. Although the whole network of structures involved in saccadic adaptation remains to be elucidated, it is clear from lesion and activation studies that the MPC is critically involved (Goldberg et al., 1993; Desmurget et al., 1998, 2000; Takagi et al., 1998; Barash et al., 1999). Interestingly, saccadic adaptation has been shown in human subjects to be highly specific to the type of saccade tested. For example, adaptation of reflexive visual saccades does not transfer to internally generated visual or memory saccades (Deubel, 1995). Given that the neural substrates of these different saccade types are partly separated (for review see Pierrot-Deseilligny et al., 1995, 2003, this volume), the cerebellar-dependent mechanisms underlying the adaptation of different saccade types supposedly occur at different sensorimotor levels.

To conclude, further investigations of the role of the cerebellum should progressively release the various degrees of freedom which are typically involved in the production of saccadic gaze shifts in the natural world. Although difficult, this task will benefit from recent developments of gaze control models and will prove necessary for a comprehensive understanding of the cerebellar role in motor control.

Abbreviations

MPC	medio-posterior cerebellum
FN	fastigial nucleus
rFN	rostral fastigial nucleus
cFN	caudal fastigial nucleus
FOR	fastigial oculomotor region
DLPN	dorsolateral pontine nucleus
NRTP	nucleus reticularis tegmenti pontis
MAO	medial accessory olive
PPRF	paramedian pontine reticular formation
MRF	mesencephalic reticular formation
EBN	excitatory burst neuron

IBN   inhibitory burst neuron
MVN   medial vestibular nucleus
IVN   inferior vestibular nucleus
SVN   superior vestibular nucleus
NPH   nucleus prepositus hypoglossi
IML   internal medullary lamina
SC   superior colliculus
dSC   deep superior colliculus
FEF   frontal eye fields

Acknowledgements

Laurent Goffart was supported by the French Ministry of Research and Technology and Alain Guillaume by the 'Fondation pour la Recherche Médicale'. We acknowledge Marie-Line Loyalle and Abdelhak Jallane for taking care of the animals, and Christian Urquizar and Marcia Riley for designing a software for data analysis. This research was supported by Institut National de la Santé et de la Recherche Médicale U94 and U534, and by a HFSP grant RG58/92B.

References

Aizenman, C.D. and Linden, D.J. (1999) Regulation of rebound depolarization and spontaneous firing patterns of deep nuclear neurons in slices of rat cerebellum. *J. Neurophysiol.*, 82: 1697–1709.

Albus, J.A. (1971) A theory of cerebellar function. *Math. Biosci.*, 10: 25–61.

Allen, G.I. and Tsukahara, N. (1974) Cerebro-cerebellar communication systems. *Physiol. Rev.*, 54: 957–1006.

Altman, J.A., Bechterev, N.N., Radionova, E.A., Shmigidina, G.N. and Syka, J. (1976) Electrical responses of the auditory area of the cerebellar cortex to acoustic stimulation. *Exp. Brain Res.*, 26: 285–298.

Andersen, R.A., Bracewell, R.M., Barash, S., Gnadt, J.W. and Fogassi, L. (1990) Eye position effects on visual, memory, and saccade-related activity in areas LIP and 7a of macaque. *J. Neurosci.*, 10(4): 1176–1196.

Aschoff, J.C. and Cohen, B. (1971) Changes in saccadic eye movements produced by cerebellar cortical lesions. *Exp. Neurol.*, 32(2): 123–133.

Barash, S., Melikyan, A., Sivakov, A., Zhang, M., Glickstein, M. and Thier, P. (1999) Saccadic dysmetria and adaptation after lesions of the cerebellar cortex. *J. Neurosci.*, 19(24): 10931–10939.

Batini, C., Buisseret, P. and Kado, R.T. (1974) Extraocular proprioceptive and trigeminal projections to the Purkinje cells of the cerebellar cortex. *Arch. Ital. Biol.*, 112: 1–17.

Batini, C., Buisseret-Delmas, C., Corvisier, J., Hardy, O. and

Jassik-Gerschenfeld, D. (1978) Brain stem nuclei giving fibers to lobules VI and VII of the cerebellar vermis. *Brain Res.*, 153: 241–261.

Batton, R.R., Jayaraman, A., Ruggiero, D. and Carpenter, M.B. (1977) Fastigial efferent projections in the monkey: an autoradiographic study. *J. Comp. Neurol.*, 174: 281–306.

Berthoz, A. and Llinas, R. (1974) Afferent neck projection to the cat cerebellar cortex. *Exp. Brain Res.*, 20: 385–401.

Blanks, R.H.I. (1988) Cerebellum. In: J.A. Büttner-Ennever (Ed.), *Neuroanatomy of the Oculomotor System*. Elsevier, Amsterdam, pp. 255–272.

Buchtel, H.A., Iosif, G., Marchesi, G.F., Provini, L. and Strata, P. (1972) Analysis of the activity evoked in the cerebellar cortex by stimulation of the visual pathways. *Exp. Brain Res.*, 15: 278–288.

Büttner, U., Fuchs, A.F., Markert-Schwab, G. and Buckmaster, P. (1991) Fastigial nucleus activity in the alert monkey during slow eye and head movements. *J. Neurophysiol.*, 65: 1360–1371.

Büttner, U., Glasauer, S., Glonti, L., Kleine, J.F. and Siebold, C. (1999) Otolith processing in the deep cerebellar nuclei. *Ann. N.Y. Acad. Sci.*, 871: 81–93.

Cajal, S.R. (1888) Estructura de los centros nerviosos de las aves, I. Cerebelo. *Revist. Trimest. Histol. Norm. Pathol.*, 1.

Carpenter, M.B. and Batton, R.R. (1982) Connections of the fastigial nucleus in the cat and monkey. In: S.L. Palay and V. Chan-Palay (Eds.), *The Cerebellum — New Vistas*. Springer, Berlin, pp. 250–295.

Cohen, B., Goto, K., Shanzer, S. and Weiss, A.H. (1965) Eye movements induced by electrical stimulation of the cerebellum in the alert cat. *Exp. Neurol.*, 13: 145–162.

Courville, J. and Diakiw, N. (1976) Cerebellar corticonuclear projection in the cat. The vermis of the anterior and posterior lobes. *Brain Res.*, 110: 1–20.

Crandall, W.F. and Keller, E.L. (1985) Visual and oculomotor signals in nucleus reticularis tegmenti pontis in alert monkey. *J. Neurophysiol.*, 54(5): 1326–1345.

Cullen, K.E. and Guitton, D. (1997) Analysis of primate IBNs spike trains using system identification techniques, I. Relationship to eye movement dynamics during head-fixed saccades. *J. Neurophysiol.*, 78: 3259–3282.

Dean, P. (1995) Modelling the role of the cerebellar fastigial nuclei in producing accurate saccades: the importance of burst timing. *Neuroscience*, 68: 1059–1077.

Desmurget, M., Pélisson, D., Grethe, J.S., Alexander, G.E., Urquizar, C., Prablanc, C. and Grafton, S.T. (2000) Functional adaptation of reactive saccades in humans: a PET study. *Exp. Brain Res.*, 132: 243–259.

Desmurget, M., Pélisson, D., Urquizar, C., Prablanc, C., Alexander, G.E. and Grafton, S.T. (1998) Functional anatomy of saccadic adaptation in humans. *Nat. Neurosci.*, 1: 524–528.

Deubel, H. (1995) Separate adaptive mechanisms for the control of reactive and volitional saccadic eye movements. *Vis. Res.*, 35: 3529–3540.

De Zeeuw, C.I., Holstege, J.C., Ruigrok, T.J.H. and Voogd, J. (1989) Ultrastructural study of the Gaba-ergic, cerebellar and mesodiencephalic innervation of the cat medial accessory olive: anterograde tracing combined with immunocytochemistry. *J. Comp. Neurol.*, 284: 12–35.

Dias, E.C. and Segraves, M.A. (1999) Muscimol-induced inactivation of monkey frontal eye field: effects on visually and memory-guided saccades. *J. Neurophysiol.*, 81(5): 2191–2214.

Dietrichs, E. and Walberg, F. (1985) The cerebellar nucleo-olivary and olivo-cerebellar nuclear projections in the cat as studied with anterograde and retrograde transport in the same animal after implantation of crystalline WGA-HRP, II. The fastigial nucleus. *Anat. Embryol.*, 173: 253–261.

Dietrichs, E. and Walberg, F. (1987) Cerebellar nuclear afferents — where do they originate? A re-evaluation of the projections from some lower braistem nuclei. *Anat. Embryol.*, 177: 165–172.

Donaldson, I.M.L. and Hawthorne, M.E. (1979) Coding of visual information by units in the cat cerebellar vermis. *Exp. Brain Res.*, 34: 27–48.

Eccles, J.C., Nicoll, R.A., Schwarz, D.W.F., Taborikova, H. and Willey, T.J. (1975) Reticulospinal neurons with and without monosynaptic input from cerebellar nuclei. *J. Neurophysiol.*, 43: 1236–1250.

Flourens, P. (1824) *Recherches expérimentales sur les propriétés et les fonctions du système nerveux central dans les animaux vertébrés*. Crevot, Paris.

Freedman, E.G. and Sparks, D.L. (1997) Activity of cells in the deeper layers of the superior colliculus of the rhesus monkey: evidence for a gaze displacement command. *J. Neurophysiol.*, 78: 1669–1690.

Freeman, J.A. (1970) Response of cat cerebellar Purkinje cells to convergent inputs from cerebral cortex and peripheral sensory systems. *J. Neurophysiol.*, 33: 697–712.

Fuchs, A.F. and Kornhuber, H.H. (1969) Extraocular muscle afferents projection to the cerebellum of the cat. *J. Physiol.*, 200: 713–722.

Fuchs, A.F., Robinson, F.R. and Straube, A. (1993) Role of the caudal fastigial nucleus in saccade generation, I. Neuronal discharge patterns. *J. Neurophysiol.*, 70: 1712–1740.

Fuchs, A.F., Robinson, F.R. and Straube, A. (1994) Participation of the caudal fastigial nucleus in smooth-pursuit eye movements, I. Neuronal activity. *J. Neurophysiol.*, 72(6): 2714–2728.

Fujikado, T. and Noda, H. (1987) Saccadic eye movements evoked by microstimulation of lobule VII of cerebellar vermis of macaque monkeys. *J. Physiol.*, 394: 573–594.

Furuya, N., Kawano, K. and Shimazu, H. (1975) Functional organization of vestibulofastigial projection in the horizontal semicircular canal system in the cat. *Exp. Brain Res.*, 24: 75–87.

Gancarz, G. and Grossberg, S. (1999) A neural model of saccadic eye movement control explains task-specific adaptation. *Vis. Res.*, 39: 3123–3143.

Gauthier, G.M. and Stark, L. (1979) Cerebellar stimulation and eye movements in cats. *Math. Biosci.*, 46: 37–58.

Gaymard, B., Rivaud, S., Amarenco, P. and Pierrot-Deseilligny, C. (1994) Influence of visual information on cerebellar saccadic dysmetria. *Ann. Neurol.*, 35: 108–112.

Gerrits, N.M. and Voogd, J. (1987) The projection of the nucleus reticularis tegmenti pontis and adjacent regions of the pontine nuclei to the central cerebellar nuclei in the cat. *J. Comp. Neurol.*, 258: 52–69.

Godschalk, M., Van der Burg, J., Van Duin, B. and De Zeeuw, C.I. (1994) Topography of saccadic eye movements evoked by microstimulation in rabbit cerebellar vermis. *J. Physiol.*, 480: 147–153.

Goffart, L. and Pélisson, D. (1994) Cerebellar contribution to the spatial encoding of orienting gaze shifts in the head-free cat. *J. Neurophysiol.*, 72(5): 2547–2550.

Goffart, L. and Pélisson, D. (1997) Changes in initiation of orienting gaze shifts after muscimol inactivation of the caudal fastigial nucleus in the cat. *J. Physiol. (Lond.)*, 503(Pt 3): 657–671.

Goffart, L. and Pélisson, D. (1998) Orienting gaze shifts during muscimol inactivation of caudal fastigial nucleus in the cat, I. Gaze dysmetria. *J. Neurophysiol.*, 79: 1942–1958.

Goffart, L. and Sparks, D.L. (1997) Saccadic dysmetria after muscimol inactivation of the caudal fastigial nucleus in the rhesus monkey. *Soc. Neurosci. Abstr.*, New Orleans, October.

Goffart, L., Guillaume, A. and Pélisson, D. (1998a) Compensation for gaze perturbation during inactivation of the caudal fastigial nucleus in the head-unrestrained cat. *J. Neurophysiol.*, 80: 1552–1557.

Goffart, L., Pélisson, D. and Guillaume, A. (1998b) Orienting gaze shifts during muscimol inactivation of caudal fastigial nucleus in the cat, II. Dynamics and eye–head coupling. *J. Neurophysiol.*, 79: 1959–1976.

Goffart, L., Sparks, D.L. and Kalesnykas, R.P. (1998c) Saccades evoked by electrical microstimulation of the fastigial saccade-related area in the head-fixed monkey. *Soc. Neurosci. Abstr.*, Los Angeles.

Goffart, L., Chen, L.L. and Sparks, D.L. (1999) Saccadic dysmetria and timed perturbation of the caudal fastigial nucleus in the rhesus monkey. *Soc. Neurosci. Abstr.*, Miami Beach.

Goffart, L., Catz, N. and Pélisson, D. (2001) Eye and head movements evoked by electrical microstimulation of the fastigial nucleus in the cat. *11th Annual Meeting of the Society Neural Control of Movement, Sevilla*.

Goffart, L., Chen, L.L. and Sparks, D.L. (2003) Saccade deficits during muscimol inactivation of the caudal Fastigial nucleus in the rhesus monkey. In preparation.

Goldberg, M.E., Musil, S.Y., Fitzgibbon, E.J., Smith, M. and Olson, C.R. (1993) The role of the cerebellum in the control of saccadic eye movements. In: N. Mano, I. Hamada and M.R. DeLong (Eds.), *Role of the Cerebellum and Basal Ganglia in Voluntary Movements*. Elsevier, Amsterdam, pp. 203–211.

Gould, B.B. (1980) Organization of afferents from the brainstem nuclei to the cerebellar cortex in the cat. *Adv. Anat., Embryol. Cell Biol.*, 62: 1–90.

Groenewegen, H.J. and Voogd, J. (1977) The parasagittal zonation within the olivo-cerebellar projection, I. Climbing fiber distribution in the vermis of cat cerebellum. *J. Comp. Neurol.*, 174: 417–488.

Gruart, A. and Delgado-Garcia, J.M. (1994) Signalling properties of identified deep cerebellar nuclear neurons related to eye and head movements in the alert cat. *J. Physiol.*, 478(1): 37–54.

Guillaume, A. and Pélisson, D. (2001) Gaze shifts evoked by electrical stimulation of the superior colliculus in the head-unrestrained cat, II. Effect of muscimol inactivation of the caudal fastigial nucleus. *Eur. J. Neurosci.*, 14(8): 1345–1359.

Guillaume, A., Goffart, L., Courjon, J.H. and Pélisson, D. (2000) Altered visuo-motor behavior during inactivation of the caudal fastigial nucleus in the cat. *Exp. Brain Res.*, 132(4): 457–463.

Guitton, D. (1992) Control of eye–head coordination during gaze shifts. *TINS*, 15(5): 174–179.

Guitton, D., Bergeron, A., Choi, W.Y. and Matsuo, S. (2003) On the feedback control of orienting gaze shifts made with eye and head movements. In: C. Prablanc, D. Pélisson and Y. Rossetti (Eds.), *Neural Control of Space Coding and Action Production. Progress in Brain Research*, Vol. 142. Elsevier, Amsterdam, pp. 55–68 (this volume).

Haas, R., Dicke, P.W. and Thier, P. (1999) Saccade-related responses of most posterior vermal Purkinje cells do not depend on the starting position of the eyes. *Soc. Neurosci. Abstr.*, 25: 1652.

Hashimoto, M. and Ohtsuka, K. (1995) Transcranial magnetic stimulation over the posterior cerebellum during visually guided saccades in man. *Brain*, 118: 1185–1193.

Helmchen, C. and Büttner, U. (1995) Saccade-related purkinje cell activity in the oculomotor vermis during spontaneous eye movements in light and darkness. *Exp. Brain Res.*, 103: 198–208.

Helmchen, C., Straube, A. and Büttner, U. (1994) Saccade-related activity in the fastigial oculomotor region of the macaque monkey during spontaneous eye movements in light and darkness. *Exp. Brain Res.*, 98: 474–482.

Hepp, K., Henn, V. and Jaeger, J. (1982) Eye movement related neurons in the cerebellar nuclei of the alert monkey. *Exp. Brain Res.*, 45: 253–264.

Hirai, T., Onodera, S. and Kawamura, K. (1982) Cerebellotectal projections studied in cats with horseradish peroxidase or tritiated amino acids axonal transport. *Exp. Brain Res.*, 48: 1–12.

Hoddevik, G.H., Brodal, A., Kawamura, K. and Hashikawa, T. (1977) The pontine projection to the cerebellar vermal visual area studied by means of the retrograde axonal transport of horseradish peroxidase. *Brain Res.*, 123: 209–227.

Homma, Y., Nonaka, S., Matsuyama, K. and Mori, S. (1995) Fastigiofugal projection to the brainstem nuclei in the cat: an anterograde PHA-L tracing study. *Neurosci. Lett.*, 23: 89–102.

Houk, J.C., Galiana, H.L. and Guitton, D. (1992) Cooperative control of gaze by the superior colliculus, brainstem and cerebellum. In: G.E. Stelmach and J. Requin (Eds.), *Tutorials in Motor Behavior*. Elsevier, Amsterdam, pp. 443–474.

Ito, M. (1984) *The Cerebellum and Neural Control*. Raven Press, New York.

Ito, M., Yoshida, M., Obata, K., Kawai, N. and Udo, M. (1970) Inhibitory control of intracerebellar nuclei by the Purkinje cells axons. *Exp. Brain Res.*, 10: 64–80.

Jimenez-Castellanos, J.J. and Reinoso-Suarez, F. (1985) Topographical organization of the afferent connections of the principal ventromedial thalamic nucleus in the cat. *J. Comp. Neurol.*, 236: 297–314.

Kanayama, R., Bronstein, A.M., Shallo-Hoffmann, J., Rudge, P. and Husain, M. (1994) Visually and memory guided saccades in a case of cerebellar saccadic dysmetria. *J. Neurol. Neurosurg. Psychiatry*, 57: 1081–1084.

Kase, M., Miller, D.C. and Noda, H. (1980) Discharges of Purkinje cells and mossy fibres in the cerebellar vermis of the monkey during saccadic eye movements and fixation. *J. Physiol.*, 300: 539–555.

Katoh, Y.Y. and Deura, S. (1993) Direct projections from the cerebellar fastigial nucleus to the thalamic suprageniculate nucleus in the cat studied with the anterograde and retrograde axonal transport of wheat germ agglutinin–horseradish peroxidase. *Brain Res.*, 617: 155–158.

Kawamura, K., Kase, M., Ohno, M., Hashikawa, T. and Kato, M. (1990) Visual inputs to the dorsocaudal fastigial nucleus of the cat cerebellum. An experimental study using single unit recordings and horseradish peroxydase labelling. *Arch. Ital. Biol.*, 128: 295–314.

Kawamura, S., Hattori, S., Higo, S. and Matsuyama, T. (1982) The cerebellar projections to the superior colliculus and pretectum in the cat: an autoradiographic and horseradish peroxidase study. *Neuroscience*, 7(7): 1673–1689.

Keating, E.G. and Gooley, S.G. (1988) Saccadic disorders caused by cooling the superior colliculus or the frontal eye field, or from combined lesions of both structures. *Brain Res.*, 438: 247–255.

Keller, E.L. (1989) The cerebellum. In: R.H. Wurtz and M.E. Golberg (Eds.), *The Neurobiology of Saccadic Eye Movements*. Elsevier, Amsterdam, pp. 391–411.

Keller, E.L., Slakey, D.P. and Crandall, W.F. (1983) Microstimulation of the primate cerebellar vermis during saccadic eye movements. *Brain Res.*, 288: 131–143.

Koella, W.P. (1959) Some functional properties of optically evoked potentials in cerebellar cortex of cat. *J. Neurophysiol.*, 22: 61–77.

Kori, A.A., Das, V.E., Zivotofsky, A.Z. and Leigh, R.J. (1998) Memory-guided saccadic eye movements: effects of cerebellar disease. *Vis. Res.*, 38(20): 3181–3192.

Kotchabhakdi, N. and Walberg, F. (1978) Primary vestibular afferent projections to the cerebellum as demonstrated by retrograde transport of horseradish peroxydase. *Brain Res.*, 142: 142–146.

Krauzlis, R.J. and Miles, F.A. (1998) Role of the oculomotor vermis in generating pursuit and saccades: effects of microstimulation. *J. Neurophysiol.*, 80(4): 2046–2062.

Kultas-Ilinsky, K., Ilinsky, I.A., Young, P.A. and Smith, K.R. (1980a) Ultrastructure of degenerating cerebellothalamic terminals in the ventral medial nucleus of the cat. *Exp. Brain Res.*, 38: 125–135.

Kultas-Ilinsky, K., Warton, S., Tolbert, D.L. and Ilinsky, I.A. (1980b) Quantitative and qualitative characteristics of dentate and fastigial afferents identified by electron microscopic autoradiography in the cat thalamus. *Brain Res.*, 201: 220–226.

Kurzan, R., Straube, A. and Büttner, U. (1993) The effect of muscimol micro-injections into the fastigial nucleus on the optokinetic response and the vestibulo-ocular reflex in the alert monkey. *Exp. Brain Res.*, 94: 252–260.

Kyuhou, S.-I. and Kawaguchi, S. (1987) Cerebellocerebral projection from the fastigial nucleus onto the frontal eye field and anterior ectosylvian visual area in the cat. *J. Comp. Neurol.*, 259: 571–590.

Laurutis, V.P. and Robinson, D.A. (1986) The vestibulo-ocular reflex during human saccadic eye movements. *J. Physiol.*, 373: 209–233.

Lefèvre, P. and Galiana, H.L. (1992) Dynamic feedback to the superior colliculus in a neural network model of the gaze control system. *Neural Networks*, 5: 871–890.

Llinas, R. and Wolfe, J.W. (1977) Functional linkage between the electrical activity in the vermal cerebellar cortex and saccadic eye movements. *Exp. Brain Res.*, 20: 1–14.

Lünenburger, L., Lindner, W. and Hoffmann, K.-P. (2003) Neural activity in the primate superior colliculus and saccadic reaction times in double-step experiments. In: C. Prablanc, D. Pélisson and Y. Rossetti (Eds.), *Neural Control of Space Coding and Action Production. Progress in Brain Research*, Vol. 142. Elsevier, Amsterdam, pp. 91–107 (this volume).

Mano, N., Ito, Y. and Shibutani, H. (1996) Context dependent discharge characteristics of saccade-related Purkinje cells in the cerebellar hemispheres of the monkey. *Prog. Brain Res.*, 112: 423–430.

Marr, D. (1969) A theory of cerebellar cortex. *J. Physiol. (Lond.)*, 202: 437–470.

Matsushita, M. and Hosoya, Y. (1978) The location of spinal projection neurons in the cerebellar nuclei (cerebellospinal tract neurons) in the cat. A study with the horseradish peroxydase technique. *Brain Res.*, 142: 237–248.

May, P.J., Hartwich-Young, R., Nelson, J.S., Sparks, D.L. and Porter, J.D. (1990) Cerebellotectal pathways in the macaque: implications for collicular generation of saccades. *Neuroscience*, 36(2): 305–324.

Mays, L.E. and Sparks, D.L. (1980) Saccades are spatially, not retinocentrically, coded. *Science*, 208: 1163–1165.

McCrea, R.A. and Baker, R. (1985) Anatomical connections of the nucleus prepositus of the cat. *J. Comp. Neurol.*, 237: 377–407.

McElligott, J.G. and Keller, E.L. (1982) In: G. Lennerstrand, D.S. Zee and E.L. Keller (Eds.), *Functional Basis of Ocular Motility Disorders*. Pergamon Press, Headington Hill Hall.

McElligott, J.G. and Keller, E.L. (1984) Cerebellar vermis involvement in monkey saccadic eye movements: microstimulation. *Exp. Neurol.*, 86: 543–558.

Middleton, F.A. and Strick, P.L. (1998) Cerebellar output: motor and cognitive channels. *TICS*, 2: 348–354.

Munoz, D.P., Guitton, D. and Pélisson, D. (1991) Control of orienting gaze shifts by the tectoreticulospinal system in the head-free cat, III. Spatiotemporal characteristics of phasic motor discharges. *J. Neurophysiol.*, 66(5): 1642–1666.

Murakami, S., Noda, H. and Warabi, T. (1991) Converging eye movements evoked by microstimulation of the fastigial nucleus of macaque monkeys. *Neurosci. Res.*, 10(2): 106–117.

Mushiake, H. and Strick, P.L. (1993) Preferential activity of dentate neurons during limb movements guided by vision. *J. Neurophysiol.*, 70: 2660–2664.

Nakano, K., Takimoto, T., Kayahara, T., Takeuchi, Y. and Kobayashi, Y. (1980) Distribution of cerebellothalamic neurons projecting to the ventral nuclei of the thalamus: an HRP study in the cat. *J. Comp. Neurol.*, 194: 427–439.

Noda, H. (1991) Cerebellar control of saccadic eye movements: its neural mechanisms and pathways. *Jpn. J. Physiol.*, 41: 351–368.

Noda, H. and Fujikado, T. (1987a) Involvement of Purkinje cells in evoking saccadic eye movements by microstimulation of the posterior cerebellar vermis of monkeys. *J. Neurophysiol.*, 57: 1247–1261.

Noda, H. and Fujikado, T. (1987b) Topography of the oculomotor area of the cerebellar vermis in macaques as determined by microstimulation. *J. Neurophysiol.*, 58(2): 359–378.

Noda, H., Murakami, S., Yamada, J., Tamaki, J. and Aso, T. (1988) Saccadic eye movements evoked by microstimulation of the fastigial nucleus of macaque monkeys. *J. Neurophysiol.*, 60(3): 1036–1052.

Noda, H., Sugita, S. and Ikeda, Y. (1990) Afferent and efferent connections of the oculomotor region of the fastigial nucleus in the macaque monkey. *J. Comp. Neurol.*, 302: 330–348.

Noda, H., Murakami, S. and Warabi, T. (1991) Effects of fastigial stimulation upon visually-directed saccades in macaque monkeys. *Neurosci. Res.*, 10: 188–199.

Ohtsuka, K. (1988) Inhibitory action of Purkinje cells in the posterior vermis on fastigio-prepositus circuit of the cat. *Brain Res.*, 455: 153–156.

Ohtsuka, K. and Noda, H. (1990) Direction-selective saccadic-burst neurons in the fastigial oculomotor region of the macaque. *Exp. Brain Res.*, 81: 659–662.

Ohtsuka, K. and Noda, H. (1991a) Saccadic burst neurons in the oculomotor region of the fastigial nucleus of macaque monkeys. *J. Neurophysiol.*, 65(6): 1422–1434.

Ohtsuka, K. and Noda, H. (1991b) The effect of microstimulation of the oculomotor vermis on discharges of fastigial neurons and visually directed saccades in macaques. *Neurosci. Res.*, 10: 290–295.

Ohtsuka, K. and Noda, H. (1992) Burst discharges of fastigial neurons in macaque monkeys are driven by vision- and memory-guided saccades but not by spontaneous saccades. *Neurosci. Res.*, 15: 224–228.

Ohtsuka, K. and Noda, H. (1995) Discharge properties of Purkinje cells in the oculomotor vermis during visually guided saccades in the macaque monkey. *J. Neurophysiol.*, 74(5): 1828–1840.

Ohtsuka, K., Edamura, M., Kawahara, K. and Aoki, M. (1987) The properties of goal-directed eye movements evoked by microstimulation of the cerebellar vermis in the cat. *Neurosci. Lett.*, 76: 173–178.

Ohtsuka, K., Sato, H. and Noda, H. (1994) Saccadic burst neurons in the fastigial nucleus are not involved in compensating for orbital nonlinearities. *J. Neurophysiol.*, 71(5): 1976–1980.

Optican, L.M. (1982) Saccadic dysmetria. In: G. Lennerstrand, D.S. Zee and E.L. Keller (Eds.), *Functional Basis of Ocular Motility Disorders*. Pergamon Press, Headington Hill Hall, pp. 441–451.

Optican, L.M. and Robinson, D.A. (1980) Cerebellar-dependent adaptive control of primate saccadic system. *J. Neurophysiol.*, 44(6): 1058–1076.

Optican, L.M., Zee, D.S. and Miles, F.A. (1986) Floccular lesions abolish adaptive control of post-saccadic ocular drift in primates. *Exp. Brain Res.*, 64(3): 596–598.

Pélisson, D., Prablanc, C. and Urquizar, C. (1988) Vestibuloocular reflex inhibition and gaze saccade control characteristics during eye–head orientation in humans. *J. Neurophysiol.*, 59(3): 997–1013.

Pélisson, D., Guitton, D. and Munoz, D.P. (1989) Compensatory eye and head movements generated by the cat following stimulation-induced perturbations in gaze position. *Exp. Brain Res.*, 78(3): 654–658.

Pélisson, D., Guitton, D. and Goffart, L. (1995) On-line compensation of gaze shifts perturbed by micro-stimulation of the superior colliculus in the cat with unrestrained head. *Exp. Brain Res.*, 106(2): 196–204.

Pélisson, D., Goffart, L. and Guillaume, A. (1998) Contribution of the rostral fastigial nucleus to the control of orienting gaze shifts in the head-unrestrained cat. *J. Neurophysiol.*, 80: 1180–1196.

Pélisson, D., Goffart, L., Guillaume, A. and Quinet, J. (2002) Visuo-motor deficits induced by fastigial nucleus inactivation. *The Cerebellum* (in press).

Phillips, J.O., Ling, L., Fuchs, A.F., Siebold, C. and Plorde, J.J. (1995) Rapid horizontal gaze movement in the monkey. *J. Neurophysiol.*, 73: 1632–1652.

Pierrot-Deseilligny, C., Amarenco, P., Roullet, E. and Marteau, R. (1990) Vermal infarct with pursuit eye movement disorders. *J. Neurol. Neurosurg. Psychiatry*, 53(6): 519–521.

Pierrot-Deseilligny, C., Rivaud, S., Gaymard, B., Müri, R.M. and Vermersch, A.I. (1995) Cortical control of saccades. *Ann. Neurol.*, 37: 557–567.

Precht, W., Volkind, R. and Blanks, R.H.I. (1977) Functional organization of the vestibular input to the anterior and posterior cerebellar vermis of cat. *Exp. Brain Res.*, 27: 143–160.

Quaia, C., Lefevre, P. and Optican, L.M. (1999) Model of the control of saccades by superior colliculus and cerebellum. *J. Neurophysiol.*, 82(2): 999–1018.

Ritchie, L. (1976) Effects of cerebellar lesions on saccadic eye movements. *J. Neurophysiol.*, 39(6): 1246–1256.

Robinson, D.A. (1975) Oculomotor control signals. In: G. Lennerstrand and P. Bach-Y-Rita (Eds.), *Basic Mechanisms of Ocular Motility and Their Clinical Implications*. Pergamon Press, Oxford, pp. 337–378.

Robinson, F.R. (2000) Role of the cerebellar posterior interpositus nucleus in saccades, I. Effect of temporary lesions. *J. Neurophysiol.*, 84(3): 1289–1302.

Robinson, F.R. and Fuchs, A.F. (2001) The role of the cerebellum in voluntary eye movements. *Annu. Rev. Neurosci.*, 24: 981–1004.

Robinson, F.R., Straube, A. and Fuchs, A.F. (1993) Role of the caudal fastigial nucleus in saccade generation, II. Effects of muscimol inactivation. *J. Neurophysiol.*, 70(5): 1741–1758.

Robinson, F.R., Straube, A. and Fuchs, A.F. (1997) Participation of caudal fastigial nucleus in smooth pursuit eye movements,

II. Effects of muscimol inactivation. *J. Neurophysiol.*, 78(2): 848–859.

Roldan, M. and Reinoso-Suarez, F. (1981) Cerebellar projections to the superior colliculus in the cat. *J. Neurosci.*, 1(8): 827–834.

Ron, S. and Robinson, D.A. (1973) Eye movements evoked by cerebellar stimulation in the alert monkey. *J. Neurophysiol.*, 36: 1004–1022.

Ruigrok, T.J.H. and Voogd, J. (1995) Cerebellar influence on olivary excitability in the cat. *Eur. J. Neurosci.*, 7: 679–693.

Sasaki, K., Kawaguchi, S., Oka, H., Sakai, M. and Mizuno, N. (1976) Electrophysiological studies on the cerebellocerebral projections in monkeys. *Exp. Brain Res.*, 24: 495–507.

Sato, H. and Noda, H. (1992) Saccadic dysmetria induced by transient functional decortication of the cerebellar vermis. *Exp. Brain Res.*, 88: 455–458.

Schiller, P.H. and Sandell, J.H. (1983) Interactions between visually and electrically elicited saccades before and after superior colliculus and frontal eye field ablations in the rhesus monkey. *Exp. Brain Res.*, 49: 381–392.

Schlag, J. and Schlag-Rey, M. (1987) Does microstimulation evoke fixed-vector saccades by generating their vector or by specifying their goal? *Exp Brain Res.*, 68: 442–444.

Schlag-Rey, M., Schlag, J. and Shook, B.L. (1989) Interactions between natural and electrically evoked saccades, I. Differences between sites carrying retinal error and motor error signals in monkey superior colliculus. *Exp. Brain Res.*, 76: 537–547.

Schmamann, J.D. (1996) *The Cerebellum and Cognition*. Academic Press, London.

Schwartz, D.W.F. and Tomlinson, R.D. (1977) Neuronal responses to eye muscle stretch in cerebellar lobule VI of the cat. *Exp. Brain Res.*, 27: 101–111.

Schweighofer, N., Arbib, M.A. and Dominey, P.F. (1996) A model of the cerebellum in adaptive control of saccadic gain, I. The model and its biological substrate. *Biol. Cybern.*, 75: 19–28.

Selhorst, J.B., Stark, L., Ochs, A.L. and Hoyt, W.F. (1976) Disorders in cerebellar ocular motor control, I. Saccadic overshoot dysmetria: an oculographic, control system and clinico-anatomical analysis. *Brain*, 99: 497–508.

Shimizu, N., Mizuno, M., Naito, M. and Yoshida, M. (1981a) The interaction between accuracy of gaze with and without head movements in patients with cerebellar ataxia. *Ann. N.Y. Acad. Sci.*, 374: 579–589.

Shimizu, N., Naito, M. and Yoshida, M. (1981b) Eye–head coordination in patients with parkinsonism and cerebellar ataxia. *J. Neurol., Neurosurg. Psychiatry*, 44: 509–515.

Siebold, C., Glonti, L., Glasauer, S. and Büttner, U. (1997) Rostral fastigial nucleus activity in the alert monkey during three-dimensional passive head movements. *J. Neurophysiol.*, 77: 1432–1446.

Sparks, D.L. and Mays, L.E. (1983) Spatial localization of saccade targets, I. Compensation for stimulation-induced perturbations in eye position. *J. Neurophysiol.*, 49: 45–63.

Sparks, D.L., Mays, L.E. and Porter, J.D. (1987) Eye movements induced by pontine stimulation: interaction with visually triggered saccades. *J. Neurophysiol.*, 58: 300–318.

Sparks, D.L. and Gandhi, N.J. (2003) Single cell signals: an oculomotor perspective. In: C. Prablanc, D. Pélisson and Y. Rossetti (Eds.), *Neural Control of Space Coding and Action Production. Progress in Brain Research*, Vol. 142. Elsevier, Amsterdam, pp. 35–53 (this volume).

Steriade, M. (1995) Two channels in the cerebellothalamocortical system. *J. Comp. Neurol.*, 354: 57–70.

Straube, A., Helmchen, C., Robinson, F.R., Fuchs, A.F. and Büttner, U. (1994) Saccadic dysmetria is similar in patients with a lateral medullary lesion and in monkeys with a lesion of the deep cerebellar nucleus. *J. Vestib. Res.*, 4(5): 327–333.

Straube, A., Deubel, H., Spuler, A. and Büttner, U. (1995) Differential effect of a bilateral deep cerebellar nuclei lesion on externally and internally triggered saccades in humans. *Neuroophthalmology*, 15: 67–74.

Sugimoto, T., Mizuno, N. and Uchida, K. (1982) Distribution of cerebellar fiber terminals in the midbrain visuomotor areas: an autoradiographic study in the cat. *Brain Res.*, 238: 353–370.

Suzuki, D.A. and Keller, E.L. (1982) Vestibular signals in the posterior vermis of the alert monkey cerebellum. *Exp. Brain Res.*, 47: 145–147.

Suzuki, D.A. and Keller, E.L. (1988a) The role of the posterior vermis of monkey cerebellum in smooth-pursuit eye movement control, I. Eye and head movement-related activity. *J. Neurophysiol.*, 59(1): 1–18.

Suzuki, D.A. and Keller, E.L. (1988b) The role of the posterior vermis of monkey cerebellum in smooth-pursuit eye movement control, II. Target velocity-related Purkinje cell activity. *J. Neurophysiol.*, 59(1): 19–40.

Takagi, M., Zee, D.S. and Tamargo, R.J. (1998) Effects of lesions of the oculomotor vermis on eye movements in primate: saccades. *J. Neurophysiol.*, 80(4): 1911–1931.

Takagi, M., Zee, D.S. and Tamargo, R.J. (2000) Effects of lesions of the oculomotor cerebellar vermis on eye movements in primate: smooth pursuit. *J. Neurophysiol.*, 83(4): 2047–2062.

Takikawa, Y., Kawagoe, R., Miyashita, N. and Hikosaka, O. (1998) Presaccadic omnidirectional burst activity in the basal interstitial nucleus in the monkey cerebellum. *Exp. Brain Res.*, 121(4): 442–450.

Thach, W.T., Goodkin, H.P. and Keating, J.G. (1992) The cerebellum and the adaptive coordination of movement. *Annu. Rev. Neurosci.*, 15: 403–442.

Thielert, C.D. and Thier, P. (1993) Patterns of projections from the pontine nuclei and the nucleus reticularis tegmenti pontis to the posterior vermis in the rhesus monkey: a study using retrograde tracers. *J. Comp. Neurol.*, 337(1): 113–126.

Thier, P., Dicke, P.W., Haas, R. and Barash, S. (2000) Encoding of movement time by populations of cerebellar Purkinje cells. *Nature*, 405(6782): 72–76.

Vahedi, K., Rivaud, S., Amarenco, P. and Pierrot-Deseilligny, C. (1995) Horizontal eye movement disorders after posterior vermis infarctions. *J. Neurol. Neurosurg. Psychiatry*, 58: 91–94.

Van Gisbergen, J.A.M., Robinson, D.A. and Gielen, S. (1981) A quantitative analysis of generation of saccadic eye movements by burst neurons. *J. Neurophysiol.*, 45: 417–442.

Van Opstal, A.J., Hepp, K., Suzuki, Y. and Henn, V. (1995) Influence of eye position on activity in monkey superior colliculus. *J. Neurophysiol.*, 74(4): 1593–1610.

Vilis, T. and Hore, J. (1981) Characteristics of saccadic dysmetria in monkeys during reversible lesions of medial cerebellar nuclei. *J. Neurophysiol.*, 46(4): 828–838.

Warton, S., Jones, D.G., Ilinsky, I.A. and Kultas-Ilinsky, K. (1983) Nigral and cerebellar synaptic terminals in the intermediate and deep layers of the cat superior colliculus revealed by lesioning studies. *Neuroscience*, 10: 789–800.

Waterhouse, B.D. and McElligott, J.G. (1980) Simple spike activity of Purkinje cells in the posterior vermis of awake cats during spontaneous saccadic eye movements. *Brain Res. Bull.*, 5: 159–168.

Wilson, V.J., Uchino, Y., Maunz, R.A., Susswein, A. and Fukushima, K. (1978) Properties and connections of cat fastigiospinal neurons. *Exp. Brain Res.*, 32(1): 1–17.

Wolfe, J.W. (1972) Responses of the cerebellar auditory area to pure tone stimuli. *Exp. Neurol.*, 36: 295–309.

Yamada, J. and Noda, H. (1987) Afferent and efferent connections of the oculomotor cerebellar vermis in the macaque monkey. *J. Comp. Neurol.*, 265(2): 224–241.

Zee, D.S., Yee, R.D., Cogan, D.G., Robinson, D.A. and Engel, W.K. (1976) Ocular motor abnormalities in hereditary cerebellar ataxia. *Brain*, 99: 207–234.

C. Prablanc, D. Pélisson and Y. Rossetti (Eds.)
Progress in Brain Research, Vol. 142
© 2003 Elsevier Science B.V. All rights reserved

CHAPTER 6

Neural activity in the primate superior colliculus and saccadic reaction times in double-step experiments

Lars Lünenburger *, Werner Lindner and Klaus-Peter Hoffmann

Allgemeine Zoologie und Neurobiologie, Ruhr-Universität Bochum, D-44780 Bochum, Germany

Abstract: Although primates including humans can do 2–3 saccades per second while observing their environment, this seems to be more complicated when the same visual target is displaced twice in brief succession. When the subject has to follow this target with its gaze, the reaction time of the second saccade is longer than that of the first. We present data from electrophysiological recordings in the superior colliculus of a monkey that is performing a double-step saccade task. Analysis of the neuronal activity shows that the fixation neurons and the saccadic neurons respond differently in single- and double-step tasks. Fixation neurons are not as active between the two saccades as could be expected from single-step trials. Therefore, the fixation neurons are not likely to cause the increase in reaction time. The recorded saccadic neurons usually showed a presumably visual activation about 70 ms after target appearance and a motor burst starting briefly before the saccade. A target-aligned response was encountered in half of the neurons about 150 ms after the second target appearance. The early visual target-aligned response is often lost before the second saccade in a double-step task with short stimulus delay. The rise of activity was slower before the second than before the first saccade. The neural latency was therefore longer before the second saccade. The motor burst coincides with the second saccade although it is delayed. Thus, the motor burst was always predictive of the occurrence of the saccade. We conclude that the fixation neurons in the superior colliculus are not likely to cause the delay of the second saccade, and that the activity in the saccadic neurons in the superior colliculus encodes the timing of the second saccade even if it is delayed.

Introduction

While exploring the external world, human subjects usually make 2–3 saccadic eye movements per second, allowing undisturbed perception between saccades for about 300 ms. In experimental conditions where a subject is asked to fixate a target that is displaced twice (double-step task), it was shown that there is a significant delay in the response to the second target step (Feinstein and Williams, 1972; Becker and Jürgens, 1979). We demonstrated that this phenomenon of an increased reaction time

for the second saccade depends on the delay between both target displacements (Lünenburger et al., 2000a). Indeed, early data (Feinstein and Williams, 1972) reveals that decreasing the stimulus delay provokes a monotonous increase in reaction time for the second saccade. Recent psychophysical findings suggest that this decrease is rather exponential (Lünenburger et al., in revision). Yet, the increase of the second reaction time, i.e. the delay of the second saccade, is not caused by an absolute refractory period of the saccadic system. While earlier studies observed inter-saccadic delays for two subsequent memory-guided saccades of down to about 50 ms (Goossens and Van Opstal, 1997), we were able to demonstrate non-increased reaction times for two subsequent visually guided saccades by use of the gap effect. Removal of the fixated visual target for

---

* Correspondence to: Lars Lünenburger, Paraplegic Center of the University Hospital Balgrist, CH-8008 Zürich, Switzerland. E-mail: lars.luenenburger@balgrist.unizh.ch

about 200 ms (gap) prior to a single target displacement is known to reduce the reaction time (Saslow, 1967) and to increase the occurrence of express saccades (Fischer and Weber, 1993). A gap before the second displacement in a double-step task abolishes the increase of the second reaction time to values sometimes even shorter than the first (Lünenburger et al., in revision).

It is well known that the generation of saccadic eye movements is controlled by neurons in the frontal eye field (FEF), lateral intraparietal area (LIP) and superior colliculus (SC) (for reviews see Sparks and Hartwich-Young, 1989; Moschovakis et al., 1996; Andersen et al., 1997; Colby and Goldberg, 1999). Damage to these areas impairs the ability to produce saccades either temporarily or permanently (Schiller et al., 1980, 1987; Lynch, 1992). However, very little, if any, is known about the brain structures and mechanisms sustaining the increased reaction time for the second saccade to double-step displaced targets. The SC appears to be the final common pathway to the brainstem saccadic system, and is thus essential for triggering all saccades (Hanes and Wurtz, 2001). In this study, we will investigate the possibility that the SC may be involved in the effect of increased reaction time of the second saccade in a double-step task.

The SC comprises both fixation and saccadic neurons and it is generally assumed that the initiation of saccadic eye movements at this level relies on the interaction between the activity of these two cell populations (Munoz and Guitton, 1991; Munoz and Wurtz, 1993a,b; Munoz et al., 2000). Although the firing rate of fixation neurons at target appearance does not predict the saccadic reaction time (Everling et al., 1998), the reduction of neural activity between the disappearance of the fixation point and the appearance the target (gap) seems to be relevant (Dorris et al., 1997) because it allows faster building up of the activity of the saccadic neurons. This build-up activity was shown to be predictive for saccadic reaction time (Dorris and Munoz, 1998) and express saccade occurrence (Sparks et al., 2000). If switching off the fixation neurons is necessary to initiate a saccade, it is possible that an increase of activity in fixations neurons, such as the 'postsaccadic enhancement' (Munoz and Wurtz, 1993a), would raise the reaction time for the subsequent saccade and even

reduce the likeliness to trigger it. We therefore investigated the possibility that activity of fixation neurons is higher before the second saccade in the double-step paradigm than before a single saccade. Saccadic neurons in the SC are known to be relevant for triggering the saccade and determining its spatial properties. Assuming an integrate-and-threshold model for the saccadic neurons a weaker activation can be hypothesized for the second compared to the first saccade. This hypothesis will be tested by comparing the activity pattern of SC fixation and saccadic neurons recorded in single- and double-step tasks.

Preliminary results have been published elsewhere in abstract form (Lünenburger et al., 2000b, 2001; Lindner et al., 2001) and are part of a doctoral thesis of LL (Lünenburger, 2002).

Methods

Data were collected from one male adult rhesus monkey (*Macaca mulatta*) trained to perform single-step and double-step saccade tasks. Details about animal surgery, experimental setup and recording techniques have been previously described (Werner, 1993; Werner et al., 1997; Stuphorn et al., 2000). All procedures were approved by a local ethics committee and followed the European and the German national regulations (European Communities Council Directive, 86/609/ECC; Tierschutzgesetz) as well as the National Institutes of Health Guidelines for Care and Use of Animals for Experimental Procedures.

In brief, the monkey was seated in a primate chair and its gaze was monitored by the search-coil technique (Judge et al., 1980). Single-cell activity was recorded with glass-insulated tungsten microelectrodes from the intermediate and deep layers of the left and the right superior colliculus (SC). The recording chamber was tilted backwards 45° from vertical and was stereotaxically placed on the midline of the skull aiming at the SC. In that configuration, the electrodes were lowered almost perpendicularly through the SC layers. The monkey was head-fixed or head-free and faced a circular translucent screen (distance 27.5 cm) on which visual targets (red LED; 1° diameter, 0.2 cd/m^2) were back-projected via mirrors mounted on galvanometers under computer control. The animal behavior was monitored by a computer which also recorded the spike events, eye and head movements. Saccade onset was defined in an off-line analysis as the first of three consecutive samples for which the horizontal eye velocity exceeded a relative velocity threshold of 25% of the peak velocity in the detection window ranging from 100 to 500 ms after target appearance.

Since the visual behavior of the animal is still being studied, histological verification of the recording sites will only be available after completion of the project. All neurons in this study exhibited the highly characteristic visual and motor properties that were previously described for the SC (Schiller and Koerner, 1971; Wurtz and Goldberg, 1971; Munoz and Wurtz, 1995a,b; for recent reviews see Munoz et al., 2000; Soetedjo et al., 2002).

Paradigms

Two paradigms were used, paradigm A to study saccadic neurons, paradigm B for fixation neurons (Fig. 1). In both paradigms, a visual target was first presented at a peripheral position on the screen after the monkey pressed a button near its hip with the hand. The monkey had to acquire and maintain fixation for 800–1200 ms in a window of 4° radius around this fixation point before the target was displaced to the center of the screen where it remained for a defined time before it was moved to another peripheral position.

In paradigm A, the target displacements were adjusted to the position of the visual receptive field that was previously determined while passing through the superficial SC layers. Since the visual and motor maps in the SC are in register (Schiller and Koerner, 1971), this part of the visual space coincides with the motor field of the saccadic neurons in the intermediate and deep layers. To allow comparison of the second saccades in trials where the first saccade had the same or the opposite direction, the second saccades must have the same head centered coordinates in all trials. Therefore, the reverse double-step started with a fixation at a target that is in the movement field relative to the center of the screen. The target was then displaced to the center of the screen, such that the first saccade had a non-preferred direction. When the target was displaced back into the movement field, the evoked second saccade had preferred direction and amplitude. The onward double-step started with fixation

at a target that was mirror symmetric to the movement field relative to the center of the screen. The target was moved first to the center of the screen and then, after the delay, to the movement field relative to the center. Therefore, both evoked saccades had preferred direction and amplitude. To trigger the second target displacement in paradigm A, the time when the monkey's gaze entered the control window (4°) was determined and after a predetermined delay of either 0 ms, 100 ms, or 200 ms the second displacement was initiated. In some blocks, only 0 ms delay was used.

In paradigm B, the spatial target arrangement was a horizontal 15° center-in and a horizontal 7.5° center-out combination. This was used because no optimal saccade vector can be assigned to fixation neurons, which were recorded using this paradigm. The second target displacement occurred with a static delay of 400 ms after the first target displacement.

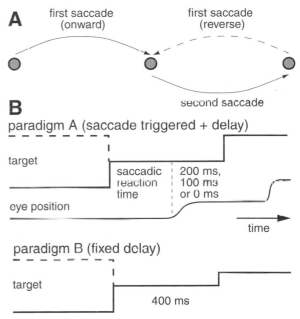

Fig. 1. Spatial setup (A) and temporal sequence (B) of the behavioral paradigms used in the present study. The target locations (schematized in A) were adapted to produce saccades for optimal activation of the recorded neurons in paradigm A. One peripheral target was always located at the optimal vector from the center of the screen, the other peripheral target mirror symmetric to this with respect to the center. In paradigm B, the first saccade was 15° center-in, the second 7.5° center-out. (B) The different timings of paradigm A (saccade triggered plus delay) and paradigm B (fixed delay) are described in detail in the methods section.

Analysis of fixation neurons

Neurons recorded in the SC were classified as fixation neurons when they showed tonic discharge during fixation and reduced or no activity during saccades. To compare the activity in a double-step trial with the activity that could be expected from the corresponding single-step trials, we calculated their average spike density functions ($\sigma = 10$ ms) when aligned to saccade onset and normalized to 1.0 (Fig. 4A and B). The resulting functions $f_{1,2}(t)$ reflect the probability of the neuron to be active at a particular time t. For each double-step trial, the appropriate two single-step responses were shifted to the onsets of the actually measured saccades and multiplied (Fig. 4C). The resulting function $g(t)$ represents the expected probability that the neuron is active in the double step. The resulting functions $g(t)$ of all trials were averaged (Fig. 4C, red curve) and compared to the recorded activity in the double step, which was also normalized (Fig. 4C, blue curve). To quantitatively compare the activities, the spike density functions were integrated over the interval between average first and second saccadic reaction times. This procedure was performed for each of the four double-step conditions in paradigm B (left/right × onward/reverse).

Analysis of saccadic neurons

Neurons with phasic spike activity during the saccade were considered as saccadic neurons and were classified into visual saccadic, purely saccadic, and purely visual neurons based on their activity patterns. An idealized visual saccadic neuron (Fig. 2) would fire a series of action potentials at a fixed latency after the appearance of the target in the receptive field. These spikes build the vertical band in the target-aligned plot of Fig. 2A. This part of the neural activation will be referred to as the target-aligned component (TAC). The reaction time of the saccade is variable. A second series of spikes varies with the start of the saccade. When we now aline the spike trains to the end of the saccade (Fig. 2B), these spikes build a vertical band in the spike rasters. This part of the neural activation will be called saccade-aligned component (SAC). It is very likely that TAC is the visual response and SAC is the motor burst.

In order to characterize the changes in neural discharge of SC saccadic neurons, we applied a burst detection analysis. The burst detection algorithms available could not be successfully applied to our neural data without changes [e.g. threshold for spike density, similar to Goossens and Van Opstal, 2000, threshold for instantaneous rate, own unpublished approach, similar to Sparks et al., 2000, an algorithm based on a Poisson spiking process (Hanes et al., 1995), and an algorithm based on an Erlang spiking process (Commenges et al., 1986; Seal et al., 1983)]. The target-aligned component (TAC) of the activity consisted often of only one or two spikes, which, of course, will be neglected by the algorithms in favor of the always much stronger saccade-aligned component (SAC). Too often the automatically detected start of activation varied with the saccade and not with the target appearance. This would have signaled a purely saccadic neuron while visual inspection was clearly revealing the consistent presence of a TAC (> 75% of trials). To circumvent this problem, we manually set the start of activity in the appropriate trials, after applying an algorithm following Commenges et al. (1986) and Seal et al. (1983) to all trials.

Results

Behavior and Psychophysics

The saccadic reaction times were calculated for the saccades in the single-step blocks and for the second saccades in the double-step blocks. Each block contained 10–20 trials per condition. Most second saccades in the double-step task had a longer reaction time than the saccades in the single-step task (Table 1, Fig. 3A, Wilcoxon rank-sum, $P < 0.01$). The reaction times of the second saccades were in general longer for shorter stimulus delays. The strongest increase was observed for second saccades in the double step with 0 ms delay between first saccade and second target displacement. Here, the differences are 103 ms for onward and 88 ms for reverse double step. Comparing the corresponding onward and reverse conditions shows a non-significantly longer reaction time in the onward double-step conditions (Wilcoxon rank-sum, $P > 0.05$). Thirteen blocks were used in paradigm B, where the delay between

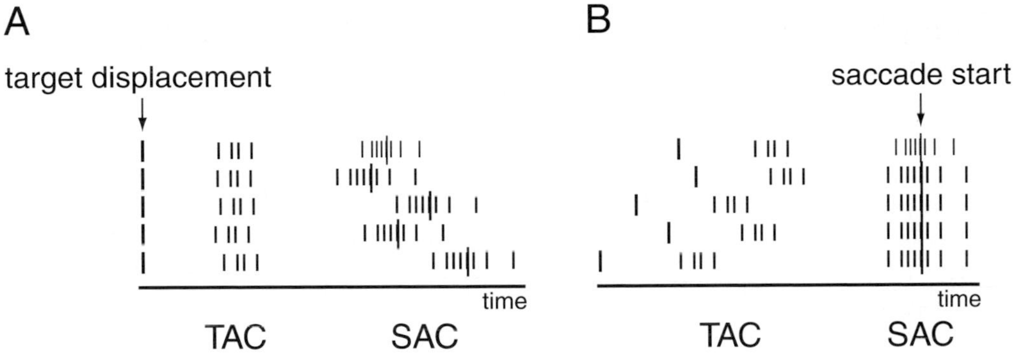

A
target displacement

TAC   SAC

B
saccade start

TAC   SAC

Fig. 2. The activity of an idealized visual saccadic neuron in a single-step saccade task is sketched for alignment to the target (A) and on the saccade (B). Long tick marks represent the target displacement and the end of the saccade. Each short tick stands for an action potential. The neuron's response consists of a target-aligned component (TAC) and a saccade-aligned component (SAC).

TABLE 1

Saccadic reaction times in the single- and double-step saccade task

Paradigm	n	Single-step	Double-step	
			onward	reverse
A: saccade-triggered				
+ 0 ms	29	171	274	259
+ 100 ms	11	–	205	172
+ 200 ms	11	–	188	182
B: 400 ms fix	13	230	264	223

The values are medians of reaction times (in ms) for all blocks. The number of blocks used to obtain this median is n.

both target displacements was 400 ms (Fig. 3B). The second reaction time was higher than the single-step reaction time for the onward, but not for the reverse double step (Wilcoxon rank-sum, $P < 0.05$ and $P > 0.05$, respectively).

Neural activation during the double-step task

In total, 77 neurons were recorded in the SC while the monkey performed double-step saccade tasks. Of these, 45 neurons were quantitatively tested for the purpose of this study. We will describe the activity of fixation neurons first and that of saccadic neurons second.

Fixation neurons in the SC

Only seven fixation neurons have been recorded in the double-step paradigm B (see Fig. 4). In these trials the target appeared 15° to the left or right,

was displaced to the center of the screen for 400 ms and displaced a second time 7.5° to the right or to the left. This delivered four different conditions with respect to the directions of the two saccades. Single-step saccades of 15° to the left and to the right were used for comparison. Of the seven fixation neurons, five provided sufficient data for the analysis. The neuron's activity pattern from the appropriate single-step tasks was combined according to the saccadic reaction times of a double-step task (see 'Methods') and compared to the actually recorded activity in the double step. According to our hypothesis the integral of simulated activity between the two saccades was compared with the real activity for all neurons in the four conditions resulting in 20 data points in Fig. 5.

In 15 of the 20 data points the ratio of actual to simulated activity ranged from 0.25 to 0.8 and therefore lie below the diagonal of the scatter plot. In four data points the activity was similar (ratio 1.0

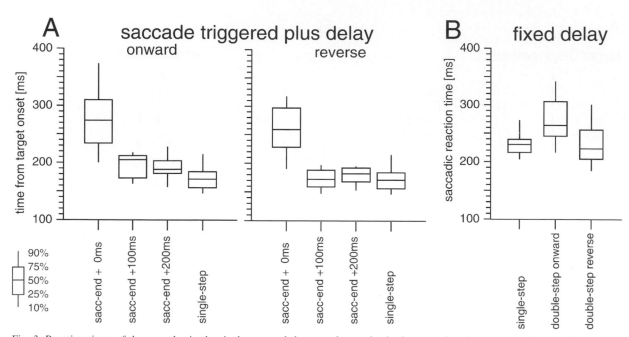

Fig. 3. Reaction times of the saccades in the single step and the second saccades in the onward and reverse double step of paradigms A and B. The boxes extend between the 25% and 75% quartiles and are separated by a line for the median. The vertical lines extend to the 10% and 90% percentiles. (A) In paradigm A, 29 recording blocks contribute to the single step and the double step with 0 ms delay, eleven of these also to the double step with 100 ms and 200 ms delay. The reaction time of the second saccade is in general longer than that of the single-step saccade. Shorter delays of the target displacement in the double step lead to longer reaction times. (B) In paradigm B, the delay between both target displacements was 400 ms. The second reaction time in the onward double step is longer than the reaction time in the single step, in the reverse double step it is not.

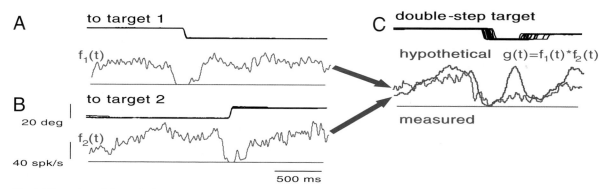

Fig. 4. Illustration of the analysis applied to collicular fixation neurons. $f_{1,2}(t)$ are the normalized spike density function representing the probability of the neuron to be active in the single step at a specific time t relative to the saccade seen in the eye traces printed above. Single-step saccades to the left (A) and to the right (B) are used to predict the neural activity of a left–right double step (C). $g(t)$ is the result of the calculation that has to be compared to the actual recording.

to 1.3), and in one data point the ratio was about 3.3. Thus over all, the fixation neurons showed less activity before the second saccade in the double-step task contrary to what the hypothesis predicted.

Saccadic neurons in the SC

Most phasic SC neurons recorded in this study were visual saccadic, i.e. they responded to the onset of a

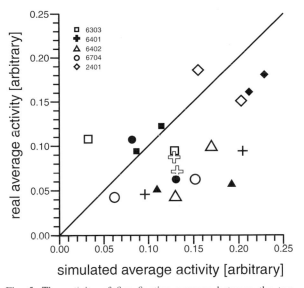

Fig. 5. The activity of five fixation neurons between the two saccades of a double-step task (measured as integral of the spike density function) is compared to the simulation results combining two single-step responses to an artificial double step. Different symbols are used for the results of the different neurons, as indicated in the upper left corner. Open symbols represent the onward conditions (both saccades same direction), closed symbols reverse conditions (opposite saccade directions). Since most data points lie below the diagonal, the neurons are less activated between the two saccades than could be expected.

visual stimulus and also before the saccade into their movement field.

Example neuron

First, we will present the activity of a representative neuron (unit SC08-2305) from the left SC that was recorded while the monkey performed paradigm A. Paradigm A contained seven conditions: three onward double-step conditions, in which both saccades had preferred directions; three reverse double-step conditions, in which only the second saccade had preferred direction; and a single step in preferred direction. The second target displacement in the double step occurred either 0 ms, 100 ms, or 200 ms after the first saccade. This series of experiments was performed when the monkey was head-free.

The three onward double steps are shown in Fig. 6, and the three reverse double steps in Fig. 7. In each figure, the instantaneous spike frequency,

spike rasters and eye position recordings are shown. The upper and lower eye position traces represent horizonal and vertical eye movements, respectively. Target displacements and saccade ends are marked by long tick marks. Short ticks represent triggered action potentials. In the onward double step (Fig. 6), the monkey made two saccades with the optimal direction and amplitude for this neuron. The three horizontal rows of subplots show the different triggering (timing) of the second target displacement. For each trial (row) three different alignments are presented (downward pointing arrows): (1) in the left column to the first target displacement; (2) in the middle column to the second target displacement (this is equivalent to the alignment to the first saccade); and (3) in the right column to the start of the second saccade. The reverse double-step conditions are presented in Fig. 7. All three reverse double-step conditions in paradigm A contained a first saccade that was opposite to the neuron's optimal direction. The neuron was never activated by this saccade, nor by the target displacement that provoked it. The second saccade is adapted to the neuron's movement field and leads to an activation of the neuron. The left column of Fig. 7 shows the alignment to the second target displacement, the right column to the second saccade.

The peak spike frequency was similar for all saccades when the plot is aligned to the appropriate saccade. However, the rise time appeared shorter for the first saccade than for any second saccade. The highest spike frequency occurred always near the start of each saccade. The activity terminated quickly after each saccade's end. Before this main activation around the start of the saccade, the neuron was activated during one or two brief phases at fixed latencies after target onset (TAC). The neuron started firing about 70 ms after the target displacement. This early activation can be seen before all first saccades, as well as all second saccades except those in the 0 ms delay trials. In these trials with very short intervals between both target displacements (or equivalently first saccade and second target displacement), the neuron is activated much later. Another phase of activation can be observed about 150 ms after the second target displacement (also a TAC). It is most prominent in the 100 ms delay onward trials (middle row of Fig. 6). However, it is not visible

98

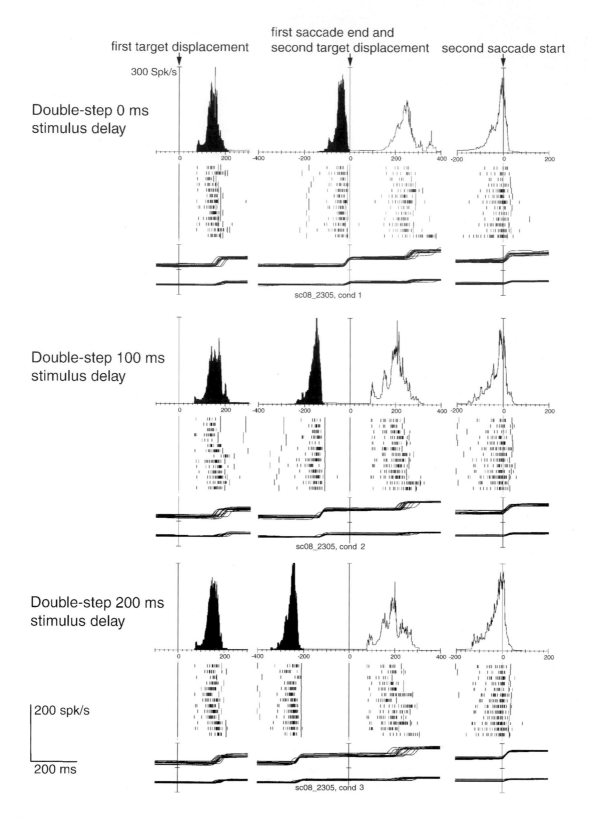

first target displacement

first saccade end and
second target displacement

second saccade start

300 Spk/s

Double-step 0 ms
stimulus delay

sc08_2305, cond 1

Double-step 100 ms
stimulus delay

sc08_2305, cond 2

Double-step 200 ms
stimulus delay

200 spk/s

200 ms

sc08_2305, cond 3

after the first target displacement, because the motor burst can be found at this time after target onset.

The patterns of activation of the 18 analyzed neurons in paradigm A were to a large extent similar to that of the neuron described above. However, the tri-phasic activation could be observed in 10 of these 18 neurons only (56%; visual inspection).

Plotting the neural latencies of an idealized visual saccadic neuron as a function of saccadic reaction time, the points of the beginning of activation will lie on a horizontal line in the scatter plot. The beginning of activation is independent of saccadic reaction time, and both do not correlate. The end of activation of such a neuron will be correlated to the saccadic reaction time and build a diagonal line in the scatter plot because of the SAC. The per-trial analysis of the discharges of the example neurons from Figs. 6 and 7 is presented in Fig. 8. For each trial, the times of burst begin are plotted against the saccadic reaction time using open symbols, the times of burst end using closed symbols. For the first saccades in the double-step task, as well as the saccade in the single-step task, the open symbols cluster along a horizontal line, signaling independence of the neural latency from the saccadic reaction time. This is also observed for the second saccades in the double steps with 100 ms and 200 ms delay. For the onward trials with 0 ms delay, the open symbols lie higher. This reflects an increase of the neural latency and a possible dependence on saccadic reaction time. For the reverse double-step trials with 0 ms delay, about half of the symbols remain on a horizontal line, i.e. neural latency is independent of saccadic reaction time and the latency is comparable to that after the first target appearance. This analysis could be performed for ten further neurons and all of them showed similar results.

Activity of saccadic neurons in the double-step task

Twenty-nine neurons recorded in paradigm A contributed to the burst detection analysis. Eighteen of

these only contributed to the single step and the double step with 0 ms delay between first saccade and second target displacement. The small proportion of analyzable neurons out of the recorded neurons is related to the delicate burst detection algorithm.

For each neuron, the medians of four events were calculated separately in four conditions (colored symbols in Fig. 9): double step with 0 ms, 100 ms, and 200 ms, respectively, as well as single step. The results of the burst detection analysis are presented separately for trials in which both saccades had the same direction (onward, Fig. 9A) and in which the saccades had opposite directions (reverse, Fig. 9B). (1) As described above, the saccadic reaction time was longer for the second saccade in the double step (black symbols) than in the single step. The population median over all neurons (black line) reveals the increase of saccadic reaction time with decreasing delay between first saccade and second target displacement. (2) The start of the activation (blue symbols) appears to depend on the stimulus delay, yet not as strongly as the saccade. For start of activation, the population median (blue line) is shorter than 100 ms for single steps as well as double steps with delays of 100 ms and 200 ms. The medians of the individual neurons comply with this (approximate) constancy. Strong changes can be found for the double steps with 0 ms delay. In these conditions, the burst begins much later for about half of the neurons (compare symbols). This leads to the increase of the population median (see line). This increase is stronger in the onward than in the reverse conditions. (3) The instant of peak activation (maximum spike density, $\sigma = 10$ ms, red lines and symbols) occurred in all conditions briefly before the saccade and varied with the saccadic reaction time. (4) The end of the detected activation (green lines and symbols) occurred on average 50 ms later than the saccade. The latter two values measure the saccade-aligned component of the activation.

The effects on the neural latency can also be shown by applying an analysis using receiver op-

Fig. 6. An example neuron from the left SC (depth 1370 μm below SC surface, tested saccade 12° right, 3° up) recorded in paradigm A. While the onward double-step conditions are presented in this figure, the three reverse double-step conditions are presented in the three rows of Fig. 7. The activation related to the first saccade can be seen in black, that related to the second in outlined. The alignments are described in detail in the text.

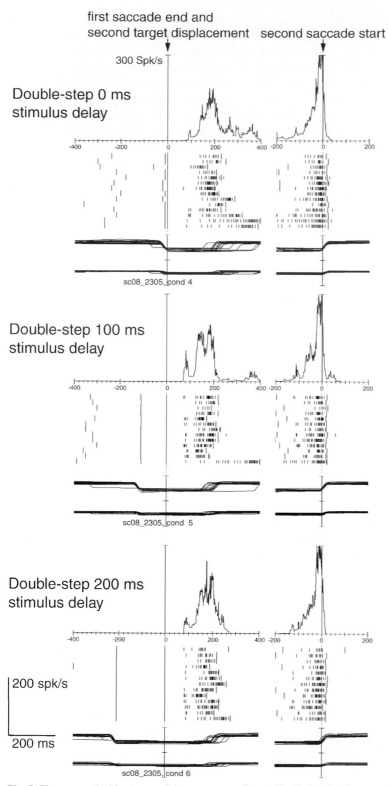

first saccade end and
second target displacement   second saccade start

300 Spk/s

Double-step 0 ms
stimulus delay

sc08_2305, cond 4

Double-step 100 ms
stimulus delay

sc08_2305, cond 5

Double-step 200 ms
stimulus delay

200 spk/s

200 ms

sc08_2305, cond 6

Fig. 7. The reverse double-step conditions corresponding to Fig. 6. See that figure and the text for further explanation.

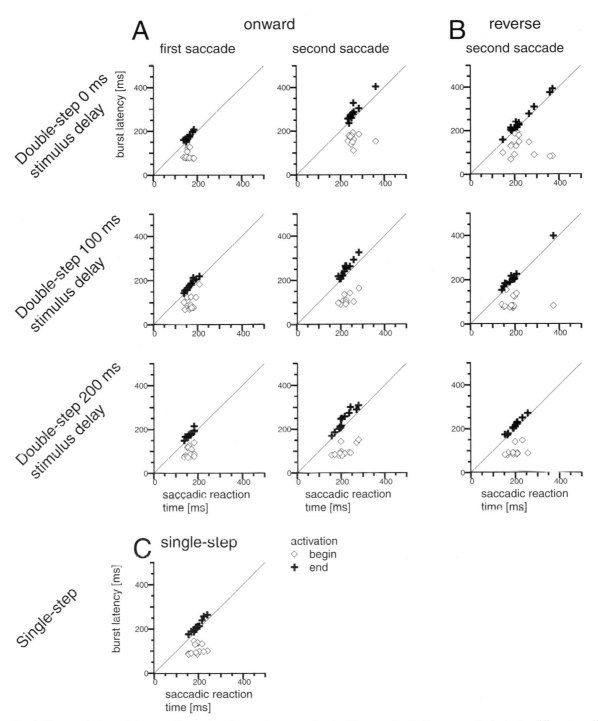

Fig. 8. The correlations of the saccadic reaction time to the start and end of the neural activation, respectively, in the different conditions is shown for the example neuron which is shown in Figs. 6 and 7. The onward double-step conditions are shown in A, reverse double-step conditions in B, and the single-step condition in C. Open symbols represent the begin of activation, closed symbols the end of activation. See text for details.

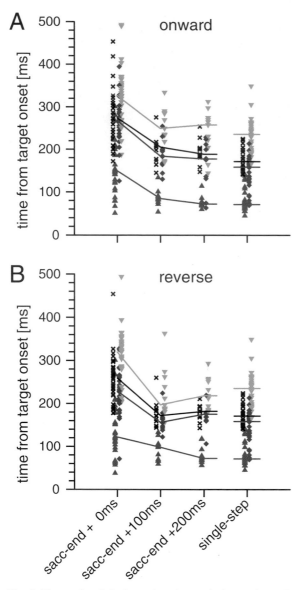

Fig. 9. The results of the burst detection analysis are shown for trials in which both saccades had the same direction (onward, A) and in which the saccades had opposite directions (reverse, B). The medians of begin of activation (blue), peak spike density (red), saccadic reaction time (black), and end of activation (green) for the recording blocks of each neuron are presented as symbols. The population median over all neurons is shown as a line. The first three columns represent the second saccades in double steps with 0 ms, 100 ms and 200 ms delay between the first saccade and the second target displacement. The fourth column represents the result from the comparable single-step saccade. Eleven neurons recorded in paradigm A contribute to all four columns, eighteen neurons in paradigm B to the first and the fourth column.

erating characteristics. This analysis (not shown) following Hanes et al. (1995) compares the probability distributions of the spike density functions at different times (5 ms bins) for two sets of trials and determines the first bin in which the distributions differ. The neural latency can be calculated by this analysis when comparing trials in which the saccade had the preferred direction to those in which the saccade had the null direction. Application of this analysis (that could be applied to 40 of the recorded neurons) supports the described effects on the start of the activation determined by the burst detection analysis.

Discussion

In the present study, we reported discharge characteristics of neurons in the superior colliculus while the monkey performed double-step and single-step saccade tasks. We showed that the reaction time of the second saccade in the double-step task is longer than for the same saccade in a single-step task. It was found that the activity of fixation neurons is lower between both saccades in a double step than could be expected from their activity in a single step. For saccadic neurons, the peak and end of activation varies in parallel to the saccadic reaction time. Yet, the beginning of activation is time-linked to the target displacement and is only notably increased when the second target displacement was triggered immediately after the first saccade. Per-trial correlation analysis supported these results. The saccadic neurons usually showed a biphasic activation after the first target displacement. The first phase was temporally coupled to the target displacement, while the second, stronger activation occurred almost simultaneously with the saccade. The same neurons sometimes showed triphasic activation after the second target displacement, the strongest, last phase again being coupled to the saccade. Because the saccade has a prolonged reaction time in this case, the corresponding neural activation is also delayed. Yet, often a weak activation was observed at a time where, after the first target displacement, the saccade and the main activation would have been observed. The earliest, target-aligned activation was only observed with long delays between both target displacements.

Behavioral equivalence to human

The increased reaction time of the monkey in the double-step saccade task corresponds well with the behavior described for human subjects in Feinstein and Williams (1972), Becker and Jürgens (1979) and Lünenburger et al. (2000a). However, the comparison of onward and reverse double-step reaction times leads to the opposite result in human and monkeys. The human results might reflect inhibition of return (Posner and Cohen, 1984; for recent reviews see Taylor and Klein, 1998; Klein, 2000). Inhibition of return prevents repeated fixation of the same location and therefore improves the efficiency of visual scanning. In contrast, the monkey shows shorter reaction times for second saccades that were in the opposite direction of the first than those with the same direction. (Dorris et al., 1999) report reaction times for the monkey which correspond to the results of the present study and therefore also differ from the human data. This discrepancy between the behavior of the two species remains to be explained.

Functional role of fixation neurons

Our initial hypothesis was that the postsaccadic enhancement of fixation neurons could be responsible for the increased reaction time of the second saccade in the double step. This hypothesis could not be supported by our data. We had assumed that a putatively higher activity of collicular fixation neurons after the first saccade would delay the second saccade. But, the recorded fixation neurons did not regain high firing rates between the two saccades. Although the number of analyzed fixation neurons is small, we speculate that the fixation neurons are not likely to cause the increased reaction time of the second saccade.

The observed low activity in the double-step task might result from a specific inhibitory input that is not yet known. The inhibition of the fixation neurons in this context might actually be useful. Without it, the fixation neurons might reactivate and therefore delay the upcoming saccade further or even prevent its triggering. Munoz and Wurtz (1995b) hypothesized that there is actually a continuum from the fixation neurons in the rostral SC to the saccadic 'build-up neurons' in the caudal SC. Given that there

is lateral inhibition in the SC (Munoz and Istvan, 1998), the activity of build-up neurons could lead to the inhibition of the fixation neurons between the two saccades in the double-step task. However, such inhibition is unlikely to happen in our experimental conditions since the target remained at the same position (fovea) for at least 100 ms after the first saccade, i.e. stimulating the central receptive fields of the rostral pole of the SC. The build-up neurons lie more caudally, a region where more eccentrically located receptive fields are represented. To these locations, the target is displaced later. In the single-step task, the re-activation of the fixation neurons happened within 100 ms after the saccade. To prevent this reactivation, it would be necessary to send a signal before the second target displacement, and this is not possible from lateral inhibition within the SC. Inhibition of fixation neurons from higher-order centers might have been possible because the double-step trials were done in blocks in paradigms B. Therefore, the monkey possibly knew at the beginning of the trial that it had to do two saccades. In paradigm A, one single-step condition was randomly interleaved. But since this condition was the only one that started with central fixation, it was predictable too. This monkey would have been able to predict a double-step trial with certainty from peripheral starting position. However, this 'cognitive' prediction requires the involvement of the cortex, most likely frontal cortex. The frontal cortex, especially frontal eye field (FEF) and supplementary eye field (SEF), can have strong influence on the basal ganglia, which efficiently inhibit the intermediate layers of the SC via the substantia nigra pars reticulata (SNpr) (Hikosaka et al., 2000).

Discharge characteristics of the saccadic neurons

In the present study, we presented results on the discharge of saccadic neurons during to subsequent visually guided saccades. Earlier recordings in the superior colliculus also described the activity of collicular neurons during sequences of two saccades. Mays and Sparks (1980) discovered the quasi-visual neurons in this way. Yet, the stimulus was only briefly flashed at the two target locations before the first saccade. In this way, it was possible to examine the collicular coding of memorized saccade targets. Actually, the effect of the increased reaction time of the second saccade could not be assessed with this visual stimulation because both saccades are memory-guided. Recent results of Goossens and Van Opstal (1997) indicate that the interval of the two saccades in this paradigm may be as short as 50 ms. This also prohibits direct comparison with our present study.

The neural inputs leading to the peak of activity about 70 ms after target onset is consistent with the visual input from the visual cortex described by Schiller et al. (1974). However, recent studies indicate that the input could also arrive via the parietal cortex. For example, area V6A has a latency for visual response of about 60 ms (Fattori et al., 2001) that could be conveyed to the SC (Shipp et al., 1998). Input from other parietal areas is also possible.

Functional role of the saccadic neurons

The main activation of recorded saccadic neurons (measured as time of peak activity) coincided well with the occurrence of the saccade evoked by the first target displacement. This was observed as well for second saccades in a double-step task, which have prolonged reaction times. Because of this temporal linkage, we assume that this is the motor activation of the neurons. To show this more convincingly, one would have to temporally separate and decouple the visual stimulation and the motor response. This could have been done by delayed saccade tasks. Yet, this tasks requires the monkey to withhold a saccade to a new, salient stimulus in the periphery. This is unnatural and needs training that, on the other hand, might influence the monkey's behavior in the usual saccade task which interests us. The temporal co-variation of this activation component with the saccade should be sufficient to identify it as the motor burst.

Express saccades have a very short reaction time. Sparks et al. (2000) report that the activation of SC neurons during express saccades shows a merged visual and motor burst around the saccade. They concluded that "the hypothesis that the motor burst of collicular neurons serves as a signal for triggering saccade onset can now be extended to express saccades". From this we can deduce that the motor burst is predictive of the saccade triggering for normal and express saccades. Our results, presented in the present study, show that when the saccade is delayed (like a second saccade in a double step) the main peak of activation is also delayed and remains temporally coupled to the saccade. We conclude that the motor burst is the trigger signal for any saccade: express, regular, or delayed saccade. The motor burst might be the signal for triggering the saccade or the feedback signal that the saccade is performed. A discrimination between these two alternatives is not possible using data from this study. Recent experiments by Soetedjo et al. (2002) indicate that it might be a feedback signal.

A possible cause of the delay of the second saccade

A second target-aligned activation (TAC), apart from the early presumably visual component, was observed about 150 ms after the second target displacement. This activation was not visible before the first saccade because the saccadic motor burst occurs approximately at that time. We suppose that this second TAC triggers the first saccade in the double-step and single-step saccades. We furthermore hypothesize that the second saccade is delayed because it is not triggered by the second TAC. The missing activation by the first TAC in the double step with 0 ms delay might increase the reaction time in this condition further. Assuming an integrate-to-threshold model, the threshold will be reached later which delays the saccade.

The substantia nigra (SNpr) has to be inhibited after the first target displacement to disinhibit the SC (Hikosaka et al., 2000). The second TAC may thus develop into the motor burst and lead to saccades with reaction times around 150 ms. Assuming that SNpr is inhibited later or less after the second target displacement, the development of the second TAC into the motor burst is prevented and the second saccade can only be triggered later. Experiments in humans that include a gap before the second target displacement show a reaction time of the second saccade that is not increased compared to the first (Lünenburger et al., in revision). It is conceivable that the gap leads to early inhibition of SNpr followed by disinhibition of the SC such that the second TAC can trigger the saccade with normal reaction time.

A possible role of the delay of the second saccade

It has been shown that the visual receptive field of neurons in the lateral intraparietal area (LIP) change before a saccade is executed. The receptive fields shift already before the saccade to the location that corresponds to the receptive field relative to the final eye position after the saccade (Kubischik et al. in preparation, Duhamel et al., 1992; Colby et al., 1995; Colby and Goldberg, 1999). We infer that this shift of all the receptive fields of LIP neurons represents a distortion of the neural map of the visual world before and during saccades, and that this distortion remains until after the saccade. Other visual brain areas might change their maps similarly. We hypothesize that the triggering of a saccade to a new target briefly after another is inhibited until the distortion in the map has sufficiently decayed and the normal maps are restored.

Conclusions

If a target is displaced two times in brief succession, the reaction time of the second saccade is longer than that of the first saccade in monkey and human. The increase in reaction time is larger when the second target displacement occurs quicker after the first saccade. In contrast to the human, the monkey has longer reaction times for second saccades that have the same direction as the first compared to those that have the opposite direction. Fixation neurons in the superior colliculus have lower activity between the two saccades in the double-step task. They are not likely to cause the delay of the second saccade, because they are not reactivated and therefore do not have to be inhibited to allow triggering the second saccade. Saccadic neurons usually showed multiphasic activation. The main activation occurred briefly before the saccade. It might thus be the trigger for saccade initiation or the feedback signal of saccade execution. The early, presumably visual activation is observed before the first and second saccades except before the second saccades in trials with 0 ms delay between the first saccade and the second target displacement. Under these conditions, the saccadic reaction time was highest. Another activation temporally coupled to the target onset is visible with a latency of about 150 ms after the second target displacement. This activation is not hidden by the main neural activation during the second saccade as it is for the first saccade. The reaction time of the second saccade might be increased because the SC is prohibited from developing this target-aligned activation into the motor burst and trigger the saccade.

Acknowledgments

We want to thank Alexander Thiele for theoretical and programming help with the burst detection algorithms. Christian Casanova, Dieter F. Kutz and Matthias Klar made helpful suggestions to earlier versions of the manuscript. Furthermore we are indebted to Stephanie Krämer and Hermann Korbmacher for their technical support. This work was supported by the Deutsche Forschungsgemeinschaft (DFG-graduate program 'KOGNET III', DFG-SPP 1001 'Sensorimotor Integration', Ho450/24, SFB-509 'Neurovision'). One of the authors (LL) wants to thank the Boehringer Ingelheim Fonds for the generous support.

References

Andersen, R.A., Snyder, L.H., Bradley, D.C. and Xing, J. (1997) Multimodal representation of space in the posterior parietal cortex and its use in planning movements. *Annu. Rev. Neurosci.*, 20: 303–330.

Becker, W. and Jürgens, R. (1979) An analysis of the saccadic system by means of double step stimuli. *Vis. Res.*, 19: 967–983.

Colby, C.L. and Goldberg, M.E. (1999) Space and attention in parietal cortex. *Annu. Rev. Neurosci.*, 22: 319–349.

Colby, C.L., Duhamel, J.-R. and Goldberg, M.E. (1995) Oculocentric spatial representation in parietal cortex. *Cereb. Cortex*, 5: 470–481.

Commenges, D., Pinatel, F. and Seal, J. (1986) A program for analysing single neuron activity by methods based on estimation of a change-point. *Comput. Methods Progr. Biomed.*, 23: 123–132.

Dorris, M.C. and Munoz, D.P. (1998) Saccadic probability influences motor preparation signals and time to saccadic initiation. *J. Neurosci.*, 18: 7015–7026.

Dorris, M.C., Paré, M. and Munoz, D.P. (1997) Neuronal activity in monkey superior colliculus related to the initiation of saccadic eye movements. *J Neuroscience*, 17: 8566–8579.

Dorris, M.C., Taylor, T.L., Klein, R.M. and Munoz, D.P. (1999) Influence of previous visual stimulus or saccade on saccadic reaction times in monkey. *J. Neurophysiol.*, 81: 2429–2436.

Duhamel, J.-R., Colby, C.L. and Goldberg, M.E. (1992) The updating of the representation of visual space in parietal cortex by intended eye movements. *Science*, 255: 90–92.

Everling, S., Paré, M., Dorris, M.C. and Munoz, D.P. (1998) Comparison of the discharge characteristics of brain stem omnipause neurons and superior colliculus fixation neurons in monkey: Implications for control of fixation and saccade behavior. *J. Neurophysiol.*, 79: 511–528.

Fattori, P., Gamberini, M., Kutz, D.F. and Galletti, C. (2001) 'Arm-reaching' neurons in the parietal area V6A of the macaque monkey. *Eur. J. Neurosci.*, 13: 2309–2313.

Feinstein, R. and Williams, W.J. (1972) Interactions of the horizontal and vertical human oculomotor systems: the saccadic systems. *Vis. Res.*, 12: 33–44.

Fischer, B. and Weber, H. (1993) Express saccades and visual attention. *Behav. Brain Sci.*, 16: 533–610.

Goossens, H.H.L.M. and Van Opstal, A.J. (1997) Local feedback signals are not distorted by prior eye movements: Evidence from visually evoked double saccades. *J. Neurophysiol.*, 78: 533–538.

Goossens, H.H.L.M. and Van Opstal, A.J. (2000) Blink perturbed saccades in monkey. II. Superior colliculus activity. *J. Neurophysiol.*, 83: 3430–3452.

Hanes, D.P. and Wurtz, R.H. (2001) Interaction of the frontal eye field and superior colliculus for saccade generation. *J. Neurophysiol.*, 85: 804–815.

Hanes, D.P., Thompson, K.G. and Schall, J.D. (1995) Relationship of presaccadic activity in frontal eye field and supplementary eye field to saccade initiation in macaque: Poisson spike train analysis. *Exp. Brain Res.*, 103: 85–96.

Hikosaka, O., Takikawa, Y. and Kawagoe, R. (2000) Role of the basal ganglia in the control of purposive saccadic eye movements. *Psychol. Rev.*, 80: 953–978.

Judge, S.J., Richmond, B.J. and Chu, F.C. (1980) Implantation of magnetic search coils for measurement of eye position: an improved method. *Vis. Res.*, 20: 535–538.

Klein, R.M. (2000) Inhibition of return. *Trends Cogn. Sci.*, 4: 138–147.

Lindner, W., Lünenburger, L. and Hoffmann, K.-P. (2001) Burst-activity during combined eye–hand movements in the superior colliculus of the macaque monkey. In: N. Elsner and G.W. Kreutzberg (Eds.), Göttingen Neurobiology Report. Thieme, Stuttgart, p. 560.

Lünenburger, L. (2002) Influence of arm movements on saccades (Einfluss von Armbewegungen auf Sakkaden). Ph.D. thesis, Ruhr-University Bochum.

Lünenburger, L., Kutz, D.F. and Hoffmann, K.-P. (2000a) Influence of arm movements on saccades in humans. *Eur. J. Neurosci.*, 12: 4107–4116.

Lünenburger, L., Kutz, D.F. and Hoffmann, K.-P. (2000b) Influence of arm movements on saccades in humans: Effects in double-step tasks. *Soc. Neurosci. Abstr.*, 26: 497.3.

Lünenburger, L., Lindner, W. and Hoffmann, K.-P. (2001) Influence of arm movements on saccades: Effects of double step tasks. *Annual Meeting of the Society for Neural Control of Movement*. (http://www-ncm.cs.umass.edu/abstracts/2001/346176.html).

Lynch, J.C. (1992) Saccade initiation and latency deficits after combined lesion of the frontal and posterior eye fields in monkeys. *J. Neurophysiol.*, 68: 1913–1916.

Mays, L.E. and Sparks, D.L. (1980) Dissociation of visual and saccade-related responses in superior colliculus neurons. *J. Neurophysiol.*, 43: 207–232.

Moschovakis, A.K., Scudder, C.A. and Highstein, S.M. 1996 The microscopic anatomy and physiology of the mammalian saccadic system. *Prog. Neurobiol.*, 50: 133–254.

Munoz, D.P. and Guitton, D. (1991) Control of orienting gaze shifts by tectoreticulospinal system in the head-free cat. II. Sustained discharges during motor preparation and fixation. *J. Neurophysiol.*, 66: 1624–1641.

Munoz, D.P. and Istvan, P.J. (1998) Lateral inhibitory interactions in the intermediate layers of the monkey colliculus. *J. Neurophysiol.*, 79: 1193–1209.

Munoz, D.P. and Wurtz, R.H. (1993a) Fixation cells in monkey superior colliculus. I. Characteristics of cell discharge. *J. Neurophysiol.*, 70: 559–575.

Munoz, D.P. and Wurtz, R.H. (1993b) Fixation cells in monkey superior colliculus. II. Reversible activation and deactivation. *J. Neurophysiol.*, 70: 576–589.

Munoz, D.P. and Wurtz, R.H. (1995a) Saccade-related activity in monkey superior colliculus I. Characteristics of burst and buildup cells. *J. Neurophysiol.*, 73: 2313–2333.

Munoz, D.P. and Wurtz, R.H. (1995b) Saccade-related activity in monkey superior colliculus II. Spread of activity during saccades. *J. Neurophysiol.*, 73: 2334–2348.

Munoz, D.P., Dorris, M.C., Paré, M. and Everling, S. (2000) On your mark, get set: Brainstem circuitry underlying saccadic initiation. *Can. J. Physiol. Pharmacol.*, 78: 934–944.

Posner, M.I. and Cohen, Y. (1984) Components of visual orienting. In: H. Bouma and D.G. Bouwhuis (Eds.), *Attention and Performance*. Vol. X, Erlbaum, London, pp. 531–556.

Saslow, M.G. (1967) Effects of components of displacement-step stimuli upon latency for saccadic eye movement. *J. Opt. Soc. Am.*, 57: 1024–1029.

Schiller, P.H. and Koerner, F. (1971) Discharge characteristics of single units in superior colliculus of the alert rhesus monkey. *J. Neurophysiol.*, 34: 920–936.

Schiller, P.H., Stryker, M., Cynader, M. and Bergman, N. (1974) Response characteristics of single cells in the monkey superior colliculus following ablation or cooling of visual cortex. *J. Neurophysiol.*, 37: 181–194.

Schiller, P.H., True, S.D. and Conway, J.L. (1980) Deficits in eye movements following frontal eye-field and superior colliculus ablations. *J. Neurophysiol.*, 44: 1175–1189.

Schiller, P.H., Sandell, J.H. and Mausnell, J.H. (1987) The effect of frontal eye field and superior colliculus lesions on saccadic latencies in the rhesus monkey. *J. Neurophysiol.*, 57: 1033–1049.

Seal, J., Commenges, D., Salamon, R. and Bioulac, B. (1983) A statistical method for the estimation of neuronal response latency and its functional interpretation. *Brain Res.*, 278: 382–386.

Shipp, S., Blanton, M. and Zeki, S. (1998) A visuo-somatomotor pathway through superior parietal cortex in the macaque monkey: cortical connections of areas V6 and V6A. *Eur. J. Neurosci.*, 10: 3171–3193.

Soetedjo, R., Kaneko, C.R.S. and Fuchs, A.F. (2002) Evidence that the superior colliculus participates in the feedback control of saccadic eye movements. *J. Neurophysiol.*, 87: 679–695.

Sparks, D.L. and Hartwich-Young, R. (1989) The deep layers of the superior colliculus. *Rev. Oculomot. Res.*, 3: 213–255.

Sparks, D.L., Rohrer, W.H. and Zhang, Y. (2000) The role of the superior colliculus in saccade initiation: a study of express saccades and the gap effect. *Vis. Res.*, 40: 2763–2777.

Stuphorn, V., Bauswein, E. and Hoffmann, K.-P. (2000) Neurons in the primate superior colliculus coding for arm movements in gaze-related coordinates. *J. Neurophysiol.*, 83: 1283–1299.

Taylor, T.L. and Klein, R.M. (1998) On the causes and effects of inhibition of return. *Psychon. Bull. Rev.*, 5: 625–643.

Werner, W. (1993) Neurons in the primate superior colliculus are active before and during arm movements to visual targets. *Eur. J. Neurosci.*, 5: 335–340.

Werner, W., Hoffmann, K.-P. and Dannenberg, S. (1997) Anatomical distribution of arm-movement-related neurons in the primate superior colliculus and underlying reticular formation in comparison with visual and saccadic cells. *Exp. Brain Res.*, 115: 206–216.

Wurtz, R.H. and Goldberg, M.E. (1971) Superior colliculus cell responses related to eye movements in awake monkeys. *Science*, 171: 82–84.

C. Prablanc, D. Pélisson and Y. Rossetti (Eds.)
Progress in Brain Research, Vol. 142
© 2003 Elsevier Science B.V. All rights reserved

CHAPTER 7

Neural control of 3-D gaze shifts in the primate

Eliana M. Klier [1], Julio C. Martinez-Trujillo [2], W. Pieter Medendorp [2],
Michael A. Smith [3] and J. Douglas Crawford [4,*]

[1] *CIHR Group for Action and Perception, Centre for Vision Research, Department of Biology, York University,
Toronto, ON M3J 1P3, Canada*
[2] *CIHR Group for Action and Perception, Centre for Vision Research, York University, Toronto, ON M3J 1P3, Canada*
[3] *CIHR Group for Action and Perception, Department of Psychology, York University, Toronto, ON M3J 1P3, Canada*
[4] *CIHR Group for Action and Perception, Departments of Psychology, Biology, and Kinesiology and Health Sciences, York University,
Toronto, ON M3J 1P3, Canada*

Abstract: The neural mechanisms that specify target locations for gaze shifts and then convert these into desired patterns of coordinated eye and head movements are complex. Much of this complexity is only revealed when one takes a realistic three-dimensional (3-D) view of these processes, where fundamental computational problems such as kinematic redundancy, reference-frame transformations, and non-commutativity emerge. Here we review the underlying mechanisms and solutions for these problems, starting with a consideration of the kinematics of 3-D gaze shifts in human and non-human primates. We then consider the neural mechanisms, including cortical representation of gaze targets, the nature of the gaze motor command used by the superior colliculus, and how these gaze commands are decomposed into brainstem motor commands for the eyes and head. A general conclusion is that fairly simple coding mechanisms may be used to represent gaze at the cortical and collicular level, but this then necessitates complexity for the spatial updating of these representations and in the brainstem sensorimotor transformations that convert these signals into eye and head movements.

The problem of 3-D gaze shifts

The term 'gaze' is loosely used in common language to denote the direction in which one is looking. We can define this more rigorously as the visual axis (i.e., the line passing from the fovea through the optical focal point toward the object of current regard). By this definition, gaze is determined by the orientation of the eye in space, which in turn will be influenced by the orientation of the eye in the head, the head on the body, and the body with respect to

the earth. Of course, when the head is immobilized, as is often the case in the laboratory, gaze control becomes synonymous with oculomotor control. At the opposite extreme, in real life situations, where very large shifts in gaze are often required, the body also contributes. But here we will consider gaze control in the manner most commonly implied in the current literature, i.e., gaze movements produced by coordinated movements of the eyes and head.

Most studies of gaze control take a 1-D or 2-D approach. From this perspective, certain fundamental findings arise, among them, that gaze shifts generally start with a rapid eye movement (saccade) toward the desired visual target, followed closely by a slightly less rapid head movement in the same general direction (Morasso et al., 1973; Guitton and Volle, 1987; Freedman et al., 1996). When gaze first reaches the target, either at the end of the saccade or through

---

*Correspondence to: J. Douglas Crawford, Department of Psychology, 209 B.S.B., York University, 4700 Keele Street, Toronto, ON M3J 1P3, Canada. Tel.: +1-416-736-2100/ext. 88621; Fax: +1-416-736-5814; E-mail: jdc@yorku.ca

a combination of the eye and head movement, the system locks gaze onto the target by engaging the vestibulo-ocular reflex (VOR). The VOR then stabilizes the gaze line by counter-rotating the eye against the movement of the head, which generally continues until the eyes are somewhat centered within the orbit (Fuller, 1996; Tweed, 1997). Most studies on the neurophysiological mechanisms for gaze control have thus focused on the mechanisms that coordinate the timing of these various stages.

However, if one is interested in the spatial aspects of gaze control, then one must seriously consider the 3-D geometry that pertains to eye movement, head movement, and their relation to the location of the visual target. The eyes and head both rotate *and* translate with respect to visual targets, where each of these types of motion have three degrees of freedom (Tweed and Vilis, 1987; Angelaki et al., 2000; Medendorp et al., 2002). Here we will mainly consider rotations and their effect on orientations of the eyes and head. These structures obviously rotate in the horizontal and vertical dimension. The third dimension is called torsion, which roughly refers to the tilting of the eyes or head about the gaze line (more rigorous definitions will be provided in the next section).

As we shall see, both the eyes and head have the musculature necessary to rotate in all three of these degrees of freedom (Simpson and Graf, 1981; Suzuki et al., 1999). So when one moves from a 2-D to a 3-D perspective, the first and most obvious question to ask is, what does torsion do, and how is it controlled? But this is only the beginning, because in 3-D (i.e., in the real world) a number of computational problems arise that are either not present or are obscure from a more abstract 2-D perspective. First, there is the degrees of freedom problem (Bernstein, 1967). Since gaze direction is inherently a 2-D variable, the eyes and head, each with their three degrees of freedom, have an infinite number of ways to contribute to the same gaze direction. For example, one could fixate a visual target and spin the eyes torsionally about the line of sight without changing gaze. Obviously we do not do this normally, but scientists in this field are interested in which choices of orientation the system actually makes, how it implements these choices and what this says about the neural mechanisms involved (Helmholtz, 1867; Nakayama, 1975; Tweed

and Vilis, 1990; Straumann et al., 1991; Hepp, 1994; Crawford and Vilis, 1995).

Another computational problem that presents itself in 3-D is the non-commutativity of rotations (Westheimer, 1957; Tweed et al., 1999). When rotations are not constrained to occur about a single fixed axis — as they never are for the eyes and head — then the order of rotation has a strong effect on the final orientation. For example, a 30° upward rotation followed by a 30° leftward rotation results in a different final orientation than the same two rotations in the reverse order. This has a number of implications for the motor control of gaze, which have been reviewed and argued to considerable extent elsewhere (Tweed and Vilis, 1987; Schnabolk and Raphan, 1994; Quaia and Optican, 1998).

Finally, the question of neural 'reference frames' and 'coordinate systems' often only becomes clearly delineated in 3-D (Soechting and Flanders, 1992). These terms are frequently used in the gaze control literature, very often inappropriately. When we define some spatial variable, we must do so with respect to some fixed reference frame. For a physiological example, the initial visual stimulus is defined in an ocular frame, where the activity of ganglion cells specifies the direction of a given target with respect to the fovea, all within a 2-D retinal map that is fixed to the eye. In comparison, the eyes move relative to the head so the eye muscles are organized in a head-centered frame, and similarly the neck muscles are organized with respect to a trunk-fixed frame.

This is separate from the concept of a coordinate system, which provides a set of axes (or more correctly basis vectors) which are useful to describe the components of a variable within some frame (Soechting and Flanders, 1992). The choice of coordinate systems is arbitrary, as long as it 'spans' the degrees of freedom of the space, but as a default most people prefer orthonormal coordinate systems. We do this all the time do describe our data, but sticking to physiology, the retina does not have a coordinate system, whereas the eye muscles and vestibular canals do specify natural coordinates in a head frame (if we imply a certain coupling between the opponent pairs of these structures) (Simpson and Graf, 1985). The question of whether the neural control system itself employs such coordinate systems is more controversial (Robinson, 1992; Crawford, 1994).

Once one has specified the reference frame and the coordinate system, one is then prepared to define a number of kinematic variables. But these are separate from the coordinate systems in which they operate. For example, one can use a given head-fixed coordinate system to define eye orientation, the angular velocity of the eye, eye rotations, displacements in eye orientation, and a number of other variables, each with a different meaning (Hepp, 1994; Crawford and Guitton, 1997). Thus, terms like 'gaze coordinates' or 'velocity coordinates' are not meaningful. In designing or understanding a control system, one must specify the frame of reference, the coordinates within this frame, and the variable being measured.

A very frequent error in the gaze control literature is to equate displacements with retinal coordinates and gaze positions with space coordinates. Or, to think that displacements are frame-free. It is true that displacements are defined with regard to a reference position, whereas positions, orientations, etc. must be defined with respect to single common zero point (i.e., a reference position). However, displacements are not frame-free (Hepp et al., 1993; Crawford and Guitton, 1997). Consider Sperry's famous experiment of surgically rotating a frog's eye by 180° (Sperry, 1943). When the frog then saw a fly displaced leftward in retinal coordinates, it flung its tongue rightward in frog head coordinates. So, the frame of reference for a displacement must be specified. This is very relevant here because many think that gaze is controlled largely through a series of internal displacement-like commands beginning with the visual target defined in the retinal frame and ending with the motor displacements of the eyes with respect to the head and the head with respect to the body (Becker and Jurgens, 1979; Van Opstal et al., 1991; Colby and Goldberg, 1999; Klier et al., 2001).

Moreover, the reference frame problem that we saw with the frog does not only occur for torsional eye orientations. We have shown that because of the geometry resulting from the way that light projects onto the retina and how this in turn depends on eye orientation, even moving the eyes up or down (left or right), changes the correspondence between the visual code and motor codes for target displacement

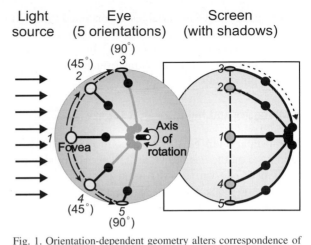

Fig. 1. Orientation-dependent geometry alters correspondence of visual and motor codes. A semi-transparent 'eye' is viewed from a behind-right perspective, where the eye is back-lit so that the shadows project onto a frontal screen. This projection system is not arbitrary, because it mirrors the geometry of the raw 2-D eye-coil signals used to measure gaze in physiological studies. At position 1, the eye is looking straight ahead, with the fovea (open disk) oriented at the back of the eye. Two sites of retinal stimulation (dot) are represented as 'retinal error' vectors emanating rightward from the fovea; one 40° right (black line) and one 80° right (gray line). These correspond to 40° and 80° rightward visual targets (dispensing with the optical inversion), as shown by the shadows projected on the screen (dot). This is the trivial situation in which a point of horizontal stimulation on the retina calls for a purely horizontal eye movement to acquire the target. But what if the eye rotates up or down about its horizontal axis by 45° or 90° (initial static eye orientations 2–5)? The stimulus vectors remain fixed anatomically on the same horizontal retinal meridian (so that from our space-fixed perspective they now appear rotated to non-horizontal lines). How do these same retinal displacements correspond to target displacements in visual space? The screen view indicates that these horizontal displacements (in retinal coordinates) now correspond to non-horizontal displacement vectors in space, the latter becoming more and more oblique as a function of the length of retinal vector and the amount of eye rotation. For example, at position 3, the 80° rightward retinal target would call for an eye movement qualitatively like the one indicated by the dashed arrow on the screen. (Adapted from Klier et al., 2001.)

in space (Fig. 1) (Crawford and Guitton, 1997; Klier et al., 2001).

The purpose of this chapter is to consider how the primate brain deals with the problems of excess degrees of freedom in gaze control and how it performs the visual–motor reference frame transformations alluded to above. We will deal first with the kinematic aspects of the behavior, followed by a consideration of what variables are encoded in which frames/coordinate systems at various points within the gaze control system, and end by considering what we know about the transformations between these representations.

Kinematics and behavior of 3-D gaze

The primary job of the gaze control system is to land gaze on the desired visual target. Although gaze itself is a 2-D variable, its main job still falls prey to the 3-D considerations summarized in the last section. In particular, the reference frame problem involved in converting a visual signal defined in the ocular frame into commands for movement relative to the head and body frames (Fig. 1). With the use of simulations, we have shown that a direct mapping of the components of the visual vector onto the components of a motor vector would produce accurate gaze shifts for small displacements, but progressively larger position-dependent errors for movements over 30° in amplitude (Crawford and Guitton, 1997; Klier and Crawford, 1998). One can appreciate this from Fig. 1 by considering what would happen if that one single horizontal retinal error were mapped onto the same horizontal gaze shift at all vertical positions, whereas the projection shows that the required gaze shift depends on initial positions. Conversely, the same simulations showed that in order to avoid these errors, the system has to take eye (and head) orientation into account. So does it?

We tested this by measuring saccades over a wide range of initial eye positions (including torsional eye positions induced by tilting the head) and found that saccades are more accurate than could be predicted by a simple displacement-to-displacement mapping (Klier and Crawford, 1998). Indeed, the predicted errors of this model become so huge within the range of head-free gaze control (up to 90°) that this hardly seems to deem further testing. Clearly, the neural control system performs a position-dependent reference frame transformation. Where and how this is done will be the subject of a later section.

Another, more extensively studied issue is the degrees of freedom problem. With the head immobilized, it is well known that the eye obeys Donders' law, i.e., for each gaze direction only one 3-D eye orientation is used (Donders, 1848). Listing's law

further specifies that the eye only assumes those orientations that can be reached by rotations about an axis in a head-fixed plane (Listing's plane) that is orthogonal to gaze at the special reference orientation called primary position (Helmholtz, 1867; Hepp, 1990; Tweed and Vilis, 1990). In other words, if we define these axes in a coordinate system where the vertical and horizontal axes are fixed in Listing's plane, and the orthogonal torsional axis is parallel to gaze at the primary position (Listing's coordinates), then Listing's law simply states that torsion is maintained at zero (Fig. 2A) (Westheimer, 1957). (Note that this is not the same as cyclotorsion about the line of sight, which shows so-called 'false torsion' at oblique eye orientations.)

Several studies in humans and monkeys have shown that a similar form of Donders' law also holds for the orientation of the eye-in-space when subjects make head-free gaze shifts (Straumann et al., 1991; Glenn and Vilis, 1992; Radau et al., 1994; Crawford et al., 1999; Ceylan et al., 2000). However, the constraint is not quite as stringent as Listing's law (i.e., the torsional standard deviations are 2–3 times higher). Moreover, instead of falling in a plane, the axes used to describe eye-in-space orientations form a twisted surface (Fig. 2B), when plotted in an orthogonal coordinate system where the forward-pointing torsional axis is fixed in space. This twist corresponds to the twist produced by rotating an object in Fick coordinates, where the vertical axis (for horizontal rotation) would be fixed in the body, the horizontal axis (for vertical rotation) would be fixed in the eye, and the third torsional axis would also be fixed in the eye and held at zero (Glenn and Vilis, 1992). (More accurately, the constraint is about half way between zero torsion in Fick and Listing's coordinates.) Orientations of the head show a similar Fick-like constraint, during gaze shifts (Fig. 2C). Obviously these are neural constraints since we can violate this rule by voluntarily rotating the head torsionally any time we want.

What about orientations of the eye relative to the head during these head-free gaze shifts? They need not show the same constraint as the eye-in-space, since the latter is the product of constraints in both the eye-in-head and head-in-space. It turns out that Listing's law is still obeyed by the eye-in-head, but only during fixations at the end of the gaze shift

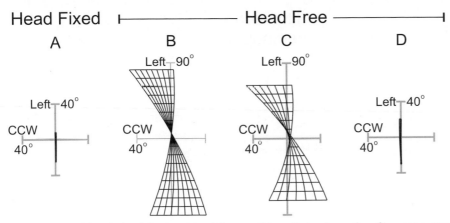

Fig. 2. Donders' law in head-fixed and head-free conditions. 2nd order surface fits were computed to fixation points (i.e., when the velocity of both the eye and head were <10°/s) during random gaze shifts. Side views of the data are presented where torsion (i.e., clockwise and counterclockwise movements) fall along the abscissa. (A) In the head-fixed condition (where eye-in-space = eye-in-head), eye positions appear to lie in a flat plane viewed edge-on (i.e., Listing's plane). (B–D) In head-free condition, the eye-in-space (B) and head-in-space (C) positions look like flat planes twisted about the center (i.e., a Fick-like surface), while the eye-in-head (D) surface resembles the head-fixed condition.

(Fig. 2D) (Tweed et al., 1998; Crawford et al., 1999). In contrast, during the gaze shift, the eye-in-head violates all forms of Donders' law (Tweed et al., 1998; Crawford et al., 1999). This is not due to sloppiness, but rather because the VOR phase of the gaze shift cannot simultaneously obey Donders' law and stabilize the retinal image. So the VOR chooses to stabilize vision, producing real torsional eye-in-head rotations (Crawford and Vilis, 1991; Misslisch and Hess, 2000). In order to counteract these effects and end up with the eye in Listing's plane rather than with some willy-nilly level of torsion, the system has also developed a rather sophisticated mechanism, generating saccades with torsional components that anticipate (in an equal an opposite way) the torsion produced by the VOR (Crawford et al., 1991; Tweed et al., 1998; Crawford et al., 1999). These movements are much too rapid and precise to be explained as any kind of passive mechanism (Seidman and Leigh, 1989). Thus, with careful measurement, one observes a continuous pattern of the eyes shooting out of and then coming back into Listing's plane by the end of the gaze shift.

Spatial updating

Every time one generates a gaze shift, it changes the spatial correspondence between the retina and the visual world. This is not a big deal for objects that are continuously in clear view, but it does pose a problem for the remembered locations of objects because a memory trace coded in a raw visual frame would no longer be valid at the new eye position. Clearly the system is not fooled by this since we are able to generate accurate saccades to remembered targets after intervening gaze shifts (Hallett and Lightstone, 1976; Herter and Guitton, 1998), including gaze shifts composed of both eye and head movement. Although a number of mechanisms have been proposed to account for this perceptual stability, the weight of the current evidence suggests that each time gaze is shifted, internal representations of retinal targets are counter-rotated within the internal eye-centered maps of the visuomotor system, such that their spatial correspondence remains correct (Goldberg and Bruce, 1990; Duhamel et al., 1992; Walker et al., 1995; Henriques et al., 1998; Batista and Andersen, 2001; Medendorp and Crawford, 2002).

In 2-D models of this process, this internal re-mapping is accomplished by subtracting a 2-D motor vector representing the gaze shift (presumably in the form of an efference copy) from the visual vector (Goldberg and Bruce, 1990; Quaia et al., 1998). However, in the real 3-D system this would not work for a couple of reasons. First, since the eyes and head (Donders' law not withstanding) do sometimes rotate torsionally, and this also changes the spatial correspondence of the retina to the world, one would

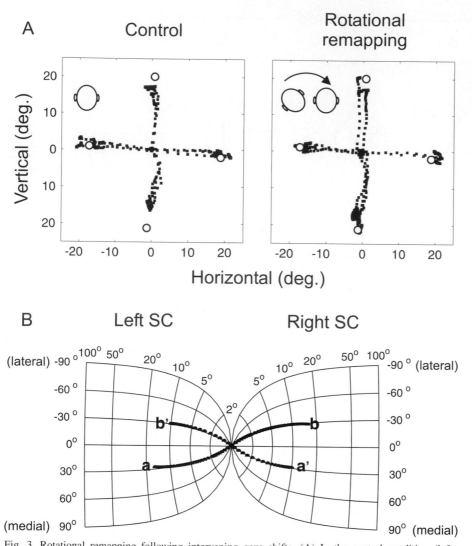

Fig. 3. Rotational remapping following intervening gaze shifts. (A) In the control condition (left panel) the subjects made no head movement before saccading to the remembered target (circle). In the 'rotational remapping' condition (right panel) the subjects perceived the target at a 45° rightward head tilt, rolled their heads upright, and subsequently made the saccade. One subject's performance to the four cardinal targets is shown. In both conditions, saccadic directions were accurate. (B) Rotational remapping on the superior colliculus map. A space-fixed target a (10° leftward and 30° upward) flashed when the eye is turned 45° counterclockwise, stimulates the left side of the retina. It is represented, therefore, on the left SC. But after the eye rotates upright, the remembered target is now to the right relative to the retina. In the collicular map its representation must cross the midline, from the left to the right SC (a′). At the same time, target b (10° rightward and 30° downward in space) should cross in the opposite direction, from the right SC to the left (b′). (Adapted from Medendorp et al., 2002.)

need a 3-D operator to provide optimal eye-centered re-mapping of the visual memory trace (Medendorp et al., 2002). Our recent experiment shows that the human system does indeed possess such an operator. Specifically, following torsional rotations of the eyes and head, subjects are still able to localize re-membered visual targets using a saccade (Fig. 3A) (Medendorp et al., 2002).

Interestingly, this requires an internal 'rotational remapping', where the amount and direction of remapping depends both on the movement itself and initial location of the representation within the internal eye-centered maps of the brain (e.g., in the superior colliculus) (Fig. 3B). Furthermore, the necessity of a 3-D feedback signal probably means that the efference copy is originating in the brainstem (and/or from vestibular feedback about head motion) before being fed back to higher visuomotor centers (Smith and Crawford, 2001a). Moreover, since such a remapping must be done as a rotation (i.e., a non-commutative process), this cannot be captured by a vector subtraction model. Our simulations further show that a non-commutative model is even required for saccades within Listing's plane, and the lack of errors observed when such saccades are tested again shows that the principles of non-commutativity are heeded in the internal re-mapping mechanism (Smith and Crawford, 2001a).

Another bit of interesting geometry that arises during head-free situations has more to do with translations. With the head free, the eye frequently translates through space as well as rotates (Medendorp et al., 1998). This again changes the correspondence between the internal eye-centered maps of space and the visual world, but this time in a way that depends on target depth (i.e., motion parallax) (Howard and Rogers, 1995). Our recent experiments show that during such translations, subjects are able to remember and saccade toward perceived target locations in a translation and depth-dependent manner (Medendorp et al., 2001). Again, this shows that the updating mechanism cannot rely on the efference feedback signal alone. Rather, the amount of internal 're-mapping' must also depend on local information content including the depth of the target.

Gaze target coding in the superior colliculus and frontal cortex

Over the last decade or two, there has been a general consensus that the superior colliculus (SC) encodes displacements in gaze, following a fairly orderly topographic map that begins with small displacements coded at the more anterior SC with subsequently larger displacements coded as one progresses toward the posterior SC (Straschill and Rieger, 1973; Guitton et al., 1980; Roucoux et al., 1980; Pare et al., 1994; see also Guitton et al., 2003, this volume). However, in light of the frame dependence of gaze displacements (Fig. 1), it is necessary to ask if these

are displacements in the ocular frame (i.e., retinal error), or displacements with respect to the body (i.e., motor error). Moreover, certain reports of gaze shifts evoked by stimulation of the posterior SC seemed to suggest that at least that portion of the structure might encode desired gaze directions (not displacement) relative to the body (Roucoux et al., 1980; Pare et al., 1994).

We tested between these options by stimulating different points of the SC in head-free monkeys and observing the position-dependencies in the evoked gaze shifts (Klier et al., 2001). Depending on the site, this produced a variety of different gaze shift sizes and directions, from small saccade-like movements, to very large gaze shifts involving both the eye and head (Fig. 4A–C). According to one model, this should have produced fixed-vector, position-independent gaze shifts, whereas at the opposite extreme one might predict movements that always converge to a common position for each site. An alternative explanation, according to the geometry illustrated in Fig. 1, holds that if the SC simply codes target direction relative to the eye (i.e., a retinal model), then this would tend to map onto relatively fixed-vector movements for smaller gaze shifts at more anterior sites, but progressively more convergent movements as one progresses more posteriorly, evoking larger movements (Klier et al., 2001).

Fig. 4D shows the results, plotting the level of position-depend convergence for gaze shifts evoked at each site as a function of the characteristic size of the gaze shifts evoked from that site. For reference the predictions of the three models are also shown. Clearly, the data followed the predictions of the retinal model. Moreover, this model explains why the anterior SC code seems to be more fixed-vector and the posterior SC more goal-directed. This pattern simply falls out of the geometry of projecting the eye-centered retinal code onto the required gaze shift from different initial gaze positions. Of course, if the SC is coding a simple target-in-retina signal, then this implies that something downstream must be implementing the position-dependencies required to map this signal onto the different gaze trajectories observed in our data, in other words, to implement the reference frame transformations required to activate eye and neck muscles which clearly are not organized in eye-fixed coordinates. This presumably

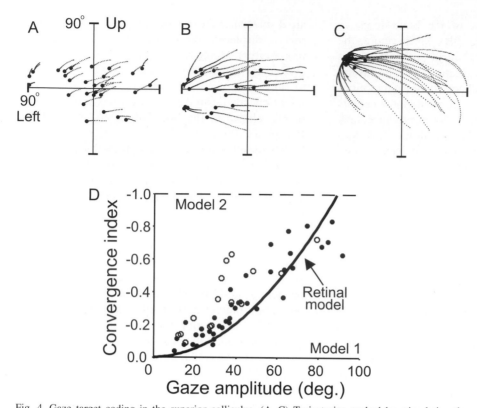

Fig. 4. Gaze target coding in the superior colliculus. (A–C) Trajectories evoked by stimulating three SC sites. Gaze plots are shown for a relatively anterior site (∼30° gaze shifts) (A), an intermediate site (∼60° gaze shifts) (B), and an extremely posterior site (∼90° gaze shifts) (C). Data are plotted in space coordinates and the final end-points of each movement are shown (dots). (D) A convergence index determines the most suitable model of SC coding. Gaze convergence indices from two monkeys (circle, dot) are plotted against the characteristic gaze amplitude for each stimulation site. One model (Model 1) predicts a fixed convergence index of 0 (slope along the abscissa) indicating fixed-vector, position-independent gaze shifts. Another model (Model 2) predicts a fixed convergence index of −1 (dashed line) indicating goal-directed, position-dependent gaze shifts. The retinal model requires that convergence indices be small for small gaze amplitudes, but then increase non-linearly for larger gaze amplitudes (continuous line). The data favor the retinal model and follow its predictions very closely. (Adapted from Klier et al., 2001.)

frees the job of the SC to deal with earlier aspects of gaze coding such as target selection and timing of the movement, within a relatively simple spatial frame. Consistent with this, the SC shows evidence of the eye-centered remapping across eye movements described in the previous section (Walker et al., 1995).

But what of the other, higher-level gaze-coding structures in the cortex? Recently, we have performed a similar series of experiments involving stimulation of the supplementary eye fields (SEF) of the frontal cortex. Again, this is a structure for which there is considerable controversy about whether it codes fixed-vector movements or goal-directed gaze shifts (or even more complex object-centered codes)

(Russo and Bruce, 1993; Tehovnik et al., 1998; Olson and Gettner, 1999). Our hypothesis was that, if a wide enough range of head-free gaze shifts could be evoked, they might be shown to follow the predictions of the retinal model. However, the results have not been as straightforward as those for the SC (Martinez-Trujillo et al., 2002). With the head free to move, stimulation of the SEF did produce gaze shifts with considerable head movement from many sites. And this did substantially change the apparent coding in these structures as compared to head-fixed controls. However, when the data were plotted as in Fig. 4D, we found sites that fit into the predictions of all three models. Thus, the SEF may be a center for integrating and providing signals for gaze shifts in a variety of different frames, but like with the SC, it very likely does not concern itself with computing the detailed kinematics of the gaze shift.

Role of the superior colliculus in 3-D eye–head coordination

As mentioned in the previous section, stimulation of the SC produces gaze shifts involving movement of both the eyes and the head. But does this mean that the SC codes separate, parallel commands for the eyes and head, or that the SC simply codes a shift in gaze, with coordination of the eye and head organized downstream? The weight of opinion and evidence from microstimulation and single-unit recording studies currently falls toward the latter option (Munoz and Guitton, 1991; Freedman et al., 1996; Freedman and Sparks, 1997; Klier et al., 2001). Consistent with this, we have recently trained monkeys to alter their patterns of eye–head coordination in a context-dependent fashion, and have found that at least some of this context-dependent behavior is retained when the SC is stimulated, as if some state-dependent coordination variable were retained downstream from the SC (Constantin et al., 2001).

So then, what happens downstream from the SC? We have already mentioned that a reference frame transformation must occur downstream, but in the current context, it is also important to consider the role of the SC in the 3-D aspects of eye–head coordination. As described in an earlier section, both the eye and head obey Donders' law, at least during fixations, and this involves a precise coordinating mechanism between torsion produced during the saccade and VOR stages of the eye-in-head movement. If the SC encodes an early 'gaze relative to eye' signal, then one would expect these neural constraints and coordination mechanisms to also be implemented downstream from the SC. In other words, one would expect that stimulation of the would produce fully formed gaze shifts (in the 3-D sense), including movements that obey Donders' law and show anticipatory torsion in the saccades. This indeed is what we found (Crawford et al., 2000), as shown in Fig. 5. Most interestingly, stimulation of one site in the SC could produce saccades with zero torsion with the head fixed, or with various amounts of torsion that correctly anticipated the oncoming VOR phase when the head was free. Since the VOR can only be predicted by knowing the intended head movement, this again suggests that a very sophisticated mechanism for coordinating the eye to-the-head is located in the neural transformations downstream from the SC.

Intrinsic coordinate systems for oculomotor control

To better understand the signal output by the SC, it is necessary to know how these signals must finally be 'read' by the downstream motor control centers for the eye (and head). In the case of the eye, it is well documented that the motor command for saccades takes the form of a velocity-like signal, whose horizontal components are largely organized in the paramedian pontine reticular formation (PPRF) (Luschei and Fuchs, 1972; Hepp and Henn, 1983), and whose vertical and torsional signals are organized in the midbrain rostral interstitial nucleus of the medial longitudinal fasciculus (riMLF) (King and Fuchs, 1979; Buttner-Ennever et al., 1982; Henn et al., 1989). It is also accepted that these velocity-like commands are then neurally integrated (in the mathematical sense) to produce the tonic signal that holds the eye in place at the end of the movement. Again, there is an anatomic division between the horizontal and vertical/torsional components, with the former organized in the region of the medial vestibular nucleus (MVN) (Cannon and Robinson, 1987; Cheron and Godaux, 1987), and the latter organized in the midbrain interstitial nucleus of Cajal (INC) (Crawford et al., 1991; Fukushima, 1991).

Interestingly, the arrangement of these signals suggests a coordinate system very similar to that observed in the vestibular canals and the extra-ocular muscles. Specifically, the PPRF/MVN corresponding to the horizontal canals/recti, and the riMLF/INC possessing neurons with tuning resembling the directions controlled by the vertical canals/muscles (Fukushima et al., 1987). In particular, the midbrain seems to separate neurons into populations encoding up/clockwise or down/clockwise directions on the right side (subjects point of view) and up/counterclockwise or down/counterclockwise directions on the left side (Crawford et al., 1991).

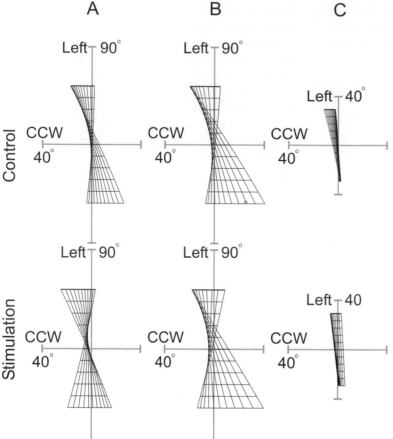

Fig. 5. 3-D eye–head coordination is implemented downstream from the SC. Best-fit surfaces for the eye-in-space (A), head-in-space (B) and eye-in-head (C) from control (top row) and SC stimulation-induced (bottom row) trials. The six variables describing 2nd order best-fit surfaces to the endpoints of control (top row) and SC stimulation-induced (bottom row) data were averaged across all random files (control data) and all sites tested (SC stimulation data). The six averaged variables produced 2nd order surfaces which are shown from a side view (torsion along the abscissa). Statistical analysis showed that the corresponding surfaces were not significantly different from one another.

This has given rise to speculation about whether these apparent intrinsic neural coordinates correspond best to those of the canals or muscles (Robinson and Zee, 1981; Robinson, 1985; Simpson and Graf, 1985; Crawford et al., 1991; Crawford and Vilis, 1992).

However, a third possibility is that, although their organization may be influenced by and optimized in similar ways to both of these, they may in fact align best with something else, i.e., Listing's plane (Crawford and Vilis, 1992; Crawford, 1994). If the oculomotor system used a canal/muscle-like coordinate system that aligned with Listing's plane,

then this would provide the advantage that symmetric bilateral activation would cancel out torsion in Listing's coordinates, specifying movements and positions in Listing's plane. Conversely, torsional movements away from Listing's plane would then require an activation pattern that was asymmetric across the two sides of the brain, either preferentially activating more 'clockwise' neurons on the right side or 'counterclockwise' neurons on the left. Observation of the eye rotations produced by stimulating the riMLF and INC, and the patterns of eye rotation or eye position holding retained after reversibly inactivating these structures are consistent with this

scheme, suggesting that these structures code head-
-fixed coordinate axes aligned with and symmetric
about Listing's plane (Crawford and Vilis, 1992;
Crawford, 1994).

Intrinsic coordinates for head control

Compared to the oculomotor system, less is known
about the brainstem circuits for control of head
movement, and how they are driven by higher-level
circuits in the SC and cortex. Structures implicated in head control include the vestibular nuclei
(Banovetz et al., 1995; Roy and Cullen, 2001),
the PPRF (Robinson et al., 1994; Sparks et al.,
2001), inhibitory oculomotor burst neurons (Cullen
and Guitton, 1997), the central mesencephalic reticular formation (cMRF) (Waitzman, 2001), and the
INC (Fukushima et al., 1987). Although evidence is
sketchy, it seems that the circuits for head movement
control might be organized along similar lines as
those for oculomotor control, perhaps even sharing
common neural signals (Grantyn and Berthoz, 1987;
Guitton, 1992). In particular, it could be that the horizontal and vertical components of the head control
signals are similarly partitioned between the pons
and midbrain, and that velocity signals derived from
gaze commands might be integrated to represent and
control final head posture.

To test the latter idea, we recently explored the
INC in the head-free monkey, with the use of microstimulation and injection of muscimol, a GABA$_A$
agonist which reversibly suppresses the activity in
local populations of cell bodies. In these experiments
(Klier et al., 2002), we confirmed that stimulation of
the right/left produced clockwise/counterclockwise
head rotations (from the subject's perspective) (Hassler and Hess, 1954), much like the oculomotor
results (Crawford et al., 1991). These head rotations
also showed signs of holding their final position
(until corrected), as if the signal had been neurally
integrated. Moreover, injection of muscimol into the
same sites produced a pattern of head drift consistent with the idea that the INC was the neural
integrator for torsional and vertical head postures.
Complimenting the stimulation data, this drift finally
settled with the head deviated in torsionally orientations (Fig. 6), i.e., clockwise for left injections and
counterclockwise for right injections. (Note, this is

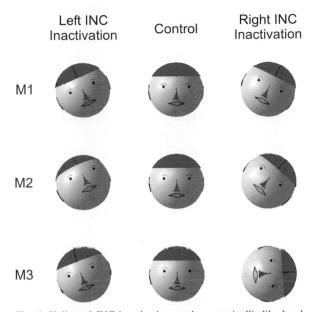

Fig. 6. Unilateral INC inactivation produces torticollis-like head
postures. In controls (center column) the head is upright and
points directly straight ahead (i.e., torsion component = vertical component = horizontal component = 0). After left INC
inactivation (left column) the head assumes unnatural CW head
orientations, whereas after right INC inactivation (right column)
the head assumes unnatural CCW head orientations. Data are
shown from three monkeys (M1, M2 and M3). (Adapted from
Klier et al., 2002.)

opposite to the directions elicited by stimulating the
same sites.) These findings suggest that the INC is
also a neural integrator for torsional/vertical head
posture, and further implicate it in the etiology of
torticollis (Sano et al., 1972), a clinical disorder that
results in head postures similar to those observed in
Fig. 6.

These data clearly implicate the INC in the 3-D
aspects of head control, but to understand this as a
control system, more detailed questions arise. For
example, supposing the basic scheme mentioned in
the preceding paragraphs is right, is there a specific
coordinate system that best describes the organization of vertical, torsional, and horizontal head control
signals in the brainstem? To follow the oculomotor
example, our head movement results suggest a coordinate system consistent with a canal-like coordinate
system (Klier et al., 1999). But whereas in the oculomotor system it made sense to align that coordinate
system with Listing's plane, here it would make

sense to align the coordinates more with the Fick strategy observed in natural behavior (i.e., so that the amount of torsion in or out of the Fick-like Donders' constraint could be determined through the bilateral balance of activity across the brainstem).

Consistent with this, our analysis suggests that head rotations elicited by stimulation of the INC often occur about axes aligning with the vertical canal sensitivity axes, and which remained head-fixed at different head positions (Klier et al., 1999), much like those of a Fick coordinate system. To complete this story, it would be necessary to explore the brainstem sites involved in the control of horizontal head rotation, and see if they employ a body-fixed vertical axis like that observed in the behavioral Fick constraint.

Where are the transformations?

The picture that emerges from the previous sections is that a fairly simple 2-D eye-centered gaze control signal emerges from the SC, which must then be used to drive 3-D brainstem control signals in coordinate systems appropriate for control of the eye and head. This leaves a considerable amount of complexity to the intervening transformations, including solutions to the problems of eye–head coordination, the degrees of freedom problems for both the eyes and head, and the reference frame transformations described in the previous section. We know remarkably little about how these transformations are performed. Although we can speculate that a number of brainstem areas are involved (i.e., NRTP, cMRF, LLBN, cerebellum, etc.), this seems to leave a lot of the job to occur across a very few serial synaptic connections.

So how could the brainstem handle this complexity, in effect asking it to do much of the job reserved for the parietal–premotor–motor cortex arc in arm movement control? One answer — demonstrated most neatly by neural network simulations — is that a large number of neurons arranged in parallel with even a modest inherent non-linearity (like thresholds and saturations) can perform quite complex operations across only a few synapses (Van Opstal and Van Gisbergen, 1989). For example, we have recently trained a three-layer neural network to transform retinotopically coded visual signals and

eye orientation signals into the correct motor error commands for accurate saccades in Listing's plane, with the latter coded in the canal-like Listing's coordinates described above (Smith and Crawford, 2001b). The network learns the transformation with only a handful of hidden units, employing a solution similar to the classic 'gain field' story (Fig. 7) (also see Krommenhoek et al., 1993; Van Opstal et al., 1995). When one considers that the real network has millions of neurons, a considerably greater diversity of computational power at the synaptic level, and re-entrant pathways through the cerebellum and other side loops, the power and complexity of this transformation is perhaps not so surprising. But it also hints that the working out the details of these transformations, as opposed to just identifying the major milestones like we have so far, will not be a straightforward task.

Conclusions and future directions

In our view, the neural control systems for 3-D gaze are organized along principles much like those proposed by founding fathers of neurophysiology like Sherrington and Bernstein. In particular, the coding of potential or desired gaze targets at the level of topographic or pseudo-topographic maps in the SC and cortex is only made possible by considerable complexity in the forward serial transformations and parallel modules of the downstream brainstem motor control mechanisms. A certain level of similarity between the brainstem oculomotor and head control mechanisms may help us to understand these transformations, and how the eye and head work together as one system to produce gaze shifts. Conversely, if detailed kinematics information is necessary for the spatial updating of the higher-level representations — as our work suggests — then a similar level of complexity is required in the reverse bottom-up transformations, which in turn must interact with local cortical representations to produce a dynamic, 3-D representation of visual space. Our future work will focus on these forward and reverse transformations, as well as continuing to understand the basic control signals for 3-D eye–head coordination and head control.

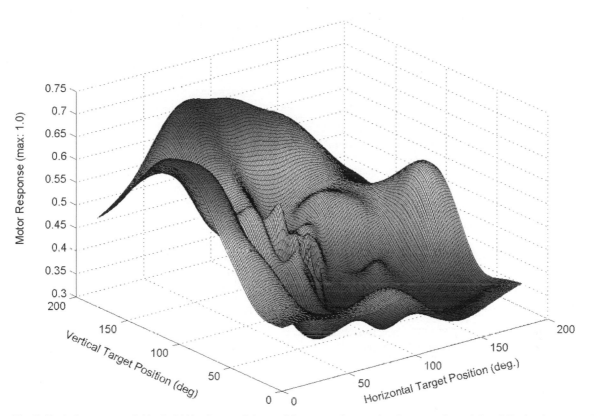

Fig. 7. Typical movement field of a hidden layer unit in our 3-layer neural networks. Our networks took in a 2-D visual target and a 3-D eye orientation and produced the correct motor output which would generate a saccade to the selected visual target. As in physiological studies, we are able to map the visual (input) and movement (output) fields of each of the hidden layer units. The movement fields were generated by stimulating all possible 2-D visual target locations and recording the output of each hidden layer unit. The floor of the graph (X and Y axes) indicate the horizontal and vertical components of possible 2-D target locations while the height of the graph (Z axis) represents the magnitude of response throughout the movement field. Although complex, these movement fields exhibited preferred (highest regions) and anti-preferred (lowest regions) areas of activity. In order to account for the eye-position-dependent modification of motor error, the neural networks used a bias mechanism whereby the entire movement field was shifted upward when eye position was in the preferred direction of the unit.

References

Angelaki, D.E., McHenry, M.Q. and Hess, B.J. (2000) Primate translational vestibuloocular reflexes. I. High-frequency dynamics and three-dimensional properties during lateral motion. *J. Neurophysiol.*, 83: 1637–1647.

Banovetz, J.M., Peterson, B.W. and Baker, J.F. (1995) Spatial coordination by descending vestibular signals. 1. Reflex excitation of neck muscles in alert and decerebrate cats. *Exp. Brain Res.*, 105: 345–362.

Batista, A.P. and Andersen, R.A. (2001) The parietal reach region codes the next planned movement in a sequential reach task. *J. Neurophysiol.*, 85: 539–544.

Becker, W. and Jurgens, R. (1979) An analysis of the saccadic system by means of double-step stimuli. *Vis. Res.*, 19: 967–983.

Bernstein, N. (1967) *The Co-ordination and Regulation of Movements.* Pergamon Press, Oxford.

Buttner-Ennever, J.A., Buttner, U., Cohen, B. and Baumgartner, G. (1982) Vertical gaze paralysis and the rostral interstitial nucleus of the medial longitudinal fasciculus. *Brain*, 105: 125–149.

Cannon, S.C. and Robinson, D.A. (1987) Loss of the neural integrator of the oculomotor system from brain stem lesions in monkey. *J. Neurophysiol.*, 57: 1383–1409.

Ceylan, M., Henriques, D.Y.P., Tweed, D.B. and Crawford, J.D. (2000) Task-dependent constraints in motor control: pinhole goggles make the head move like an eye. *J. Neurosci.*, 20: 2719–2730.

Cheron, G. and Godaux, E. (1987) Disabling of the oculomotor neural integrator by kainic acid injections in the prepositus–vestibular complex of the cat. *J. Physiol.*, 394: 267–290.

Colby, C.L. and Goldberg, M.E. (1999) Space and attention in parietal cortex. *Annu. Rev. Neurosci.*, 22: 319–349.

Constantin, A.G., Wang, H., Klier, E.M. and Crawford, J.D. (2001) Role of the superior colliculus (SC) in adaptive eye–head coordination. *Soc. Neurosci. Abstr.*, 27: 405.8.

Crawford, J.D. (1994) The oculomotor neural integrator uses a behavior-related coordinate system. *J. Neurosci.*, 14: 6911–6923.

Crawford, J.D. and Guitton, D. (1997) Visual–motor transformations required for accurate and kinematically correct saccades. *J. Neurophysiol.*, 78: 1447–1467.

Crawford, J.D. and Vilis, T. (1991) Axes of eye rotation and Listing's law during rotations of the head. *J. Neurophysiol.*, 65: 407–423.

Crawford, J.D. and Vilis, T. (1992) Symmetry of oculomotor burst neuron coordinates about Listing's plane. *J. Neurophysiol.*, 68: 432–448.

Crawford, J.D. and Vilis, T. (1995) How does the brain deal with the problems of rotational movement? *J. Motor Behav.*, 27: 89–99.

Crawford, J.D., Cadera, V. and Vilis, T. (1991) Generation of torsional and vertical eye position signals by the interstitial nucleus of Cajal. *Science*, 252: 1551–1553.

Crawford, J.D., Ceylan, M.Z., Klier, E.M. and Guitton, D. (1999) Three-dimensional eye–head coordination during gaze saccades in the primate. *J. Neurophysiol.*, 81: 1760–1782.

Crawford, J.D., Klier, E.M. and Wang, H. (2000) Listing's and Donders' law of the eye and head are coordinated downstream of the superior colliculus. *Soc. Neurosci. Abstr.*, 26: 292.

Cullen, K.E. and Guitton, D. (1997) Analysis of primate IBN spike trains using system identification techniques. II. Relationship to gaze, eye, and head movement dynamics during head-free gaze shifts. *J. Neurophysiol.*, 78: 3283–3306.

Donders, F.C. (1848) Beitrag zur Lehre von den Bewegungen des menschlichen Auges. *Hollandische Beitrage zu den anatomischen und physiologischen Wissenschaften*, 1: 105–145.

Duhamel, J.-R., Colby, C.L. and Goldberg, M.E. (1992) The updating of the representation of visual space in parietal cortex by intended eye movements. *Science*, 255: 90–92.

Freedman, E.G. and Sparks, D.L. (1997) Activity of cells in the deeper layers of the superior colliculus of the rhesus monkey: evidence for a gaze displacement command. *J. Neurophysiol.*, 78: 1669–1690.

Freedman, E.G., Stanford, T.R. and Sparks, D.L. (1996) Combined eye–head gaze shifts produced by electrical stimulation of the superior colliculus in rhesus monkeys. *J. Neurophysiol.*, 76: 927–952.

Fukushima, K. (1991) The interstitial nucleus of Cajal in the midbrain reticular formation and vertical eye movements. *Neurosci. Res.*, 10: 159–187.

Fukushima, K., Fukushima, J. and Terashima, T. (1987) The pathways responsible for the characteristic head posture produced by lesions of the interstitial nucleus of Cajal in the cat. *Exp. Brain Res.*, 68: 88–102.

Fuller, J.H. (1996) Eye position and target amplitude effects on human visual saccadic latencies. *Exp. Brain Res.*, 109: 457–466.

Glenn, B. and Vilis, T. (1992) Violations of Listing's law after large eye and head gaze shifts. *J. Neurophysiol.*, 68: 309–318.

Goldberg, M.E. and Bruce, C.J. (1990) Primate frontal eye fields. III. Maintenance of a spatially accurate saccade signal. *J. Neurophysiol.*, 64: 489–508.

Grantyn, A. and Berthoz, A. (1987) Reticulo-spinal neurons participating in the control of synergic eye and head movements during orienting in the cat. I. Behavioral properties. *Exp. Brain Res.*, 66: 339–354.

Guitton, D. (1992) Control of eye–head coordination during orienting gaze shifts. *Trends Neurosci.*, 15: 174–179.

Guitton, D. and Volle, M. (1987) Gaze control in humans: eye–head coordination during orienting movements to targets within and beyond the oculomotor range. *J. Neurophysiol.*, 58: 427–459.

Guitton, D., Crommelinck, M. and Roucoux, A. (1980) Stimulation of the superior colliculus in the alert cat. I. Eye movements and neck EMG activity evoked when the head is restrained. *Exp. Brain Res.*, 39: 63–73.

Guitton, D., Bergeron, A., Choi, W.Y. and Matsuo, S. (2003) On the feedback control of orienting gaze shifts made with eye and head movements. In: C. Prablanc, D. Pélisson and Y. Rossetti (Eds.), *Neural Control of Space Coding and Action Production. Progress in Brain Research*, Vol. 142. Elsevier, Amsterdam, pp. 55–68 (this volume).

Hallett, P.E. and Lightstone, A.D. (1976) Saccadic eye movements towards stimuli triggered by prior saccades. *Vis. Res.*, 16: 99–106.

Hassler, R. and Hess, W.R. (1954) Experimentelle und anatomische Befunde über die Drehbewegungen und ihre nervosen Apparate. *Arch. Psychiatr. Nervenkr.*, 192: 488–526.

Helmholtz, H. (1867) *Handbuch der Physiologischen Optik*. Leopold Voss, Leizpig. [English translation: Treatise on Physiological Optics. Translated by J.P.C. Southall, Opt. Soc. Am., Rochester, NY, 1925, vol. 3, pp. 44–51.]

Henn, V., Hepp, K. and Vilis, T. (1989) Rapid eye movement generation in the primate. Physiology, pathophysiology, and clinical implications. *Rev. Neurol. (Paris)*, 145: 540–545.

Henriques, D.Y.P., Klier, E.M., Smith, M.A., Lowy, D. and Crawford, J.D. (1998) Gaze-centered remapping of remembered visual space in an open-loop pointing task. *J. Neurosci.*, 18: 1583–1594.

Hepp, K. (1990) On Listing's law. *Commun. Math. Phys.*, 132: 285–292.

Hepp, K. (1994) Oculomotor control: Listing's law and all that. *Curr. Opin. Neurobiol.*, 4: 862–868.

Hepp, K. and Henn, V. (1983) Spatio-temporal recoding of rapid eye movement signals in the monkey paramedian pontine reticular formation (PPRF). *Exp. Brain Res.*, 52: 105–120.

Hepp, K., Van Opstal, A.J., Straumann, D., Hess, B.J. and Henn, V. (1993) Monkey superior colliculus represents rapid eye movements in a two-dimensional motor map. *J. Neurophysiol.*, 69: 965–979.

Herter, T.M. and Guitton, D. (1998) Human head-free gaze saccades to targets flashed before gaze-pursuit are spatially accurate. *J. Neurophysiol.*, 80: 2785–2789.

Howard, I.P. and Rogers, B.J. (1995) *Binocular Vision and Stereopsis*. Oxford University Press, New York.

King, W.M. and Fuchs, A.F. (1979) Reticular control of vertical saccadic eye movements by mesencephalic burst neurons. *J. Neurophysiol.*, 42: 861–876.

Klier, E.M. and Crawford, J.D. (1998) Human oculomotor system accounts for 3-D eye orientation in the visual–motor transformation for saccades. *J. Neurophysiol.*, 80: 2274–2294.

Klier, E.M., Wang, H. and Crawford, J.D. (1999) Stimulation of the interstitial nucleus of Cajal (INC) produces torsional and vertical head rotations in Fick coordinates. *Soc. Neurosci. Abstr.*, 25: 1650.

Klier, E.M., Wang, H. and Crawford, J.D. (2001) The superior colliculus encodes gaze commands in retinal coordinates. *Nat. Neurosci.*, 4: 627–632.

Klier, E.M., Wang, H., Constantin, A.G. and Crawford, J.D. (2002) Midbrain control of three-dimensional head orientation. *Science*, 295: 1314–1316.

Krommenhoek, K.P., Van Opstal, A.J., Gielen, C.C. and Van Gisbergen, J.A. (1993) Remapping of neural activity in the motor colliculus: a neural network study. *Vis. Res.*, 33: 1287–1298.

Luschei, E.S. and Fuchs, A.F. (1972) Activity of brainstem neurons during eye movements of alert monkeys. *J. Neurophysiol.*, 35: 445–461.

Martinez-Trujillo, J.C., Klier, E.M., Wang, H. and Crawford, J.D. (2002) The contribution of head movements to visuospatial coding in frontal cortex and superior colliculus of the macaque monkey. *Neural Control of Movement Abstr.*, A-02.

Medendorp, W.P. and Crawford, J.D. (2002) Visuospatial coding of reaching targets in near and far space. *NeuroReport*, 13: 633–636.

Medendorp, W.P., Melis, B.J., Gielen, C.C. and Van Gisbergen, J.A. (1998) Off-centric rotation axes in natural head movements: implications for vestibular reafference and kinematic redundancy. *J. Neurophysiol.*, 79: 2025–2039.

Medendorp, W.P., Smith, M.A., Tweed, D.B. and Crawford, J.D. (2001) Representation and remapping of 3-D visual space during head-free gaze shifts. *Soc. Neurosci. Abstr.*, 27: 237.3.

Medendorp, W.P., Smith, M.A., Tweed, D.B. and Crawford, J.D. (2002) Rotational remapping in human spatial memory during eye and head motion. *J. Neurosci.*, 22: RC196.

Misslisch, H. and Hess, B.J. (2000) Three-dimensional vestibuloocular reflex of the monkey: optimal retinal image stabilization versus Listing's law. *J. Neurophysiol.*, 83: 3264–3276.

Morasso, P., Bizzi, E. and Dichgans, J. (1973) Adjustment of saccade characteristics during head movements. *Exp. Brain Res.*, 19: 492–500.

Munoz, D.P. and Guitton, D. (1991) Control of orienting gaze shifts by the tectoreticulospinal system in the head-free cat. II. Sustained discharges during motor preparation and fixation. *J. Neurophysiol.*, 66: 1624–1641.

Nakayama, K. (1975) Coordination of extraocular muscles. In: P. Bach-y-Rita and G. Lennerstrand (Eds.), *Basic Mechanisms of Ocular Motility and their Clinical Implications*. Pergamon, Oxford, pp. 193–207.

Olson, C.R. and Gettner, S.N. (1999) Macaque SEF neurons encode object-centered directions of eye movements regardless of the visual attributes of instructional cues. *J. Neurophysiol.*, 81: 2340–2346.

Pare, M., Crommelinck, M. and Guitton, D. (1994) Gaze shifts evoked by stimulation of the superior colliculus in the head-free cat conform to the motor map but also depend on stimulus strength and fixation activity. *Exp. Brain Res.*, 101: 123–139.

Quaia, C. and Optican, L.M. (1998) Commutative saccadic generator is sufficient to control a 3-D ocular plant with pulleys. *J. Neurophysiol.*, 79: 3197–3215.

Quaia, C., Optican, L.M. and Goldberg, M.E. (1998) The maintenance of spatial accuracy by perisaccadic remapping of visual receptive fields. *Neural Networks*, 11: 1229–1240.

Radau, P., Tweed, D. and Vilis, T. (1994) Three-dimensional eye, head and chest orientations following large gaze shifts and the underlying neural strategies. *J. Neurophysiol.*, 72: 2840–2852.

Robinson, D.A. (1985) The coordinates of neurons in the vestibulo-ocular reflex. In: A. Berthoz and G. Melvill Jones (Eds.), *Adaptive Mechanisms in Gaze Control. Facts and Theories*. Elsevier, Amsterdam, pp. 297–311.

Robinson, D.A. (1992) Implications of neural networks for how we think about brain function. *Behav. Brain Sci.*, 15: 644–655.

Robinson, D.A. and Zee, D.S. (1981) Theoretical considerations of the function and circuitry of various rapid eye movements. In: A. Fuchs and W. Becker (Eds.), *Progress in Oculomotor Research*. Elsevier/North Holland, New York, pp. 3–9.

Robinson, F.R., Phillips, J.O. and Fuchs, A.F. (1994) Coordination of gaze shifts in primates: brainstem inputs to neck and extraocular motoneuron pools. *J. Comp. Neurol.*, 346: 43–62.

Roucoux, A., Guitton, D. and Crommelinck, M. (1980) Stimulation of the superior colliculus in the alert cat. II. Eye and head movements evoked when the head is unrestrained. *Exp. Brain Res.*, 39: 75–85.

Roy, J.E. and Cullen, K.E. (2001) Selective processing of vestibular reafference during self-generated head motion. *J. Neurosci.*, 21: 2131–2142.

Russo, G.S. and Bruce, C.J. (1993) Supplementary eye field: representation of saccades and relationship between neural response fields and elicited eye movements. *J. Neurophysiol.*, 69: 800–818.

Sano, K., Sekino, H., Tsukamoto, Y., Yoshimasu, M. and Ishijima, B. (1972) Stimulation and destruction of the region of the interstitial nucleus in cases of torticollis and see-saw nystagmus. *Confin. Neurol.*, 34: 331–338.

Schnabolk, C. and Raphan, T. (1994) Modeling three-dimensional velocity-to-position transformation in oculomotor control. *J. Neurophysiol.*, 71: 623–638.

Seidman, S.H. and Leigh, R.J. (1989) The human torsional vestibulo-ocular reflex during rotation about an earth-vertical axis. *Brain Res.*, 504: 264–268.

Simpson, J.I. and Graf, W. (1981) Eye–muscle geometry and compensatory eye movements in lateral-eyed and frontal-eyed animals. *Ann. N.Y. Acad. Sci.*, 374: 20–30.

Simpson, J.I. and Graf, W. (1985) The selection of reference frames by nature and its investigators. In: A. Berthoz and G. Melvill Jones (Eds.), *Adaptive Mechanisms in Gaze Control. Facts and Theories*. Elsevier, Amsterdam, pp. 297–311.

124

Smith, M.A. and Crawford, J.D. (2001a) Implications of ocular kinematics for the internal updating of visual space. *J. Neurophysiol.*, 86: 2112–2117.

Smith, M.A. and Crawford, J.D. (2001b) Network properties in a physiologically realistic model of the 2D to 3D visuomotor transformation for saccades. *Soc. Neurosci. Abstr.*, 27: 71.38.

Soechting, J.F. and Flanders, M. (1992) Moving in three-dimensional space: frames of reference, vectors and coordinate systems. *Annu. Rev. Neurosci.*, 15: 167–191.

Sparks, D.L., Freedman, E.G., Chen, L.L. and Gandhi, N.J. (2001) Cortical and subcortical contributions to coordinated eye and head movements. *Vis. Res.*, 41: 3295–3305.

Sperry, R.W. (1943) Visuomotor coordination in the newt (*Triturus viridescens*) after regeneration of the optic nerve. *J. Comp. Neurol.*, 79: 33–55.

Straschill, M. and Rieger, P. (1973) Eye movements evoked by focal stimulation of the cat's superior colliculus. *Brain Res.*, 59: 211–227.

Straumann, D., Haslwanter, T., Hepp-Reymond, M.C. and Hepp, K. (1991) Listing's law for eye, head and arm movements and their synergistic control. *Exp. Brain Res.*, 86: 209–215.

Suzuki, Y., Straumann, D., Simpson, J.I., Hepp, K., Hess, B.J. and Henn, V. (1999) Three-dimensional extraocular motoneuron innervation in the rhesus monkey. I: Muscle rotation axes and on-directions during fixation. *Exp. Brain Res.*, 126: 187–199.

Tehovnik, E.J., Slocum, W.M., Tolias, A.S. and Schiller, P.H. (1998) Saccades induced electrically from the dorsomedial frontal cortex: evidence for a head-centered representation. *Brain Res.*, 795: 287–291.

Tweed, D. (1997) Visual–motor optimization in binocular control. *Vis. Res.*, 37: 1939–1951.

Tweed, D. and Vilis, T. (1987) Implications of rotational kinematics for the oculomotor system in three dimensions. *J. Neurophysiol.*, 58: 832–849.

Tweed, D. and Vilis, T. (1990) Geometric relations of eye position and velocity vectors during saccades. *Vis. Res.*, 30: 111–127.

Tweed, D.B., Haslwanter, T. and Fetter, M. (1998) Optimizing gaze control in three dimensions. *Science*, 281: 1363–1366.

Tweed, D.B., Haslwanter, T.P., Happe, V. and Fetter, M. (1999) Non-commutativity in the brain. *Nature*, 399: 261–263.

Van Opstal, A.J. and Van Gisbergen, J.A. (1989) A nonlinear model for collicular spatial interactions underlying the metrical properties of electrically elicited saccades. *Biol. Cybern.*, 60: 171–183.

Van Opstal, A.J., Hepp, K., Hess, B.J., Straumann, D. and Henn, V. (1991) Two- rather than three-dimensional representation of saccades in monkey superior colliculus. *Science*, 252: 1313–1315.

Van Opstal, A.J., Hepp, K., Suzuki, Y. and Henn, V. (1995) Influence of eye position on activity in monkey superior colliculus. *J. Neurophysiol.*, 74: 1593–1610.

Waitzman, D. (2001) Signals related to movements of the head and eyes in the mesencephalic reticular formation (MRF) of primates. *Soc. Neurosci. Abstr.*, 27: 405.14.

Walker, M.F., Fitzgibbon, J. and Goldberg, M.E. (1995) Neurons of the monkey superior colliculus predict the visual result of impeding saccadic eye movements. *J. Neurophysiol.*, 73: 1998–2003.

Westheimer, G. (1957) Kinematics of the eye. *J. Opt. Soc. Am.*, 47: 967–974.

Motor Programming and Control

C. Prablanc, D. Pélisson and Y. Rossetti (Eds.)
Progress in Brain Research, Vol. 142
© 2003 Elsevier Science B.V. All rights reserved

CHAPTER 8

From 'acting on' to 'acting with': the functional anatomy of object-oriented action schemata

Scott H. Johnson and Scott T. Grafton [*]

Center for Cognitive Neuroscience, and the Department of Psychological and Brain Sciences, Dartmouth College, Hanover, NH 03755, USA

Abstract: In this chapter it is proposed that object-based actions can be broadly classified into types. In the first, objects are 'acted on' without a specific purpose. In the second, objects are 'acted with'. In the latter case the grasp reflects the subsequent goal of the subject. Recent evidence from human functional imaging suggests different neural substrates for acting on an object (dorsal parietal cortex) and for acting with an object. Specifically, it is argued that conceptual knowledge of tool use and the pragmatics of action rely on an inferior parieto-medial frontal network in the left hemisphere.

Introduction

How we acquire, retrieve and execute motor skills are core questions in neuroscience. Although the computational structure of a well-learned skill remains unknown, enormous progress has been made in defining the functional anatomy of brain systems involved in action representation. In parallel, computational and psychophysical studies have provided theoretical models of how actions might be represented. Underlying these theories is the concept of the action schema. First proposed by Head in 1926, and elaborated by Bartlett in 1932, the schema can be thought of as an abstract memory representation, plan or script for action (Head, 1926; Bartlett, 1932). From a computational perspective, the schema is a command set that has a finite number of parameters that can be modified to meet task demands (Arbib, 1981). The idea of parameter setting has proven indispensable to computational models, and associated psychophysical investigations, of specific

motor behaviors (Iberall et al., 1986). The notion of a schema as a rule, concept or generalization is also used to characterize motor learning (Schmidt, 1975), where it has proven useful for understanding skill acquisition in different behavioral contexts.

Despite the conceptual utility of this approach, few links between schema theory and the functional neuroanatomy of motor control exist. A noteworthy exception is the characterization of reach-to-grasp (Arbib et al., 1985; Arbib, 1990; Iberall and Arbib 1990). Here, grasp affordances of the target object and the timing of hand preshaping with respect to limb transport have been shown to be critical components of a larger prehension schema that can be characterized by a limited set of parameters (Jeannerod, 1984). As discussed below, links between computational models of reach-to-grasp and underlying neural mechanisms have been established in non-human primates. A major challenge is to extend schemata to more abstract motor actions, where parameters must be adjusted to fit task demands of greater complexity, such as tools usage. In this chapter, we consider the problem of tool use as a logical extension of reaching-to-grasp (Johnson, 2003). Based on recent work in functional neuroimaging, we propose that hand–object interactions can be understood in terms of two broad classes of schemata that involve disso-

---

[*] Correspondence to: Scott T. Grafton, HB 6162, Moore Hall, Dartmouth College, Hanover, NH 03755, USA. Tel.: +1-603-646-0038; Fax: +1-603-646-1181; E-mail: Scott.T.Grafton@Dartmouth.edu

ciable parietofrontal systems: (1) *acting on* objects (reaching, grasping and manipulation) is supported by schemata resulting from on-line, sensorimotor transformations; (2) *acting with* objects (tool use) involves separate schemata arising from distributed practice of skilled actions. We can *act on* an object as when moving a scissors from one place to another on our desk. This involves schemata for transforming sensory information concerning the attributes of the scissors into one of a potentially large set of postures appropriate for achieving the goal of a stable grip for transportation. Of critical importance in selecting the appropriate action are the physical properties of the target object. For instance, we typically select grasps that allow the opposing forces of the fingers to cancel through objects' centers of mass (Goodale et al., 1994). Or, we can *act with* an object as when grasping and manipulating a scissors to clip an article from the newspaper. Here too sensorimotor transformations play an indispensable role in controlling the action. However, selection is guided by a schema that consists of parameters for grasping and manipulating the scissors in the precise and over-learned postures necessary to achieve the goal of dexterous clipping. Consequently, for scissors and many other objects, actions generated by application of *acting with* schemata often differ dramatically from those arising from schemes for *acting on*. More precisely, when using objects as tools we often grasp and manipulate them in ways that are not predicted by their physical properties; i.e., with expertise, schemata for acting with come to take precedence over the more stimulus-driven acting on schemata. We argue that these broad behavioral distinctions reflect the operation of two functionally and anatomically dissociable parieto-frontal systems specialized for computing these respective schemata.

On the one hand, sensorimotor transformations involved in acting on objects occur in bilaterally organized parietofrontal circuits that have been extensively mapped in non-human primates and recently extended to humans. On the other hand, a century of neuropsychological studies and recent functional imaging data suggest that acting with tools is supported by a left-lateralized system involving the inferior parietal lobule (IPL) and medial frontal gyrus. Both the human proclivity for tool use and inter-species differences in cortical architecture within

the IPL raise the possibility that this later system may be unique to human beings. We begin with an overview of relevant anatomic pathways defined in the non-human primate and then review recent human functional imaging studies of tool-related actions.

Neuroanatomy of parieto-frontal action circuits

Numerous conventions have been used for parceling parietal and premotor areas in non-human primates, and these are being continuously revised and debated as new data become available (Pandya and Seltzer, 1982; Marconi et al., 2001; Rizzolatti and Luppino, 2001). Posterior parietal cortex (PPC) is separated by the intraparietal sulcus (IPs) into superior (SPL) and inferior parietal (IPL) lobules. In the monkey, SPL consists of several areas that have been defined based on their anatomical and/or functional characteristics including: subdivisions of Brodmann's area (BA) 5 (PE, PEa and PEc) mesial BA 7 (7m), PEci, medial intraparietal (MIP) within the IPs and a portion of the ventral intraparietal (VIP) area located on the rostral bank of the fundus of the IPs. The IPL includes: BA 7a, 7b, PFG (a portion of BA 7), the anterior intraparietal (AIP) and lateral intraparietal (LIP) areas within the IPs, and a portion of the ventral intraparietal (VIP) area located in the caudal bank of the IPs.

Areas within the SPL and IPL are directly and reciprocally interconnected with premotor cortex, and also provide indirect input to dorsal premotor areas vis-a-vis prefrontal cortex. Premotor cortex can be grossly divided into dorsal (PMd) and ventral (PMv) regions, which appear not to be densely interconnected (Kurata, 1991). Further, PMd is subdivided into rostral (F7) and caudal (F2) regions, while PMv consists of F4 and F5. Area F2 is reciprocally interconnected with primary motor area (F1), and is also known to project to the spinal cord directly (He et al., 1993; Wise et al., 1997).

Most of the direct visual input to area PMd in the monkey originates in the SPL (Caminiti et al., 1996); however, area PO (V6a) also provides direct visual input to F7. This is relevant to manual actions because PO is the only known visual area that lacks foveal magnification, and its response properties suggest that it may be important for detecting and localizing objects in ambient vision (Wise et al., 1997; Battaglia-Mayer et al., 2001). Area MIP receives visual input from PO and projects to both F2 and F7. As discussed below, these circuits appear to be specialized for visuomotor transformations for the control of reaching. The portion of area VIP within SPL also projects to F2. It is important to recognize that many areas within the IPL are also connected directly to PMd (Tanne et al., 1995), albeit less densely (Marconi et al., 2001). These areas include VIP, LIP, PFG, 7a and 7b. Somatosensory information concerning limb position is provided to PMd via a circuit interconnecting PEc/PEip-F2 (Matelli et al., 1998). Recent data suggest that cells in PEc are involved in the integration of eye–hand information for coordinated movements (Ferraina et al., 2001). Although not considered part of PM, it is also worth noting that the frontal eye fields (FEF, BA8) receive input from area LIP, a region known to represent coordinate transformations involved in planning and control of eye movements (Andersen et al., 1997).

The rostral portion of the IPL (7b) provides the major source of afferent projections to area PMv (Godschalk et al., 1984a; Kurata, 1991; Luppino et al., 1999). Area PMv contains two functional subdivisions, areas F4 and F5. Area F5 primarily receives input from AIP, and — as detailed below — appears to be concerned with visuomotor transformations involved in grasping. Area F4 is directly interconnected with VIP and — as elaborated below — this circuit may play a role in constructing representations of the limbs and surrounding peripersonal space (Graziano and Gross, 1998). Anterior IPL (7b) projects to PMv, including the caudal bank of the lower branch of the arcuate sulcus (F5). The middle inferior parietal lobule (areas PFG and PG) projects to the ventral part of area 46 and area 8, while the posterior IPL (7a) is connected with 46v, 46d, and BA8, as well as the anterior PMd (F7) (Petrides and Pandya, 1984).

The SPL and IPL also project to distinct regions of prefrontal cortex, which in turn provide indirect parietal input to PMd (Cavada and Goldman-Rakic, 1989). The IPL projects to dorsolateral prefrontal cortex (Cavada and Goldman-Rakic, 1989), while SPL projects to dorsomedial prefrontal cortex (Petrides and Pandya, 1984). These prefrontal

areas then project to dorsal and medial premotor cortex, respectively (Barbas, 1988). Prefrontal inputs to PMd are more concentrated in F2, and appear to provide an indirect route for visual information from both IPL and SPL (Wise et al., 1997). From a behavioral perspective, the important point is that electrophysiological investigations conducted over the past decade have revealed that several of these parietofrontal circuits are specialized for computing specific sensorimotor transformations that support different object-oriented actions.

Parietofrontal circuits for acting on objects

Dorsal pathways in reaching

Reaching and pointing are actions in which the task goal is usually linked to a specific spatial target. Thus, the underlying action representation, or schema, is relatively rigid with respect to the overall goal. As long suggested by psychophysical evidence (Jeannerod, 1981), sensorimotor transformations underlying reaching appear to involve parietofrontal circuits that are dissociable from those involved in computing the relatively more flexible schema necessary for grasping (Jeannerod and Decety, 1995). Reaching toward a target involves transforming a representation of objects' extrinsic spatial properties (i.e., location, orientation), and knowledge of the limb's position into a motor plan. Electrophysiological evidence suggests that the visuomotor transformations for reaching are accomplished within a circuit interconnecting MIP and PMd (Johnson et al., 1993; Caminiti et al., 1996; Johnson and Ferraina, 1996). Cells within area MIP appear to represent the intention to move the arm along a specific trajectory in space. Area PMd also receives direct visual (Caminiti et al., 1996) and higher-level proprioceptive (Lacquaniti et al., 1995) input from the SPL. Neurons in PMd use this input to compute representations of both the location of visual targets and the direction of intended forelimb movements needed to acquire targets, even under conditions of non-standard mappings (Shen and Alexander, 1997). Furthermore, a sub-population of PMd neurons respond to specific combinations of sensory cues specifying target location and which limb to use during a manual pointing task (Hoshi and Tanji, 2000). In other words, single PMd units appear to represent specific schemata for specific reaching actions. From the perspective of schema theory, these are highly specific, stimulus-locked action representations that require a distinct mapping of the limb onto target coordinates.

A number of PET studies have identified extensive activation of PMd, IPs and SPL during reaching, pointing and finger tracking movements (Colebatch et al., 1991; Deiber et al., 1991; Grafton et al., 1992; Kertzman et al., 1997). Recent imaging studies with more refined tasks are beginning to identify putative homologues of monkey areas and in particular, area MIP. Three will be described. In the first, subjects performed pointing movements during PET imaging (Desmurget et al., 2001). During each trial subjects made a lateral saccade from a fixation point to a target LED accompanied by a pointing movement, which — due to inertial differences between the limb versus the eyes — began after the saccade was complete. The task was performed without vision of the hand. Unknown to the subjects, targets were moved during peak saccade velocity, when saccadic suppression made subjects transiently blind. Nevertheless, they made appropriate corrective saccades and early, smooth corrections to reaching movements. After subtracting out corrections related to eye movements, a comparison between reaching scans with error correction versus those with stationary targets revealed activation in the contralateral IPs. As shown in Fig. 1, this site is centered on the medial bank of the IPs, but extends into the lateral bank. The site is a putative homologue of monkey MIP, and appears to be involved in on-line correction of the unfolding reaching schema. This interpretation is supported by results of a separate study using the same task. Here, transcranial magnetic stimulation (TMS) of this same intraparietal area, coincident with hand movement onset, completely blocked on-line error correction without dramatically altering reaches to the original target location (Desmurget, 1999). Because the eyes were already centered on the new target location prior to TMS delivery, lack of reach correction was not due to a failure to detect a shift in target location. Rather, it is attributable to TMS blocking feedback-based revision of an already unfolding motor schema for reaching.

Together, these findings show that this area within the IPs is critical for revising motor schemata in

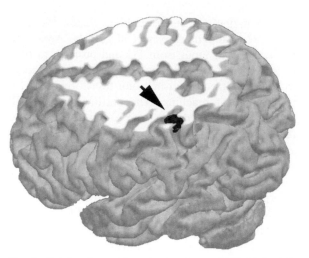

Fig. 1. Putative human homologue of area MIP (defined in non-human primates). The black area (indicated by black arrow) is activated during on-line correction of reaching movements of the contralateral hand (Desmurget et al., 2001). The site is also active during imagined movements when subjects must select the correct hand orientation to grasp an object. In both cases, the activation (Talairach coordinates −40, −49, 53) lies on the medial wall of the intraparietal sulcus.

the context of shifting task goals. Specifically the early corrections observed in this task imply that this intraparietal site is involved in computing a dynamic motor error signal for use in updating ongoing reaching actions (see also Prablanc et al., 2003, this volume).

In addition to bringing the hand to the target location, reaching for 3-D objects also involves properly orienting the limb to enable appropriate grasping. This depends both on successful integration of sensory information concerning the target object's disposition in space with representations of the effector's biomechanical properties. To investigate areas involved in this computation, we developed an event-related fMRI paradigm where subjects plan object-oriented reaching movements without overt execution (Johnson et al., in press). In this implicit motor imagery paradigm, subjects were required to select whether an under- or overhand posture would be the most comfortable way to grip a handle appearing in a variety of different 3-D orientations. For these choices to be consistent with grip preferences displayed on a comparable task that involved actually grasping handles, subjects must accurately represent both the stimulus' orientation and biomechanical constraints on pronation and supination of the hand (Johnson, 2000). In contrast to the reaching task described above, these grip selection judgments were made in the absence of overt hand movements and therefore without the benefit of sensory feedback. Nevertheless we reasoned that solving this task should still involve areas that compute schemata for reaching, i.e., a homologue of the MIP–PMd pathway.

Consistent with earlier psychophysical studies (Johnson, 2000), subjects performed these tasks in a manner highly consistent with the biomechanical constraints of the two arms. Grip selection judgments based on either hand induced bilateral activation of PMd in the region of the precentral gyrus. This observation supports the hypothesis that caudal PMd is involved in preparation and selection of conditional motor behavior (Passingham, 1993; Iacoboni et al., 1996; Grafton et al., 1998). In contrast to the bilateral effects observed in PMd, activations within PPC were dependent, in part, on the hand on which grip decisions were based. Left and right hand grip selection each activated regions located within the medial extent of the IPS of the hemisphere contralateral to the involved hand. The site was located less than 5 mm from the area that was activated during on-line correction of reaching movements described above. On the basis of both their locations and functional involvement in reach planning, we believe that this site may be homologous to monkey area MIP. Consistent with this interpretation, responses of cells within area MIP are known to be most pronounced when actions will involve the contralateral hand (Colby and Duhamel, 1991; Colby, 1998). An important point here is that the putative human MIP site was selectively activated by both on-line correction and imagined reaching, the latter of which provided no opportunity for sensory feedback. This suggests that, along with interconnected regions of PMd, the medial IPs is part of a circuit involved in computing motor schemata for both the planning and control of reaching.

Mid-parietal pathways for grasping

In contrast to pointing or reaching to a location in space, the goal of grasping an object can usually be achieved in numerous ways. Regardless of the final posture, grasping involves transforming intrinsic properties of an object (e.g., shape, size, texture) into a specific configuration of the hand and fingers. In the monkey, this transformation is accomplished in a more ventral circuit connecting areas AIP and F5. Area AIP is part of the IPL and contains several sub-populations of 'manipulation' cells that represent specific types of hand postures necessary for grasping objects (Taira et al., 1990; Sakata et al., 1995). Motor dominant neurons require no visual input and therefore discharge in either the light or dark. Visuomotor neurons respond more strongly in light, but also in dark when neither the hand nor target remain visible. Finally, visual neurons only respond in the light, and some appear to selectively represent the 3-D shapes of graspable objects (Murata et al., 1996).

Area F5 contains interleaved representations of the fingers, hands, and mouth. Cells within F5 appear to be involved in the preparation and execution of visually guided grasping actions (Rizzolatti et al., 1988). This area is subdivided into F5ab, in the posterior bank of the inferior arcuate sulcus, and area F5c, located in the dorsal convexity (Rizzolatti and Luppino, 2001). Both subdivisions receive major inputs from secondary somatosensory cortex (area SII), and IPL area PF (Godschalk et al., 1984b), the latter of which also contains a representation of the face and arm. Area F5ab also receives a major projection from AIP. Like visual neurons in AIP, some F5ab units respond selectively to 3-D shapes even when no hand movements are involved (Sakata et al., 1997). Effective stimuli are typically of a shape that is compatible with a cell's preferred hand configuration (Rizzolatti et al., 1996a). It has been suggested that these visual units code objects' 3-D features and are involved in the selection of appropriate grasping and manipulation movements (Luppino et al., 1999, p. 181). Similar to cells in the anterior superior temporal sulcus (STS) (Jellema et al., 2000), many F5c units appear to represent body movements. Specifically, many cells in F5c selectively represent specific hand configurations, e.g., power or precision gripping. However, unlike STS neurons, F5c cells do not code arbitrary postures or movements. Instead, they appear to represent the goal of, rather than the specific movements involved in, manual actions, e.g., holding, grasping, or tearing an object, and in this sense are context dependent. For instance, if the same hand movement is made in the context of a different action, say grooming instead of feeding, F5c units' responses will be weak or absent (Rizzolatti and Luppino, 2001). In short, together with area AIP, F5c neurons appear to represent schemata for particular grasping actions.

Until recently, identification of a putative AIP–F5 homologue associated with grasping in humans has proven challenging. Many of the early positron emission tomography (PET) studies observed that grasping was associated with a site in the superior frontal gyrus (BA6) that is a putative homologue of area PMd in the monkey (Grafton et al., 1996; Rizzolatti et al., 1996b). Grafton et al. (1996) suggested that difficulties identifying an AIP–F5 homologue may be related to methodological limitations including use of relatively undemanding tasks and/or reliance on the limited spatiotemporal resolution of PET. More recent work in fMRI appears to support this interpretation. Binkofski and colleagues observed significant bilateral activations within the anterior IPs (putative AIP homologue) when subjects grasped vs. pointed at rectangular visual objects. Likewise, lesions in this region were also shown to produce deficits in configuring the hand to engage objects (Binkofski et al., 1998). Moreover, haptic exploration of complex vs. simple shapes without vision induced significant activations in putative AIP as well as BA44 (putative F5) (Binkofski et al., 1999). This observation raises the possibility that the circuit is involved in visuomotor and somatomotor transformations during grasping. Put differently, schemata for grasp may be poly-modal.

In an attempt to more closely approximate task demands that activate monkey AIP–F5 neurons, we recently undertook an fMRI study of visually guided grasping using a more varied set of stimuli that have geometrically irregular bounding contours. Using similar objects, Goodale and colleagues demonstrated that subjects adopt stable precision grasps where opposing forces of the thumb and forefinger pass directly through objects' centers of mass (Goodale et al., 1994). Our subjects also showed this pattern when they were required to grasp visually presented versions with their dominant right hands. Compared with a task where subjects pointed at the

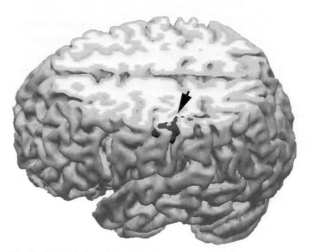

Fig. 2. Probable location of human homologue of area AIP (defined in non-human primates). The black area (indicated by the arrow) is activated during grasping of objects compared to pointing at objects. The area shown represents the overlap of 90% of subjects ($n = 12$) performing the task with the contralateral right hand. The site is located in the most anterior portion of the intraparietal sulcus, near the junction with the post-central sulcus (Talairach coordinates -45, -35, 43).

same objects, grasping activated a putative AIP site in the anterior region of the contralateral IPs as well as the secondary somatosensory region (SII), which also projects directly to F5 in monkey. The center of the AIP site was within 3 mm of what Binkofski et al., observed in their smaller study group. We found remarkable consistency across subjects suggesting that this function is highly localized (Fig. 2). Notably absent in our study are activations in inferior frontal gyrus (GFi, putative homologue of F5). The reason(s) for this is/are unclear but may have to do with the subtractive comparisons used between pointing and grasping. It is also worth noting that unlike Binkofski et al., we only observed IPs activation in the contralateral hemisphere. Further work on this problem is clearly needed; however, these results suggest that like monkeys, the transformation of objects' intrinsic spatial properties into hand configurations for grasping visual objects in humans involves a highly localized region of the anterior IPs.

To summarize, results of electrophysiology and functional imaging studies converge on the hypothesis that schemata for reaching versus grasping are constructed in two separate parietofrontal circuits in the primate brain. Further support for this hypothesis comes from observations of patients with parietal lesions resulting in optic ataxia (OA) vs. ideomotor (IM) apraxia.

Patients with optic ataxia (OA) tend to have troubles *acting on* perceptually available objects. Most investigations suggest that the common locus of damage across OA patients is the SPL, and that the deficit can occur following unilateral lesions in either hemisphere. Patients with left SPL lesions tend to show a 'visual field effect': misreaching when they are required to engage objects positioned in the contralesional hemispace. By contrast, patients with right SPL lesions often display a 'hand effect': misreaching when using the contralesional hand to acquire objects located in either hemispace (Perenin and Vighetto, 1988).

Consistent with observations in monkeys that reaching and grasping are controlled by separate parietofrontal circuits, some OA patients display deficits in visually guided reaching, while still retaining the ability to correctly preshape the hand when grasping (Tzavaras and Masure, 1976). Conversely, grasping can also be affected while reaching remains intact (Jakobson et al., 1991). Recent work in monkey electrophysiology suggests that misreaching resulting from SPL lesions may reflect a failure of parietal neurons to integrate eye and hand position signals (Battaglia-Mayer et al., 2001). Normally, this combined information would be available to premotor areas involved in action planning that receive SPL projections. However, as a result of their SPL lesions, OA patients fail when tasks demand combining eye and hand position information in order to manually engage visual objects. These lesions may therefore impair not just parietal functions, but also the complex interplay between parietal and premotor areas during reaching and grasping actions.

Parietofrontal circuits for acting with objects

Representing the workspace

Reaching and grasping are but the first steps in object, or tool, utilization. It is also essential to relate one's limbs to the proximal environment. Work suggests that visuotactile representations of peripersonal space may be constructed in a circuit connecting IPL area VIP with PMv area F4 (Fogassi et al.,

1992, 1996). Area F4 contains a representation of the face, neck, trunk, and limbs and lies caudal to F5. The majority of units in F4 are bimodal, having tactile receptive fields (RFs) that are in register with 3-D visual RFs of space immediately adjacent to the animal. Importantly, these representations are unaffected by variations in gaze direction. Similar RF properties can be found in area VIP neurons (Colby et al., 1993; Duhamel et al., 1998), which provide direct afferent input to F4 (Luppino et al., 1999). These observations have prompted the hypothesis that the VIP–F4 circuit represents peripersonal space in a frame of reference centered on the body part involved in a given visually guided action (Graziano et al., 1994, 1997; Fogassi et al., 1996).

In point of fact, there are neurons distributed throughout the IPs that appear to have visuotactile properties similar to those observed in area F4. Interestingly, the visual RFs of these units appear to *increase* when monkeys use tools to retrieve other objects (i.e., food pellets). Visual RFs normally in register with tactile RFs of the hand expand to encompass peripersonal space occupied by the tool. Such expansion is not observed when tools are merely manipulated, only when they are actively used to accomplish an intentional action (retrieval of food) (Iriki et al., 1996). Similarly, a recent PET study of monkeys showed increased activation that included VIP and PMv, as well as basal ganglia, pre-SMA, and cerebellum when monkeys used a tool to retrieve food (Obayashi et al., 2001). In a recent pilot study, we used fMRI to compare areas activated when performing a repetitive object transfer task using either the right hand or a handheld set of tongs, as shown in Fig. 3. Using tongs to transfer a set of rings from one peg to another resulted in increased activation within the contralateral inferior frontal gyrus (GFi, putative PMv, i.e., F4). This may reflect an expansion in the representation of the hand to encompass peripersonal space covered by the tool, and additional work is underway to investigate this possibility.

Representing the task

The ultimate challenge of tool use is to retrieve an action representation that matches the specific goal of a task. Over a century of evidence in the neurological

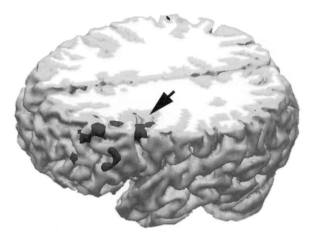

Fig. 3. Acting with tools: remapping the peripersonal workspace. The black area, indicated by the black arrow is within the inferior precentral sulcus. This site was activated during fMRI when a subject transferred objects with a set of tongs that extended the reach of the subject, compared to a control scan of transferring the objects with the fingers. This area may correspond to the ventral premotor area as defined in non-human primates. Neurons in this area in monkeys represent visuotactile properties (Graziano et al., 1997).

literature suggests that retrieval of actions associated with tools involves a system that is functionally and anatomically dissociable from that which controls dexterous prehension, i.e., the acting on system. As elaborated above, patients with OA have difficulties using visual information to control manual actions, regardless of their familiarity with the task. Despite substantial difficulties with on-line prehension to arbitrary objects, however, at least some patients may still accurately acquire familiar objects (Jeannerod, 1994). This astounding observation suggests that the areas involved in reach and grasp can be damaged without disrupting the retrieval and execution of learned skills. In other words, schemata for *acting on* might appear abnormal, while those for *acting with* a familiar object can be relatively intact! This finding has been interpreted as evidence that dorsal and ventral visual streams are interactive; that stored representations of familiar objects' physical properties could be used as cues for prehension by the damaged dorsal stream via their reciprocal interconnections. However, we suggest that this evidence might instead reflect the existence of two dissociable systems of action schemata within the parietal lobe: the acting on system that relies exclusively on

the physical properties of objects (acting on) and is impaired in OA, and the acting with system that has access to stored utilization information, and may remain intact following SPL damage. The fact that patients with ideomotor apraxia (IM) manifest the reverse dissociation, suggests that intact use of familiar objects in some OA patients is not simply a matter of differences in task difficulty.

Patients with ideomotor (IM) apraxia often appear relatively normal when controlling movements on-line, but are selectively impaired at tasks that require accessing representations of skilled actions, most notably tool use. IM apraxia patients have difficulties that may include one or more of the following: pantomiming tool-use actions, gesturing to command, imitating movements, and in some instances actually using tools or objects (for a comprehensive review see Heilman and Rothi, 1997). At the turn of the previous century, Leipmann showed that right hemisphere damage did not result in apraxia, while a large number of left hemisphere patients were apraxic even when performing movements with the non-hemiplegic, left hand (Leipmann, 1900; Geschwind, 1965; see review in Leiguarda and Marsden, 2000). In contrast to OA patients, IM apraxics commonly exhibit intact reaching and grasping (acting on), while failing to correctly retrieve actions associated with familiar tools. For instance, Sirigu et al. reported that left parietal patient LL, committed errors when grasping common objects in order to use them. However, the same objects were grasped correctly when she was simply asked to reach for and grasp them. In other words, LL was capable of performing the visuomotor transformations necessary for accurate prehension. Nevertheless, she could not control her actions based on schemata associated with objects' functions (Sirigu et al., 1995). In short, the contrasting deficits displayed by OA vs. IM apraxic patients suggest the existence of two functionally independent systems for mediating intentional actions (e.g., Buxbaum, 2002). From the perspective of schema theory, these disorders support the existence of two systems of schemata subserving object-oriented actions: one for *acting on* and another for *acting with* objects.

In his original work on IM apraxia, Leipmann hypothesized that schemata, or 'engrams', for skilled action are stored in the left IPL, specifically the supramarginal gyrus (BA40). A recent analysis of patients with IM apraxia, revealed that damage tended to co-occur within and adjacent to the left IPs including BA 7, angular (BA 39), and supramarginal (BA 40) gyri. In addition, some patients showed damage within the medial frontal gyrus as well (Haaland et al., 2000). Inferring functional localization from lesions is limited by the fact that nature's experiments' do not respect functional boundaries. Therefore, it is difficult to know whether patterns of overlap include tissue that is not directly associated with the behavioral impairment of interest, but instead happens to be damaged along with critical areas as a result of quirks in the cerebral vasculature. In an attempt to overcome these limitations, we recently undertook to evaluate Leipmann's classic hypothesis with fMRI (Johnson et al., 2002).

Common bedside screening for IM involves having the patient attempt to pantomime familiar actions including tool use. For instance, the patient might be asked to demonstrate how she would use a comb, or a hammer. Success on this task demands (1) processing linguistic stimuli in order to recognize the stimulus object, (2) identifying the action associated with the tool, (3) accessing the proper movement representations corresponding to that tool use action, and (4) implementing the correct manual action. We attempted to duplicate this test with the goal of isolating those brain areas specifically involved in accessing representations involved in tool use. Each trial in this randomized, event-related, design consisted of the following three components: (1) an instructional cue (IC); (2) a delay period of either 3 or 5 s; and (3) a movement cue (MC). On 50% of trials, ICs named familiar items that were commonly manipulated in a characteristic way with the dominant hand (e.g., knife, hammer, or pencil). When hearing one of these object ICs, subjects used the delay interval to prepare to pantomime the associated action. If the subsequent MC was a go signal, they executed the pantomime. If the MC was a no-go signal, they merely relaxed until the next IC occurred. An equal number of randomly intermixed trials began with the IC 'move'. During the delay interval on these control trials, subjects simply prepared to move their hand in a random fashion. If the MC was a go signal, they would then execute the random movements. If it was a no-go signal they would do

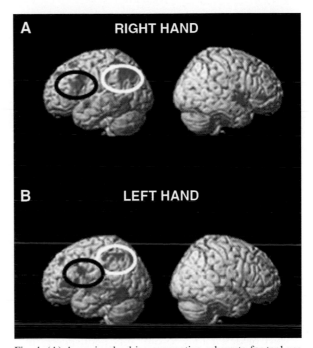

Fig. 4. (A) Areas involved in representing schemata for tool use involving the right hand. When subjects plan tool use actions involving the right hand, substantial activation of the left IPL (white circle) and GFm (black circle) are observed. Homotopic areas are not significantly activated in the right hemisphere. (B) Areas involved in representing schemata for tool use involving the left hand. Planning tool use actions involving the left hand also activate left IPL and GFm, but not homotopic regions in the right hemisphere. Together these results indicate a left hemisphere specialization for representing tool use actions.

nothing. All cues were auditory, and eyes remained closed throughout the task.

In our initial experiment, subjects used their dominant right hands to produce all pantomimes and movements. Of primary interest were those areas activated during the delay interval when subjects were retrieving a tool-associated schemata vs. preparing a random, non-meaningful, hand movement. As predicted by Leipmann over a century ago, Fig. 4A shows that we observed significant activation of the left IPL. However, this included not only BA40 but also extended into the angular gyrus (BA 39) and IPs. This pattern is generally consistent with Leipmann's claim that the left IPL plays a key role in storage of schemata for skilled actions. In addition, as reported in the lesion localization literature (Haaland et al., 2000) we also observed activation of left GFm in the majority of subjects. This pattern suggests that schemata for tool use may be distributed within this parietofrontal network, which is distinct from the more dorsal pathways involved in reaching and grasping discussed above. The involvement of GFm is particularly interesting as this area is closely linked to categorical knowledge about tools (Martin et al., 1996; Grafton et al., 1997; Chao and Martin, 2000). One possibility is that the action representations are stored within the parietal cortex but accessed via computations performed in the premotor regions of the frontal lobe.

A potential limitation of our initial experiment is that subjects always prepared and sometimes produced gestures using their dominant right hands. Consequently, left-lateralized activations in IPL and GFm may reflect a contralaterally organized system for representing tool use, rather than a true left hemisphere specialization. If so, then requiring subjects to prepare gestures for the left hand should induce a shift of activations to the right hemisphere. In a follow-up experiment we replicated the first study except that subjects were now required to prepare and produce gestures with their non-dominant left hands. If the left IPL stores schemata for skilled actions regardless of the effector system, then we should observe a pattern of activity that is very similar to the initial study, i.e., left parietofrontal activations during action retrieval. Fig. 4B shows that our data are highly consistent with this prediction. Both left IPL and GFm were activated during gesture preparation for the left hand. However, there does appear to be some segregation of left- and right-hand related activations within these general regions.

To summarize, our fMRI studies suggest that the left cerebral hemisphere of right-handers is functionally specialized for representing tool use. We are presently investigating whether this is true of left-handers as well. These representations are realized in a network of areas distributed across frontal and parietal cortex. Importantly, this network overlaps minimally with areas of parietal and premotor cortex involved in the online control of reaching, grasping and manipulating objects on the basis of their perceptual attribute. In short, we establish the existence of functionally and anatomically dissociable systems involved in the control of acting with vs. acting on objects. A key point here is that in the course of actually using tools, we would expect both systems to be involved. As noted at the outset, effective tool use requires both the visuomotor transformations of the acting on system as well as the representations for skilled action computed within the acting with system.

Conclusions

In this chapter we have argued for the applicability of schema theory for understanding the functional substrates of object-oriented actions. Specifically, we proposed that object-oriented actions are guided by two functionally and anatomically distinct representational systems, each specialized for computing different schemata. The *acting on* system involves contralaterally organized, parietofrontal circuits specialized for performing the visuomotor transformations necessary for reaching, grasping, and manipulation of objects on the basis of their perceptual attributes. This system appears to be similarly organized in human and non-human primates. By contrast, the *acting with* system involves the IPL and GFm of the left cerebral hemisphere and represents schemata for skilled tool use that have been acquired gradually over extended periods of time. This later system may be a specialization of the human brain. Like all models of complex behavior, this proposal is guilty of considerable oversimplification. However, our hope is that it effectively illustrates how the long-lived notion of the action schema might still have relevance today for researchers seeking to integrating knowledge across various disciplines in order to understand better how the brain represents action.

Acknowledgements

This work was supported in part by grants from the James S. McDonnell Foundation to SHJ and STG and to Public Health Service grant NS33504 to STG.

References

Andersen, R.A., Snyder, L.H., Bradley, D.C. and Xing, J. (1997) Multimodal representation of space in the posterior parietal cortex and its use in planning movements. *Annu. Rev. Neurosci.*, 20: 303–330.

Arbib, M.A. (1981) Perceptual structures and distributed motor control. In: V.B. Brooks (Ed.) *Handbook of Physiology, Section 2: The Nervous System, Vol. II, Motor Control, Part 1*. American Physiological Society, Bethesda, MD, pp. 1449–1480.

Arbib, M.A. (1990) Programs, schemas, and neural networks for control of hand movements: Beyond the RS framework. In: M. Jeanncrod (Ed.), *Attention and Performance XIII*. Erlbaum, Hillsdale, NJ, pp. 111–138.

Arbib, M.A., Iberall, T. and Lyons, D. (1985) Coordinated control program for movements of the hand. *Exp. Brain Res. Suppl.*, 10: 111–129.

Barbas, H. (1988) Anatomic organization of basoventral and mediodorsal visual recipient prefrontal regions in the rhesus monkey. *J. Comp. Neurol.*, 276: 313–342.

Bartlett, F.C. (1932) *Remembering*. Cambridge University Press, London, 1932.

Batista, A.P., Buneo, C.A., Snyder, L.H. and Andersen, R.A. (1999) Reach plans in eye-centered coordinates. *Science*, 285: 257–260.

Battaglia-Mayer, A., Ferraina, S., Genovesio, A., Marconi, B., Squatrito, S., Molinari, M., Lacquaniti, F. and Caminiti, R. (2001) Eye–hand coordination during reaching. II. An analysis of the relationships between visuomanual signals in parietal cortex and parieto-frontal association projections. *Cereb. Cortex*, 11: 528–544.

Binkofski, F., Dohle, C., Posse, S., Stephan, K.M., Hefter, H., Seitz, R.J. and Freund, H.J. (1998) Human anterior intraparietal area subserves prehension: a combined lesion and functional MRI activation study. *Neurology*, 50: 1253–1259.

Binkofski, F., Buccino, G., Posse, S., Seitz, R.J., Rizzolatti, G. and Freund, H. (1999) A fronto-parietal circuit for object manipulation in man: evidence from an fMRI-study. *Eur. J. Neurosci.*, 11: 3276–3286.

Boussaoud, D., Ungerleider, L.G. and Desimone, R. (1990) Pathways for motion analysis: cortical connections of the medial superior temporal and fundus of the superior temporal visual areas in the macaque. *J. Comp. Neurol.*, 296: 462–495.

Buxbaum, L.J. (2002) Ideomotor apraxia: a call for action. *Neurocase*, 7: a445–458.

Caminiti, R., Ferraina, S. and Johnson, P.B. (1996) The sources of visual information to the primate frontal lobe: a novel role for the superior parietal lobule. *Cereb. Cortex*, 6: 319–328.

Cavada, C. and Goldman-Rakic, P.S. (1989) Posterior parietal cortex in rhesus monkey: II Evidence for segregated corticocortical networks linking sensory and limbic areas with the frontal lobe. *J. Comp. Neurol.*, 287: 422–445.

Chao, L.L. and Martin, A. (2000) Representation of manipulable man-made objects in the dorsal stream. *Neuroimage*, 12: 478–484.

Colby, C.L. (1998) Action oriented spatial reference frames in cortex. *Neuron*, 20: 15–30.

Colby, C.L. and Duhamel, J.R. (1991) Heterogeneity of extrastriate visual areas and multiple parietal areas in the macaque monkey. *Neuropsychologia*, 29: 517–537.

Colby, C.L., Duhamel, J.R. and Goldberg, M.E. (1993) Ventral intraparietal area of the macaque: anatomic location and visual response properties. *J. Neurophysiol.*, 69: 902–914.

Colebatch, J.G., Adams, L., Murphy, K., Martin, A.J., Lammerstsma, A.A., Tochon-Danguy, H.J., Cark, J.C., Friston, K.J. and Guz, A. (1991) Regional cerebral blood flow during volitional breathing in man. *J. Physiol.*, 443: 91–103.

Deiber, M.P., Passingham, R.E., Colebatch, J.G., Friston, K.J., Nixon, P.D. and Frackowiak, R.S. (1991) Cortical areas and the selection of movement: a study with positron emission tomography. *Exp. Brain Res.*, 84: 393–402.

Desmurget, M., Epstein, C.M., Turner, R.S., Prablanc, C., Alexander, G.E. and Grafton, S.T. (1999). Role of the posterior parietal cortex in updating reaching movements to a visual target. *Nat. Neurosci.*, 2: 563–567.

Desmurget, M., Grea, H., Grethe, J.S., Prablanc, C., Alexander, G.E. and Grafton, S.T. (2001) Functional anatomy of non-visual feedback loops during reaching: a positron emission tomography study. *J. Neurosci.*, 21: 2919–2928.

Duhamel, J.R., Colby, C.L. and Goldberg, M.E. (1998) Ventral intraparietal area of the macaque: congruent visual and somatic response properties. *J. Neurophysiol.*, 79: 126–136.

Eidelberg, D. and Galaburda, A.M. (1984) Inferior parietal lobule. Divergent architectonic asymmetries in human brain. *Arch. Neurol.*, 41: 843–852.

Ferraina, S., Battaglia-Mayer, A., Genovesio, A., Marconi, B., Onorati, P. and Caminiti, R. (2001) Early coding of visuomanual coordination during reaching in parietal area PEc. *J. Neurophysiol.*, 85: 462–467.

Fogassi, L., Gallese, V., di Pellegrino, G., Fadiga, L., Gentilucci, M., Luppino, G., Matelli, M., Pedotti, A. and Rizzolatti, G. (1992) Space coding by premotor cortex. *Exp. Brain Res.*, 89: 686–690.

Fogassi, L., Gallese, V., Fadiga, L., Luppino, G., Matelli, M. and Rizzolatti, G. (1996) Coding of peripersonal space in inferior premotor cortex (area F4). *J. Neurophysiol.*, 76: 141–157.

Geschwind, N. (1965) Disconnexion syndromes in animals and man II. *Brain*, 88: 585–644.

Godschalk, M., Lemon, R.N., Kuypers, H.G. and Ronday, H.K. (1984a) Cortical afferents and efferents of monkey postarcuate area: an anatomical and electrophysiological study. *Exp. Brain Res.*, 56: 410–424.

Godschalk, M., Lemon, R.N., Kuypers, H.G.J.M. and Ronday, H.K. (1984b) Cortical afferents and efferents of monkey postarcuate area: an anatomical and electrophysiological study. *Exp. Brain Res.*, 56: 410–424.

Goodale, M.A., Meenan, J.P., Bulthoff, H.H., Nicolle, D.A., Murphy, K.J. and Racicot, C.I. (1994) Separate neural pathways for the visual analysis of object shape in perception and prehension. *Curr. Biol.*, 4: 604–610.

Grafton, S.T., Mazziotta, J.C., Woods, R.P. and Phelps, M.E. (1992) Human functional anatomy of visually guided finger movements. *Brain*, 115: 565–587.

Grafton, S.T., Arbib, M.A., Fadiga, L. and Rizzolatti, G. (1996) Localization of grasp representations in humans by positron emission tomography, 2. Observation compared with imagination. *Exp. Brain Res.*, 112: 103–111.

Grafton, S.T., Fadiga, L., Arbib, M.A. and Rizzolatti, G. (1997) Premotor cortex activation during observation and naming of familiar tools. *Neuroimage*, 6: 231–236.

138

Grafton, S.T., Fagg, A.H. and Arbib, M.A. (1998) Dorsal premotor cortex and conditional movement selection: A PET functional mapping study. *J. Neurophysiol.*, 79: 1092–1097.

Graziano, M.S. and Gross, C.G. (1998) Spatial maps for the control of movement. *Curr. Opin. Neurobiol.*, 8: 195–201.

Graziano, M.S., Yap, G.S. and Gross, C.G. (1994) Coding of visual space by premotor neurons. *Science*, 266: 1054–1057.

Graziano, M.S., Hu, X.T. and Gross, C.G. (1997) Visuospatial properties of ventral premotor cortex. *J. Neurophysiol.*, 77: 2268–2292.

Haaland, K.Y., Harrington, D.L. and Knight, R.T. (2000) Neural representations of skilled movement. *Brain*, 123: 2306–2313.

He, S.-Q., Dum, R.P. and Strick, P.L. (1993) Topographic organization of corticospinal projections from the frontal lobe: motor areas on the lateral surface of the hemisphere. *J. Neurosci.*, 13: 952–980.

Head, H. (1926) *Aphasia and Kindred Disorders of Speech.* Cambridge University Press, Cambridge.

Heilman, K.M. and Rothi, L.J.G. (1997) Limb apraxia: A look back. In: Hailman, K.M. and Roth, L.J. (Eds.), *Apraxia: The Neuropsychology of Action.* Psychology Press, Sussex, pp. 7–28.

Hoshi, E. and Tanji, J. (2000) Integration of target and body-part information in the premotor cortex when planning action. *Nature*, 408: 466–470.

Iacoboni, M., Woods, R.P. and Mazziotta, J.C. (1996) Brain–behavior relationships: evidence from practice effects in spatial stimulus–response compatibility. *J. Neurophysiol.*, 76: 321–331.

Iberall, T., Arbib, M.A. (1990) Schemas for the control of hand movements: an essay on cortical localization. In: M.A. Goodale (Ed.), *Vision and Action: the Control of Grasping.* Ablex Publishing Corp., New York, pp. 204–242.

Iberall, T., Bingham, G. and Arbib, M.A. (1986) Opposition space as a structuring concept for the analysis of skilled hand movements. *Exp. Brain Res.*, 15: 158–173.

Iriki, A., Tanaka, M. and Iwamura, Y. (1996) Coding of modified body schema during tool use by macaque postcentral neurones. *Neuroreport*, 7: 2325–2330.

Jakobson, L.S., Archibald, Y.M., Carey, D.P. and Goodale, M.A. (1991) A kinematic analysis of reaching and grasping movements in a patient recovering from optic ataxia. *Neuropsychologia*, 29: 803–809.

Jeannerod, M. (1981) *The Neural and Behavioral Organization of Goal-directed Movements.* Oxford Science Publishers, New York, 1981.

Jeannerod, M. (1984) The timing of natural prehension movements. *J. Mot. Behav.*, 16: 235–254.

Jeannerod, M. (1986) Mechanisms of visuomotor coordination: a study in normal and brain-damaged subjects. *Neuropsychologia*, 24: 41–78.

Jeannerod, M. (1994) The hand and the object: the role of posterior parietal cortex in forming motor representations. *Can. J. Physiol. Pharmacol.*, 72: 535–541.

Jeannerod, M. and Decety, J. (1995) Mental motor imagery: a window into the representational stages of action. *Curr. Opin. Neurobiol.*, 5: 727–732.

Jellema, T., Baker, C.I., Wicker, B. and Perrett, D.I. (2000) Neural representation for the perception of the intentionality of actions. *Brain Cogn.*, 44: 280–302.

Johnson, P.B. and Ferraina, S. (1996) Cortical networks for visual reaching: intrinsic frontal lobe connectivity. *Eur. J. Neurosci.*, 8: 1358–1362.

Johnson, P.B., Ferraina, S. and Caminiti, R. (1993) Cortical networks for visual reaching. *Exp. Brain Res.*, 97: 361–365.

Johnson, S.H. (1998) Cerebral organization of motor imagery: contralateral control of grip selection in mentally represented prehension. *Psychol. Sci.*, 9: 219–222.

Johnson, S.H. (2000) Thinking ahead: The case for motor imagery in prospective judgments of prehension. *Cognition*, 74: 33–70.

Johnson, S.H. (2003) Cortical representations of tool use. In: S.H. Johnson (Ed.), *Taking Action: Cognitive Neuroscience Perspectives on Intentional Movements.* MIT Press, Cambridge, MA.

Johnson, S.H., Newland-Norlund, R. and Grafton, S.T. (2002) Beyond the dorsal stream: a distributed left hemisphere system for the representation of skilled action. *9th Annual Meeting of the Cognitive Neuroscience Society*, San Francisco, CA.

Johnson, S.H., Rotte, M., Grafton, S.T., Hinrichs, H., Gazznaga, M.S. and Heinze, H.-J. Selective activation of a parietofrontal circuit during implicitly imagined prehension. *Neuroimage*, in press.

Kertzman, C., Schwarz, U., Zeffiro, T.A. and Hallett, M. (1997) The role of posterior parietal cortex in visually guided reaching movements in humans. *Exp. Brain Res.*, 114: 170–183.

Kurata, K. (1991) Corticocortical inputs to the dorsal and ventral aspects of the premotor cortex of macaque monkeys. *Neurosci. Res.*, 12: 263–280.

Lacquaniti, F., Guigon, E., Bianchi, L., Ferraina, S. and Caminiti, R. (1995) Representing spatial information for limb movement: role of area 5 in the monkey. *Cereb. Cortex*, 5: 391–409.

Leiguarda, R.C. and Marsden, C.D. (2000) Limb apraxias. Higher-order disorders of sensorimotor integration. *Brain*, 123: 860–879.

Leipmann, H. (1900) Das Krankheitsbild der Apraxie (motorischen/Asymbolie). *Monatsschr. Psychiatr. Neurol.*, 8: 15–44, 102–132, 182–197.

Luppino, G., Murata, A., Govoni, P. and Matelli, M. (1999) Largely segregated parietofrontal connections linking rostral intraparietal cortex (areas AIP and VIP) and the ventral premotor cortex (areas F5 and F4). *Exp. Brain Res.*, 128: 181–187.

Marconi, B., Genovesio, A., Battaglia-Mayer, A., Ferraina, S., Squatrito, S., Molinari, M., Lacquaniti, F. and Caminiti, R. (2001) Eye–hand coordination during reaching. I. Anatomical relationships between parietal and frontal cortex. *Cereb. Cortex*, 11: 513–527.

Martin, A., Wiggs, C.L., Ungerleider, L.G. and Haxby, J.V. (1996) Neural correlates of category-specific knowledge. *Nature*, 379: 649–652.

Matelli, M., Govoni, P., Galletti, C., Kutz, D.F. and Luppino,

G. (1998) Superior area 6 afferents from the superior parietal lobule in the macaque monkey. *J. Comp. Neurol.*, 402: 327–352.

Milner, A.D., Goodale, M.A. (1995) *The Visual Brain in Action*. Oxford University Press, New York, 1995.

Morel, A. and Bullier, J. (1990) Anatomical segregation of two cortical visual pathways in the macaque monkey. *Vis. Neurosci.*, 4: 555–578.

Murata, A., Gallese, V., Kaseda, M. and Sakata, H. (1996) Parietal neurons related to memory-guided hand manipulation. *J. Neurophysiol.*, 75: 2180–2186.

Obayashi, S., Suhara, T., Kawabe, K., Okauchi, T., Maeda, J., Akine, Y., Onoe, H. and Iriki, A. (2001) Functional brain mapping of monkey tool use. *Neuroimage*, 14: 853–861.

Oram, M.W. and Perrett, D.I. (1996) Integration of form and motion in the anterior superior temporal polysensory area (STPa) of the macaque monkey. *J. Neurophysiol.*, 76: 109–129.

Pandya, D.N. and Seltzer, B. (1982) Intrinsic connections and architectonics of posterior parietal cortex in the rhesus monkey. *J. Comp. Neurol.*, 204: 196–210.

Passingham, R.E. (1993) *The Frontal Lobes and Voluntary Action*. Oxford University Press, Oxford, 1993.

Perenin, M.-T. and Vighetto, A. (1988) Optic ataxia: A specific disruption in visuomotor mechanisms. *Brain*, 111: 643–674.

Petrides, M. and Pandya, D.N. (1984) Projections to the frontal cortex from the posterior parietal region in the rhesus monkey. *J. Comp. Neurol.*, 228: 105–116.

Povinelli, D. (2000) *Folk Physics for Apes: The Chimpanzee's Theory of How the World Works*. Oxford University Press, New York.

Prablanc, C., Desmurget, M. and Gréa, H. (2003) Neural control of on-line guidance of hand reaching movements. In: C. Prablanc, D. Pélisson and Y. Rossetti (Eds.), *Neural Control of Space Coding and Action Production*. Progress in Brain Research, Vol. 142. Elsevier, Amsterdam, pp. In: C. Prablanc, D. Pélisson and Y. Rossetti (Eds.), *Neural Control of Space Coding and Action Production*. Progress in Brain Research, Vol. 142. Elsevier, Amsterdam, pp. 155–170 (this volume).

Rizzolatti, G., Camarda, R., Fogassi, L., Gentilucci, M., Luppino, G. and Matelli, M. (1988) Functional organization of inferior area 6 in the macaque monkey: II Area F5 and the control of distal movements. *Exp. Brain Res.*, 71: 491–507.

Rizzolatti, G., Fadiga, L., Gallese, V. and Fogassi, L. (1996a) Premotor cortex and the recognition of motor actions. *Brain Res. Cogn. Brain Res.*, 3: 131–141.

Rizzolatti, G., Fadiga, L., Matelli, M., Bettinardi, V., Paulesu, E., Perani, D. and Fazio, F. (1996b) Localization of grasp representations in humans by PET: 1. Observation versus execution. *Exp. Brain Res.*, 111: 246–252.

Rizzolatti, G. and Luppino, G. (2001) The cortical motor system. *Neuron*, 31: 889–901.

Sakata, H., Taira, M., Murata, A. and Mine, S. (1995) Neural mechanisms of visual guidance of hand action in the parietal cortex of the monkey. *Cereb. Cortex*, 5: 429–438.

Sakata, H., Taira, M., Kusunoki, M., Murata, A. and Tanaka, Y. (1997) The TINS Lecture. The parietal association cortex in depth perception and visual control of hand action [see comments]. *Trends Neurosci.*, 20: 350–357.

Schmidt, R.A. (1975) A schema theory of discrete motor skill learning. *Psychol. Rev.*, 82: 225–260.

Shen, L. and Alexander, G.E. (1997) Preferential representation of instructed target location versus limb trajectory in dorsal premotor area. *J. Neurophysiol.*, 77: 1195–1212.

Sirigu, A., Cohen, L., Duhamel, J.R., Pillon, B., Dubois, B. and Agid, Y. (1995) A selective impairment of hand posture for object utilization in apraxia. *Cortex*, 31: 41–55.

Taira, M., Georgopolis, A.P., Murata, A. and Sakata, H. (1990) Parietal cortex neurons of the monkey related to the visual guidance of hand movement. *Exp. Brain Res.*, 79: 155–166.

Tanne, J., Boussaoud, D., Boyer-Zeller, N. and Rouiller, E.M. (1995) Direct visual pathways for reaching movements in the macaque monkey. *Neuroreport*, 7: 267–272.

Tzavaras, A. and Masure, M.C. (1976) Aspects différents de l'ataxie optique selon la latéralisation hémispherique de la lésion. *Lyon Med.*, 236: 673–683.

Wise, S.P., Boussaoud, D., Johnson, P.B. and Caminiti, R. (1997) Premotor and parietal cortex: corticocortical connectivity and combinatorial computations. *Annu. Rev. Neurosci.*, 20: 25–42.

C. Prablanc, D. Pélisson and Y. Rossetti (Eds.)
Progress in Brain Research, Vol. 142
© 2003 Elsevier Science B.V. All rights reserved

CHAPTER 9

Interactions between ocular motor and manual responses during two-dimensional tracking

Kevin C. Engel and John F. Soechting [*]

Department of Neuroscience, University of Minnesota, Minneapolis, MN 55455, USA

Abstract: Tracking of a moving target usually involves coordinated movements of the eye and the hand. To study the extent to which one behavior influences the other, eye and hand movements were recorded during three conditions (eye alone, hand alone, and eye and hand together) where subjects tracked a target that initially moved in a straight line and then made an abrupt and unpredictable change in direction. The response latencies of the eye and hand were influenced by the presence of the other tracking modality. More specifically, the latency for the hand was decreased during concomitant ocular tracking, whereas the latency for the eye was increased during combined hand–eye tracking. Moreover, the velocity profile of the smooth pursuit component of ocular tracking was different when the hand also tracked the target. Taken together, these observations support the hypothesis that at least part of the neural substrate underlying tracking is shared by the two modalities.

Introduction

In addition to the ongoing effort devoted to understanding the control of hand movement and of eye movement, the question of how the two systems are coordinated is receiving increasing attention in recent years (see also Vercher et al., 2003, this volume). In one of the first studies of alert behaving primates, Mountcastle et al. (1975) described a small subset of neurons in parietal areas 5 and 7 whose activity was related to the coordination of visual fixation with reaching. More recently, Andersen and colleagues found that hand-movement related activity of cells in the 'parietal reach region' (PRR) was modulated by gaze position, implying that the reach was coded in retinal coordinates (Batista et

al., 1999). In addition, they found that a small percentage of cells in the PRR had a firing rate that was influenced by saccadic eye movements. Moreover, the tuning of these neurons appeared to be the same for the direction of saccades made without reaches and for reaches made without saccades. This again suggests that saccades and reaches are coded in the same coordinate system, and that during a saccade a "plan is formed in the PRR that would carry the arm to the same target" (Snyder et al., 2000). Furthermore, Caminiti and colleagues studied cell activity in area 7m during a reaching task and found that it was related to eye position for a subset of cells and to hand position and movement for another subset. However, the majority of cells in area 7m responded to a combination of 'hand–eye' information (Ferraina et al., 1997). Further support for the involvement of posterior parietal cortex in visuomotor coordination is provided by the observation of Desmurget et al. (1999) that transcranial magnetic stimulation of this area disrupts corrections of reaching movements to targets that underwent step displacements. PET imaging provided further

---

[*] Correspondence to: J.F. Soechting, Department of Neuroscience, 6-145 Jackson Hall, 321 Church Street S.E., Minneapolis, MN 55455-0250, USA. Tel.: +1-612-625-7961; Fax: +1-612-626-5009;
E-mail: john@shaker.med.umn.edu

support for the idea that this region was involved in processing visual error signals (Desmurget et al., 2001).

Behavioral studies have also provided a considerable amount of information regarding the coordination between the eye and the arm. It has been shown that a subject's ocular tracking is more accurate when the movement of the target is coupled to the subject's own hand movement, as compared to cases in which the experimenter moves the target (Steinbach and Held, 1968; Gauthier and Hofferer, 1976; Mather and Lackner, 1980). In addition, by experimentally deviating a non-viewing eye during a hand-pointing task, Gauthier and colleagues could induce an error in final hand position in the direction of the perturbation (Gauthier et al., 1990). This suggests that the proprioceptive information from the eye may be used in the coding of a target position in space for the hand.

Further evidence supporting the idea that the motion of the eye is linked to the motion of the hand comes from an experiment in which subjects were asked to make rapid pointing movements to successive visual targets. In this experiment, Neggers and Bekkering (2000) showed that participants could not initiate saccades to a second target until the hand had reached the first target. This result was observable even when the subject did not have vision of the moving arm, indicating that the underlying mechanism was internal and not directly linked to vision (Neggers and Bekkering, 2001). When the gain of ocular motor pursuit was modified adaptively, subsequent manual tracking responses were influenced as well, implying that this adaptation occurs at a level common to the two motor systems (Van Donkelaar et al., 1994b). They (Van Donkelaar et al., 1994a) have also demonstrated that during manual tracking without visual feedback of hand position, subjects were able to match target speed, but were not able to fully reduce positional error. This suggests that there may be two separate inputs for manual tracking, analogous to the error signals found to drive smooth pursuit and saccade production during ocular tracking.

We have conducted a series of studies on the tracking of objects in two dimensions (Engel et al., 1999; Engel and Soechting, 2000). In these studies, subjects were asked to track a target that initially moved at a constant speed and in a constant direction, and then underwent a step change in direction. For manual tracking, after a reaction time, subjects gradually changed direction and then moved roughly in a straight line to reintercept the target (Engel and Soechting, 2000; see also Fig. 1). The time to intercept did not depend on the amount by which target motion changed, nor did it depend on the target's speed. Before the hand changed direction, it decelerated and then accelerated beyond the target speed to reacquire the target's trajectory. We showed that we could model the hand's motion by assuming that speed and direction were the controlled variables, and that they were controlled separately, with different time delays. The rate of change in hand speed was governed by the component of the positional and velocity errors along the direction of instantaneous hand motion. The rate of change in hand direction was governed by the difference between the instantaneous hand direction and a vector that pointed to the target's predicted location.

We also recorded ocular motion while subjects tracked targets following the same trajectory (Engel et al., 1999, 2000). Eye movements differ from hand movements in that they exhibit saccades as well as periods of smooth pursuit. In agreement with prior results (Rashbass, 1961), the saccades tended to reduce the positional error of gaze, whereas smooth pursuit appeared to match eye velocity to target velocity. Focussing on the smooth pursuit eye movements evoked in that experiment, we found them to be remarkably similar to the hand movements evoked by the same stimulus (Engel et al., 2000). In both cases, in response to a step change in direction, the direction of the tracking movement changed gradually, at a rate that was proportional to the magnitude of the change in target direction. The slope of the relation between the rate of change of tracking direction and the amplitude of the change in target direction was statistically identical for smooth pursuit eye movement and for hand movement.

Furthermore, the speed of smooth pursuit decreased before the eye changed direction. Thus, the latency for a change in direction was greater than the latency for a change in speed, for smooth pursuit as well as for manual tracking. Whereas the hand accelerated to a speed exceeding that of the target's, the eye generally did not. We attributed this difference

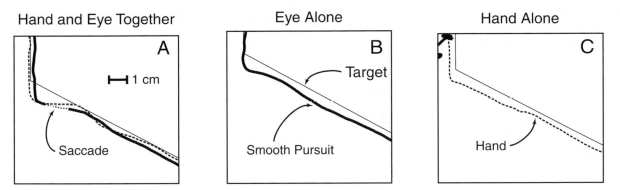

Hand and Eye Together — A

Eye Alone — B

Hand Alone — C

⊢1 cm⊣

Saccade

Target

Smooth Pursuit

Hand

Fig. 1. Representative results from the three tracking conditions. In each case, the target initially moved downward and then changed by 60° to the subject's right. Smooth pursuit gaze position is denoted by the heavy solid line, and the saccade (in A) is indicated by the dotted line. The position of the hand is defined by the dashed traces. In C, the subject attempted to maintain fixation on a point slightly above and to the left of the location at which the target changed direction.

to the fact that a position error signal accounts for the hand's acceleration beyond the target speed, and that this component of the error signal is lacking for smooth pursuit.

However, given the remarkable similarities in the responses of the eye and of the hand to target motion, we suggested that common neural mechanisms may be governing the response of both systems. In the previous experiments, we always studied eye and hand movements separately. To further explore our hypothesis, we devised a set of tasks to explore the interaction between manual and ocular tracking and in this paper, we report the results of these experiments.

Methods

We asked four subjects to participate in an experiment involving simultaneous ocular motor and manual tracking of a visual target. For these experiments, subjects gave their informed consent to the experimental procedures, which were approved by the Institutional Review Board of the University of Minnesota. In this study, subjects were asked to track a target that moved at a constant speed and made a single abrupt change in direction.

Data recording

Subjects were seated in front of a vertically mounted 20 inch touch sensitive video monitor (Elo Touch Systems, Tennessee). Seat position was adjusted such that each subject was comfortable in reaching all areas of the video screen with the index finger. Room lighting was dimmed so that objects on the screen appeared with high contrast. The touch screen recorded the position of the finger at a rate of 100 Hz and with a spatial resolution of 0.08 mm. The target for tracking was round and large enough so as not to be completely occluded by the finger (1.6 cm in diameter, 2°). Its location was updated at a rate of 60 Hz, the refresh rate of the monitor. Before each experiment, the touch screen was calibrated by having the subject touch a series of targets on a reference grid displayed on the touch screen.

The gaze position of the eyes was recorded using an infrared high speed video system (EyeLink System, SensoMotoric Instruments, Teltow, Germany). The EyeLink system consists of two head-mounted video cameras used to track eye position. A third head-mounted camera tracked the position of four infrared LED markers that were mounted along the periphery of the touch screen. Consequently, the position of the head relative to the monitor could be calculated, permitting the subject to perform without the need for the head to be fixed in space. The EyeLink system provided a spatial resolution of better than 0.01° and a sampling rate of 250 Hz. It was calibrated by having the subject fixate a series of targets on a reference grid displayed on the touch screen. Before each trial, the subject fixated a single point on the screen to remove any drift in the system. Gaze position signals from the two eyes were then averaged to reduce noise.

Experimental conditions

Throughout the experiment, three tracking conditions were presented in a random sequence. For all three conditions, the motion of the target was the same. It appeared at the middle of the top border of the screen and moved downward at a constant speed of 6.5 cm/s (7.4°/s). When the target was within ±8 cm of the center of the screen, it made a single abrupt change in direction to one of 24 evenly spaced directions encompassing 360°. The precise location of the shift in direction was randomized.

In the 'together' condition, subjects were asked to track the target with the eyes and hand concurrently. In the second condition, 'eye alone', subjects tracked the target with their eyes while keeping their index finger at a fixed point located at the lower right hand corner of the screen. In the third condition, 'hand alone', subjects tracked the target with their index finger while maintaining gaze at a fixation point on the screen. This point was placed near the center of the screen such that the target changed direction when it was at or near the foveal region (within 5° of the fixation point). Subjects were allowed to practice each type of trial before the experimental session, and were informed of the upcoming trial type before the start of the trial. All subjects completed a total of 360 trials (3 conditions × 24 directions × 5 replications).

Data analysis

Since we had previously established that there is symmetry in responses about the mid-line, and that the results are invariant under a rotation (Engel and Soechting, 2000), data from trials in which the target deviated by the same amount to the left and to the right were combined. For the eye, to average the smooth pursuit component of tracking across trials, saccades were removed from individual records by determining the time of the onset and end of each saccade and interpolating through this region (Barnes, 1982; see also Engel et al., 1999). Desaccading was performed independently for the X and Y components of velocity. For both the hand and the eye, the X and Y components of velocity were calculated by numerically differentiating the position data and then digitally smoothing them using a two-sided

exponential filter with a cutoff frequency of 12 Hz for hand velocity and 30 Hz for eye velocity. Data were averaged by aligning the trials on the point at which the target changed direction. The direction (θ) and speed (v) of tracking were computed from the X and Y components of velocity:

$$v = \sqrt{\dot{x}^2 + \dot{y}^2} \qquad \theta = \tan^{-1}\dot{x}/\dot{y}$$

To determine the latency for changes in direction and speed, the average and standard deviation were computed over the interval from 150 ms before the change in target direction to 100 ms after. Latency was defined as the time at which the trace surpassed two standard deviations around this average. On rare occasions, this method would produce an early latency due to a spike in the data. These cases were corrected by choosing the next time point that exceeded the threshold.

Results

As discussed above, previous results have shown that there appear to be numerous similarities and possible interactions between oculomotor and manual tracking. To better characterize these interactions, we recorded from both modalities simultaneously (see Methods section). To this end, we adopted a paradigm with three conditions (Fig. 1). In the 'hand and eye together' condition, the hand and the eye tracked the target simultaneously. Fig. 1A shows the results from one trial of this experimental condition. In this trial, the target initially moved downward at a constant speed and then made a change in direction of 60° to the subject's right side. The thin solid line denotes the path of the target. The path of the hand is shown by the dashed line, while the path of the eye is shown by the solid black line. A saccade occurred after the change in target direction; it is depicted by a short dotted interval in the path of the eye. Fig. 1B presents an example of the second condition ('eye alone'), in which the eyes tracked the target, while the hand remained stationary at the lower right hand corner of the screen. Notice that in Fig. 1B, not all of the positional error was reduced. This was primarily due to the size of the target, which was 1.6 cm in diameter. For this trial, the subject tracked the lower edge of the target. This example also demonstrates a case in which there was no saccade after the target changed direction. Finally, the response to the 'hand alone' condition is illustrated in Fig. 1C. In this condition, the eyes remained stationary, focused on a fixation point displayed near the middle of the screen throughout the trial (solid trace). Concurrently, the hand tracked the moving target (dashed trace).

In Fig. 1, the gaze position of the eyes on the touch screen is reported, gaze position being the combination of the position of the eye in the head, and the position of the head in space. On the basis of qualitative observations of the subjects throughout the experiment, it did not appear that there was appreciable head motion during the task. This observation was borne out by quantitative comparisons of eye and gaze trajectories. Fig. 2A shows the direction of ocular movement following a 90° change in the direction of target motion. The solid trace represents the direction of gaze position while the dashed trace represents eye position in head fixed coordinates. Each trace is the average of the same 10 trials from one subject. The correlation between the two traces is 0.998, indicating that there was little to no head movement as the subject tracked the target. The average speed of the eye and the gaze velocity were also highly correlated (Fig. 2B). These results are typical, with the average correlation for direction being 0.977 and the average correlation in speed being 0.964 for all of the data from three out of the four subjects. (Eye-in-head position was not recorded from one subject.) Therefore, for the rest

of the results, we will report gaze position, assuming that the changes in gaze result almost entirely from changes in eye position relative to the head.

The temporal evolution of the speed and the direction of eye and hand tracking were different for different experimental conditions. This can be appreciated in Fig. 3, where we present the average results of one subject for a change in target direction of 105°. The direction of the eye and the hand are shown in the left column and speed is shown in the right column. All traces begin 200 ms before the target changed direction, with the time of the directional change denoted by a vertical hash mark. Before averaging, saccades were removed from the individual eye movement records so that the entire time course of the smooth pursuit response could be visualized (see Methods). For both speed and direction, the 'eye and hand together' condition is shown as a bold trace, while the 'alone' conditions are represented by thin traces. In the following, we will take up the results for direction and speed separately.

Let us begin by considering the directional change of the eye and hand resulting from an abrupt change in target direction (left column of Fig. 3). We have previously shown that for both the hand and the eye, the direction of motion slowly changes from the original direction of travel to the new direction at a rate that varies with the amount by which the target changed direction (Engel et al., 2000). The rates at which the eye and the hand changed direction

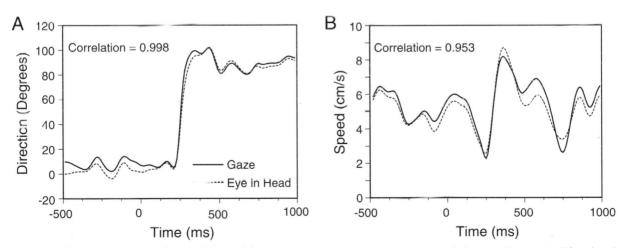

Fig. 2. Comparison of gaze and motion of the eyes relative to the head as a subject tracked a target changing direction by 90° at time 0. Gaze and eye in head motion are represented by direction (A) and speed (B). Traces represent the averages of 10 trials. The coefficients of determination between the pairs of traces are indicated in each panel.

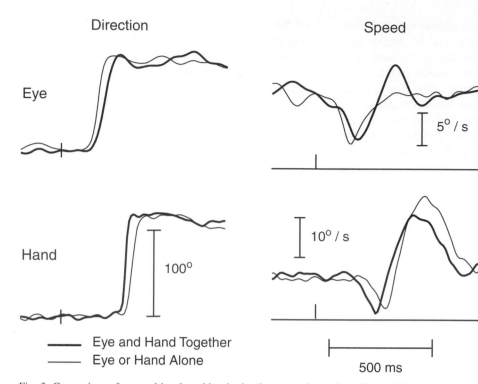

Direction   Speed

Eye

Hand

—— Eye and Hand Together
—— Eye or Hand Alone

5° / s

10° / s

100°

500 ms

Fig. 3. Comparison of eye and hand tracking in the three experimental conditions. The results are averaged data from one subject, for target motion changing direction by 105° at the time indicated by the vertical hash marks. The heavy solid lines denote a speed of zero. Note that the latencies of the changes in direction and speed of eye tracking are delayed when the eye and hand track the target, whereas those for the hand are advanced. Note also the overshoot in smooth pursuit speed, following the initial deceleration, in the 'eye and hand together' condition.

were found to be the same, with the latency for the eye being shorter than that of the hand. The rates at which the eye and the hand changed direction did not depend on the experimental condition in the present experiments. However, the latencies did. In the example in Fig. 3, the latency for a change in the direction of eye movement was 145 ms for the 'eye alone' condition and 160 ms for the 'eye and hand together' condition. For the hand, the latency for a directional change was 320 ms in the 'hand alone' condition and 300 ms in the 'eye and hand together' condition.

Averaging across all subjects and all directions, the latency for a change in eye direction was 152 ± 36 ms in the 'together' condition, and 133 ± 30 in the 'eye alone' condition. ANOVA showed this difference to be significant ($F(1,63) = 11.61, p < 0.01$). For the hand, the latency was 271 ± 31 ms in the 'together' condition, and 275 ± 40 ms in the 'hand alone' condition, a difference that was not

statistically significant ($p > 0.05$). There also was no statistical difference in the two conditions for the maximum amount by which direction changed for either the hand or the eye. In addition, the slope, or rate at which direction changed did not vary statistically for either the hand or the eye across the two conditions.

Modulations in the speed of the hand and eye were also affected by the experimental condition (right column, Fig. 3). Following an abrupt change in the direction of the target, the speed of the hand decelerated by an amount proportional to the magnitude of the change in target direction (Engel and Soechting, 2000). Subsequently, the hand changed direction and accelerated to a speed exceeding that of the target (see heavy trace in lower right panel of Fig. 3). This acceleration served to reduce the accumulated error in position. Quantitatively, we have shown that this profile can be accounted for by a model in which tangential hand acceleration is proportional to the sum of positional and velocity error terms. Specifically, the overshoot in speed results from the positional error term.

For eye alone tracking, the smooth pursuit component also decelerates by an amount proportional to the amount by which target motion changes direction. However, unlike the hand, the speed of pursuit tracking generally does not exceed the speed of the target (Engel et al., 2000; see light trace in upper right panel of Fig. 3). Accordingly, the pursuit system appears to be driven by errors in velocity, while the saccadic system reduces the accumulated errors in position (Rashbass, 1961; Lisberger et al., 1987).

By considering the speed profiles of the eye and the hand both during separate as well as during concurrent tracking, interactions between the two may be observed. For this subject, the eye began to slow down after 120 ms in the 'eye alone' condition, in contrast to a latency of 140 ms for the 'together' condition. The hand began to slow down after 270 ms in the 'hand alone' condition. This latency decreased to 220 ms in the 'together' condition. For the hand, the temporal profiles of the variations in speed were similar except for the shift in latency. However, this was not the case for smooth pursuit. When the eye was tracking with the hand, the speed of the smooth pursuit overshot the target speed by a substantial amount.

Fig. 4 depicts the modulation in the speed of the eye and hand, starting 500 ms before the target changed direction. Each trace represents the average across all subjects. Smooth pursuit velocity is plotted on the right half of the circle, with the traces arranged according to the amount by which the target changed direction. Results for the hand are shown in the left half of the circle. Results from the 'together' condition are plotted with the heavier lines, and results from the 'hand or eye alone' conditions are illustrated with the lighter traces.

The latencies for changes in speed showed the same trends with experimental conditions as did the latencies for changes in direction. On average, the latency for smooth pursuit speed was 136 ± 27 ms in the 'together' condition, compared to a latency of 117 ± 23 ms in the 'eye alone' condition. This difference was significant ($F(1,62) = 14.631, p < 0.01$). For the hand, the latency for a change in speed was 232 ± 35 ms in the 'together' condition, and 242 ± 29 ms in the 'hand alone' condition ($F(1,48) = 5.210, p < 0.05$). (Latencies could not be computed reliably in instances in which target direction changed by 30° or less and these were omitted from the analysis.) The times at which speeds reached maxima and minima followed the same trend, with these times being shorter for the hand and longer for the eye in the 'together' condition (Table I). While there might appear to be an effect of direction on latency for the hand and the eye in Fig. 4, this observation was not borne out statistically ($p > 0.05$).

The temporal profiles of the speed of the hand were similar in the two conditions (left panel, Fig. 4). This was not the case for the modulation in smooth pursuit speed (right panel, Fig. 4). The initial deceleration of smooth pursuit was similar in the two conditions, but the subsequent acceleration was not. The difference was most apparent for those directions between 30° and 135°, with the maximum speed of the eye being considerably higher in the 'eye and hand together' condition (Fig. 5). ANOVA showed the difference between the two conditions to be significant ($F(1,59) = 19.662, p < 0.01$). There was no difference in the minimum speed of the eye for the two conditions. Rather, the minimum speed of smooth pursuit could be described as a linear function of the change in target direction, with a slope of −0.02 cm/s per degree ($r^2 = 0.73$). Furthermore, there were no differences for either the minimum or maximum speed of the hand between

TABLE I

Time of maximum and minimum speeds for the eye and the hand (in ms) for the three experimental conditions

	Eye minimum[**]	Eye maximum	Hand minimum	Hand maximum[**]
Hand and eye together	200 ± 26	425 ± 89	301 ± 27	501 ± 78
Hand or eye alone	183 ± 21	404 ± 53	305 ± 62	550 ± 99

Values are means ± standard deviations; [**] denotes statistically significant differences in means ($p < 0.05$).

148

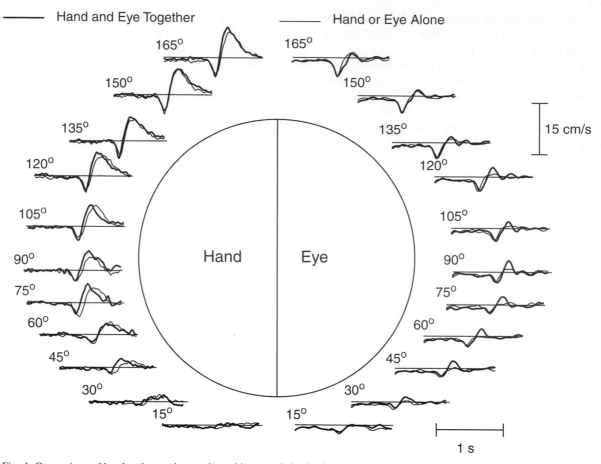

Fig. 4. Comparison of hand and smooth pursuit tracking speeds in the three experimental conditions. The traces, which are averages for all four subjects, are arrayed around the circle according to the amount by which the target changed direction. Hand speed is plotted on the left; smooth pursuit speed is shown on the right. Each trace begins 500 ms before the target changed direction.

the two conditions. Again, these data could both be described as a linear function of target direction. For the minimum speed of the hand, the slope was found to be -0.03 cm/s per degree ($r^2 = 0.85$). For the maximum speed of the hand, the slope was found to be 0.06 cm/s per degree ($r^2 = 0.62$).

Saccadic latencies and saccadic directions were also different in the two tracking conditions. Fig. 6 shows the average time of saccade onset plotted as a function of target direction for both conditions; error bars show the standard error of the mean. On average, the latency for a saccade was 44 ± 6 ms shorter in the eye alone condition. The time of saccade onset tended to be slightly larger when the target changed direction by less than 60°. This was probably due to

the slower rate at which error accumulated between the position of gaze and target direction for small angular changes in target direction.

Furthermore, as shown in Fig. 7, the direction of the saccade was affected by whether the tracking was performed by the eye alone, or simultaneously with the hand. Regression analysis showed a significant difference in the slopes representing the two conditions. For the 'hand and eye together' condition, regression gave a slope of 0.84 ± 0.02 ($r^2 = 0.99$). For the 'eye alone' condition, the slope was 0.70 ± 0.02 ($r^2 = 0.96$).

It is generally accepted that the primary error signal used during saccade planning is the positional error between the current position of gaze and the

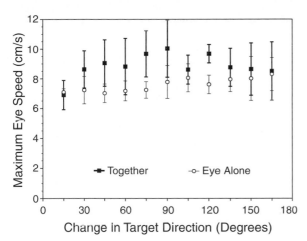

Fig. 5. Maximum smooth pursuit eye speed following a change in target direction. The data points denote the mean ± one standard deviation. Data are from all subjects for trials in which the target was tracked with the eyes alone or with eyes and hand together.

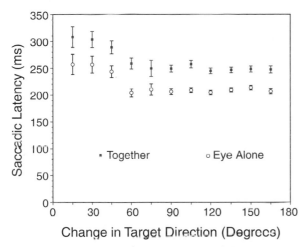

Fig. 6. Average latency of saccadic onset relative to time at which the target changed direction. The data points denote the means and error bars indicate the standard error of the mean across the four subjects.

target position (Rashbass, 1961; Bergeron and Guitton, 2000). However, it has previously been shown that the direction of saccades can best be characterized by considering the position of the target at the end of the saccade (Engel et al., 1999). As the latency for saccade initiation is nearly 50 ms longer in the 'hand and eye together' condition, the question arises as to whether the change observed in saccadic

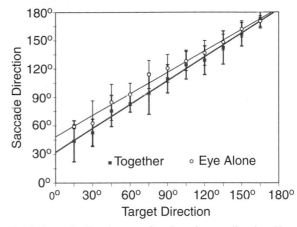

Fig. 7. Saccadic direction as a function of target direction. Note that saccadic direction (relative to the vertical) was less when eyes and hand tracked the target.

direction can be fully explained by the increased distance traveled by the target due to the longer latency. We addressed this question with a very simple model of saccadic direction. In the period before the initiation of a saccade, pursuit velocity decreases rapidly as it changes direction (see Figs. 3 and 4). Therefore, the difference in gaze position due to the increased saccadic latency is small. For both the 'eye and hand together' and 'eye alone' conditions, we assumed that saccades were initiated at a constant locus relative to the point at which the target changed direction. However, since the speed of the target was constant throughout the trial, there was a significant difference in target location, due to the altered latency for saccade initiation.

The model is illustrated schematically in Fig. 8A. We show the path of the target, making a 45° change in direction to the right (bold). The dashed line represents the distance traveled by the eye during the reaction interval, taken as constant in the two conditions. For the 'eye alone' condition, the direction from the final gaze position to the position of the target 200 ms after the directional change is shown by the light vector. The heavier vector shows the direction from the gaze position to the position of the target 250 ms after the directional change.

This model gave a reasonable account of the experimental data. Fig. 8B shows the angular difference between the direction of the saccade and the heading of the target plotted as a function of target

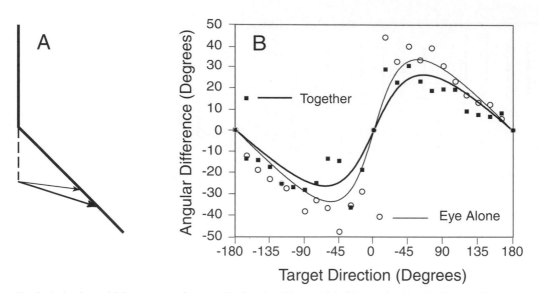

Fig. 8. A simple model that accounts for saccadic direction. The model is illustrated schematically in A, for a target motion undergoing a change in direction of 45°. Saccades are directed to the target's present location at two different latencies (200 and 250 ms). They depart from the same point because smooth pursuit speed has declined substantially following the change in target direction. (B) Comparison of the model's prediction with experimental data. The symbols represent the average difference between the saccade direction and the direction of target motion. The solid lines represent the fit of the model to the data, assuming a saccadic latency of 200 ms for the 'eye alone' condition and a latency of 250 ms for the 'together' condition. Data are averaged results for all subjects.

direction. The circles represent the average saccadic direction of all subjects for the 'eye alone' condition. The squares represent the 'eye and hand together' condition. Overlaid on this plot are the results from the model illustrated in the left hand panel, plotted across all target directions and assuming latencies of 200 ms for the 'eye alone' condition and 250 ms for the 'together' condition. The models fit the data with an r^2 value of 0.92 ('eye alone') condition, and an r^2 value of 0.86 ('eye and hand together').

Finally, we quantified the distinction between these two models. The model associated with the 'eye and hand together' data fit the 'eye alone' data with a value of 0.82; the goodness of fit was significantly diminished ($F(24, 24) = 2.21, p < 0.05$). Conversely, the model associated with the 'eye alone' data fit the 'eye and hand together' data with an r^2 value of 0.82; however, this was not a significant difference ($F(24, 24) = 1.26, p > 0.05$). This demonstrates that the difference in saccadic direction observed in the two conditions could potentially be explained by the motion of the target during the increased time required for saccade initiation.

Discussion

To assess the interactions between the manual and oculomotor systems, we recorded from both simultaneously, using a paradigm in which the two modalities tracked the target separately, as well as in combination. We found that the latency of the ocular motor system to a step change in target direction increased during concomitant manual tracking, and that the latency for the hand decreased (Figs. 3 and 4). The finding that the latencies were affected in an opposite fashion indicates that the interaction between the two systems is reciprocal. The fact that the latency of the eye was increased during simultaneous tracking indicates that the gaze position of the eyes is not merely utilized by the manual tracking system, but that the combination of manual and oculomotor tracking significantly alters the characteristics of oculomotor tracking as well. The fact that the latency of the hand decreases during simultaneous tracking does suggest that the observed changes in timing are not strictly caused by an increase in the amount of processing required by a portion of the neural architecture shared by the two tracking systems.

In a similar study, where subjects tracked targets moving in a sinusoidal trajectory in one dimension, no difference in tracking latency was found (Koken and Erkelens, 1992). However, in that study, the motion of the target was predictable. Furthermore, the authors reported that the addition of manual tracking decreased the number of saccades and increased the gain of the smooth pursuit tracking. In a recent study by Sailer et al. (2000), the authors found that there was a high amount of correlation in the latencies of eye and hand movements across a variety of tasks, with the difference between the two latencies remaining fairly constant. They suggested that the two systems rely on a set of common information. It is also possible that their results might reflect coupling between the two systems, or an internal synchronization, such that a certain amount of motor planning is accomplished before both systems are 'triggered'.

In addition to the change in the latencies of ocular and manual tracking during combined and individual tracking, the speed profile of the eye is considerably different in the two tracking conditions. In the 'hand and eye together' condition, the maximum speed of the eye during target reacquisition is much greater than it is in the 'eye alone' condition (see Figs. 3–5). In previous work, we showed that during the tracking of a target that undergoes an abrupt change in direction, the speed of the eye during 'eye alone' tracking was always less than the speed of the target during the reacquisition period (from about 200 ms to 500 ms) (Engel et al., 2000). In general, it is thought that the smooth pursuit system does not tend to reduce positional error between the gaze position and the target (Rashbass, 1961; Lisberger et al., 1987; Keller and Heinen, 1991). Rather, the intervening saccades tend to reduce any accumulated positional error. In contrast, during manual tracking, the speed of the hand must, by necessity, exceed the speed of the target for the reduction of positional error (Engel and Soechting, 2000).

In Fig. 5, we showed that for the 'eye alone' condition, the speed of the eye *did* tend to surpass target speed for large angles. For this experiment, the speed of the target was 7.4°/s, compared with target speeds of 15° and 30°/s used previously (Engel et al., 1999). Therefore differences may be due to the

increased gain of the pursuit system at low target velocities (Koken and Erkelens, 1992). However, for the 'hand and eye together' condition, the maximum speed of the eye was greater than the speed of the target for nearly all directions (Fig. 5). This pattern is similar to that seen for the hand (compare left and right sides of Fig. 4), again suggesting a linkage between the two systems. In the present experiment, the three experimental conditions were interleaved. It is possible that there were carryover effects from one trial to the next (Kowler et al., 1984). Such effects could also account for the differences in smooth pursuit velocity in the 'eye alone' condition observed in the present experiment and our previous results (Engel et al., 2000).

In a previous paper, we presented an analytical model of hand tracking in which the tangential acceleration was driven by positional as well as velocity error signals (Engel and Soechting, 2000). The overshoot in speed relative to the speed of the target results from the presence of a positional error term. This suggests that this term is negligible when only the eye tracks a target and that it becomes appreciable when the eye and the hand track the target together. If the gaze position of the eye is being used as a target reference signal by the hand during simultaneous tracking, this might be facilitated by having a control signal for the eye that was also appropriate to control the hand.

One might question whether the change in the speed profile of the eye might be explained by the eye tracking the finger during the reacquisition phase. A comparison of the right hand panels of Fig. 3 rules out this possibility: the eye was accelerating to a level above the speed of the target at the point in time that the hand had reached its minimum speed.

In addition to the changes observed in the latencies of smooth pursuit and manual tracking, the saccadic system exhibited a change in latency between the two tracking conditions, with saccade onset occurring later when tracking was performed simultaneously with the hand (Fig. 6). In addition, the direction of the saccade was altered in the two conditions (Fig. 7). In the 'hand and eye together' condition, the direction of the saccade was to a location farther away from the point at which the target changed direction. Fig. 8 demonstrates that this change in saccadic direction may be a direct consequence of the increased saccadic latency observed when both modalities are tracking together. Whether an additional difference in direction exists could not be established. This is at least in part due to complications in the experimental design. In the present experiments, the target had a diameter of approximately 2°. This target size was chosen so that the target could not be completely occluded by the finger while tracking it on the touch screen. However, this target size led to problems in accurately determining the position of the eye relative to the target as the eye tended to track multiple points on the periphery of the target in any one trial.

We have shown that there are similarities and couplings between oculomotor and manual tracking. The rate at which the eye and the hand change direction in response to a step change in target direction is similar across all directions and a wide range of target speeds. The two systems coordinate speed and direction in a very comparable manner. For both, the presence or absence of the other tracking modality affects the latency to a step change in direction. Coordinated tracking between the eye and the hand also alters the speed profile of smooth pursuit, such that it appears to include a positional error term, in a manner very similar to the hand. Finally, the latency and direction of saccades are altered in the two conditions. These similarities, along with the influences of one modality on the other, strongly suggest that the two systems share at least part of the underlying neural substrate. In addition, the fact that the smooth pursuit appears to reduce positional error when tracking simultaneously with the hand suggests that the gaze signal of the eye may be modified during combined tracking in order to be used as a reference signal to drive manual tracking (Soechting et al., 2001).

Acknowledgements

This work was supported by USPHS Grant NS 15018. The authors thank Dr. Martha Flanders for helpful criticisms.

References

Barnes, G.R. (1982) A procedure for the analysis of nystagmus and other eye movements. *Aviat. Space Environ. Med.*, 53: 676–682.

Batista, A.P., Buneo, C.A., Snyder, L.H. and Andersen, R.A. (1999) Reach plans in eye-centered coordinates. *Science*, 285: 257–260.

Bergeron, A. and Guitton, D. (2000) Fixation neurons in the superior colliculus encode distance between current and desired gaze positions. *Nat. Neurosci.*, 3: 932–939.

Desmurget, M., Epstein, C.M., Turner, R.S., Prablanc, C., Alexander, G.E. and Grafton, S.T. (1999) Role of the posterior parietal cortex in updating reaching movements to a visual target. *Nat. Neurosci.*, 2: 563–567.

Desmurget, M., Grea, H., Grethe, J.S., Prablanc, C., Alexander, G.E. and Grafton, S.T. (2001) Functional anatomy of nonvisual feedback loops during reaching: a positron emission tomography study. *J. Neurosci.*, 21: 2919–2928.

Engel, K.C. and Soechting, J.F. (2000) Manual tracking in two dimensions. *J. Neurophysiol.*, 83: 3483–3496.

Engel, K.C., Anderson, J.H. and Soechting, J.F. (1999) Oculomotor tracking in two dimensions. *J. Neurophysiol.*, 81: 1597–1602.

Engel, K.C., Anderson, J.H. and Soechting, J.F. (2000) Similarity in the response of smooth pursuit and manual tracking to a change in the direction of target motion. *J. Neurophysiol.*, 84: 1149–1156.

Ferraina, S., Johnson, P.B., Garasto, M.R., Battaglia-Mayer, A., Ercolani, L., Bianchi, L., Lacquaniti, F. and Caminit, R. (1997) Combination of hand and gaze signals during reaching: activity in parietal area 7 m of the monkey. *J. Neurophysiol.*, 77: 1034–1038.

Gauthier, G.M. and Hofferer, J.M. (1976) Eye tracking of self--moved targets in the absence of vision. *Exp. Brain Res.*, 26: 121–139.

Gauthier, G.M., Nommay, D. and Vercher, J.L. (1990) The role of ocular muscle proprioception in visual localization of targets. *Science*, 249: 58–61.

Keller, E.L. and Heinen, S.J. (1991) Generation of smooth-pursuit eye movements: neuronal mechanisms and pathways. *Neurosci. Res.*, 11: 79–107.

Koken, P.W. and Erkelens, C.J. (1992) Influences of hand movements on eye movements in tracking tasks in man. *Exp. Brain Res.*, 88: 657–664.

Kowler, E., Martins, A.J. and Pavel, M. (1984) The effect of expectations on slow oculomotor control. IV. Anticipatory smooth eye movements depend on prior target motions. *Vis. Res.*, 24: 197–210.

Lisberger, S.G., Morris, E.J. and Tychsen, L. (1987) Visual motion processing and sensory–motor integration for smooth pursuit eye movements. *Annu. Rev. Neurosci.*, 10: 97–129.

Mather, J.A. and Lackner, J.R. (1980) Visual tracking of active and passive movements of the hand. *Q. J. Exp. Physiol.*, 32: 307–315.

Mountcastle, V.B., Lynch, J.C., Georgopoulos, A., Sakata, H. and Acuna, C. (1975) Posterior parietal association cortex of the monkey: command functions for operations within extrapersonal space. *J. Neurophysiol.*, 38: 871–908.

Neggers, S.F. and Bekkering, H. (2000) Ocular gaze is anchored to the target of an ongoing pointing movement. *J. Neurophysiol.*, 83: 639–651.

Neggers, S.F. and Bekkering, H. (2001) Gaze anchoring to a pointing target is present during the entire pointing movement and is driven by a non-visual signal. *J. Neurophysiol.*, 86: 961–970.

Rashbass, C. (1961) The relationship between saccadic and smooth tracking eye movements. *J. Physiol. (Lond.)*, 159: 326–338.

Sailer, U., Eggert, T., Ditterich, J. and Straube, A. (2000) Spatial and temporal aspects of eye–hand coordination across different tasks. *Exp. Brain Res.*, 134: 163–173.

Snyder, L.H., Batista, A.P. and Andersen, R.A. (2000) Saccade-related activity in the parietal reach region. *J. Neurophysiol.*, 83: 1099–1102.

Soechting, J.F., Engel, K.C. and Flanders, M. (2001) The Duncker illusion and eye–hand coordination. *J. Neurophys*

iol., 85: 843–854.

Steinbach, M.J. and Held, R. (1968) Eye tracking of observer-generated target movements. *Science*, 161: 187–188.

Van Donkelaar, P., Fisher, C. and Lee, R.G. (1994a) Adaptive modification of oculomotor pursuit influences manual tracking responses. *Neuroreport*, 5: 2233–2236.

Van Donkelaar, P., Lee, R.G. and Gellman, R.S. (1994b) The contribution of retinal and extraretinal signals to manual tracking movements. *Exp. Brain Res.*, 99: 155–163.

Vercher, J.-L., Sarès, F., Blouin, J., Bourdin, C. and Gauthier, G. (2003) Role of sensory information in updating internal models of the effector during arm tracking. In: C. Prablanc, D. Pélisson and Y. Rossetti (Eds.), *Neural Control of Space Coding and Action Production. Progress in Brain Research*, Vol. 142. Elsevier, Amsterdam, pp. 203–222 (this volume).

C. Prablanc, D. Pélisson and Y. Rossetti (Eds.)
Progress in Brain Research, Vol. 142
© 2003 Elsevier Science B.V. All rights reserved

CHAPTER 10

Neural control of on-line guidance of hand reaching movements

Claude Prablanc *, Michel Desmurget and Hélène Gréa

Espace et Action, INSERM Unité 534, 16 avenue Doyen Lépine, 69676 Bron, France

Abstract: Orienting one's gaze towards a peripheral target is usually composed of a hypometric primary saccade followed by a secondary 'corrective saccade' triggered automatically (without conscious perception) by the retinal error at the end of the primary saccade and characterised by a short latency. Due to visual suppression during the saccade, the artificial introduction of a random small target jump during that short period remains undetected and triggers after the end of the primary saccade a normal 'corrective saccade'. As a result this procedure simulates an error in the planning of the primary saccade. On the other hand optimum hand pointing (trade-off between movement time and accuracy) is considered classically to involve a natural parallel initiation of saccade and hand response based on a poor peripheral retinal location, and a further amendment of the hand motor response based on the retinal error provided by the simultaneous vision of target and hand during the movement home phase. To test the hypothesis that the retinal feedback at the end of the primary saccade is used to update the visual target position and amend the ongoing hand motor response, we developed a paradigm involving both an optimum hand pointing and an undetected random target perturbation during the orienting saccade. In order to show that the amendments were controlled by a loop comparing the perceived target location with the dynamic hand position signal, vision of the limb was removed at movement onset. Results showed that the movement was smoothly monitored on-line without additional time processing demands. This functional property of flexibility of the ongoing hand motor response, was generalized from movement extent to movement direction. The undetectability of the perturbation at a conscious level was not a prerequisite for motor flexibility, which was further shown to depend on a critical phase of the limb movement beyond which the latter was no longer amendable, even when the limb was visible.

The hand pointing flexibility was further generalised from pointing to the more complex hand reaching and grasping process. It was shown that the flexibility of both the transport and the grasp components were closely coupled. A careful analysis of the data suggested the controlled variable to be the general posture of the upper limb, reaching Bernstein's intuitions about redundancy reduction in skeletomotor systems with degrees of freedom in excess.

A kinematics study of the motor flexibility of reaching and grasping in a patient with a bilateral optic ataxia favoured the idea of a posterior parietal cortex involvement in the error processing underlying motor flexibility, reaching the same conclusions as other recent studies using either Positron Emission Tomography or Transcranial Magnetic Stimulation.

Introduction

One of the major problems encountered in understanding the variables responsible for the accuracy of visually guided behaviour such as pointing or grasping is whether the main factors influencing movement accuracy arise from perceptual errors, non-linearity in visual to motor transformations or from motor errors. A natural visually guided behaviour involves generally an oculomotor response and an eye–head (gaze) orienting to foveate the object to reach or grasp, which may influence the ongoing hand pointing response. Thus many potential sources contribute to the improvement or the deterioration of the response accuracy. In the following investigations we will focus on those movements

* Correspondence to: C. Prablanc, Espace et Action, IN-SERM Unité 534, 16 avenue Doyen Lépine, 69676 Bron, France. Tel.: +33-472-913411; Fax: +33-472-913401; E-mail: prablanc@lyon.inserm.fr

which require a good compromise between response time and accuracy of hand reaching or grasping movement. The following chapter follows the logics of a series of studies aimed at understanding both the mechanisms responsible for an optimum response of the eye–hand coordination in a reaching or grasping task and their underlying neural structures.

Properties of the oculomotor system

In order to have some insights in the understanding of the functional organisation of the visuomotor channel, it will be taken advantage of some peculiarities of the oculomotor system in the following. The oculomotor response to a double-step stimulus is known to induce a so called 'refractory period', lengthening the reaction time to the second step. And its relationship with the superior colliculus (the main subcortical structure controlling the execution of saccades) is considered in Lünenburger et al. (2003, this volume). However, when a stimulus light is presented within the peripheral visual field, it elicits a reactive primary saccade with a latency of about 200–250 ms which amplitude is systematically hypometric by about 10%. This primary saccade is followed by a very short latency corrective saccade (about 120–150 ms), which has then a very different status from the long reaction time to the second step of a double-step stimulus. The main difference between those two situations is that in the latter one the subject is unaware of the error of his primary saccade and has no consciousness of executing a corrective saccade: this point is crucial for the following experiments. This behavioural property of two successive saccades in response to a stimulus beyond 10 to 15 degrees eccentricity is known since Becker and Fuchs (1969), and has been documented in further studies (Prablanc and Jeannerod, 1975; Deubel et al., 1982; Eggert et al., 1999). Because the accuracy of the peripheral retina diminishes with the eccentricity, it has been proposed that an optimisation of the system would require a systematic undershoot of the primary saccade to make sure that the post-saccadic stimulus falls within the same hemisphere as the initial one. This idea was supported by saccadic adaptation experiments (Henson, 1979; Deubel et al., 1986) in which an initially

hypermetric saccade induced by systematically moving the stimulus back during this ongoing saccade was after some hundreds of adaptation trials compensated in such a way that the final oculomotor response still became hypometric. This could explain why corrective saccades have such a short latency, their area being highly predictable, thus allowing an immediate triggering without any need for an interhemispherical transfer and decision. Several other explanations have been proposed. Becker (1976) suggested that the corrective saccade was internally prepared and triggered on the basis of a comparison between the very short-term stored target location and the efference copy of the primary saccade, the post-saccadic retinal error estimation being just used as a triggering go signal. This explanation accounted well for experiments performed with subjects having highly hypometric saccades (Shebilske, 1976). Harris (1995) proposed that saccadic undershoot would be consistent with an adaptive controller that attempts to minimize total saccadic flight time rather than retinal error. However, the link between the hypometry of the primary saccade and the short latency of the corrective saccade has never been clearly established. Indeed Prablanc and Jeannerod (1975) showed (through feedback stimulation) that whatever the hemifield where the stimulus fell at the end of the initial primary saccade, the elicited corrective saccade exhibited the same short latency provided the second stimulus was not too eccentric with respect to the direction of gaze and perceived as identical to the initial stimulus. As a consequence, although the normal hypometria of saccades may have had some purposive functionality, the short latency of the corrective saccade did not dependent from the hemifield where it appeared at the end of the saccade, provided the error was not exceeding some 10 to 15%. Other investigations showed that within the normal physiological variability of the primary saccade the latency of the corrective saccades was inversely proportional to the retinal error. Even shorter corrective saccade latencies have been described in highly hypometric saccades, at the limit of pathology, whose latency could be as low as 50 ms and thus suggesting they were internally triggered (Bahill et al., 1975).

One of the explanations for a relatively long latency of the primary saccade has been eluded from experiments with gap paradigms in which the fixation could be disengaged by turning the fixation stimulus off some tens of ms before the onset of the peripheral target (Fischer and Ramsperger, 1984;). The role of the fixation cells within the rostral part of the deep layers of the superior colliculus is now acknowledged as one of the main mechanisms responsible for the phenomenon of the so called 'express saccades' observed both in man and monkey with latencies ranging from 70 to 120 ms. During the saccade it is commonly admitted that there are both central and retinal inhibitory mechanisms which prevent to see a blurred image (Campbell and Wurtz, 1978; Li and Matin, 1997). In a study dealing with the onset of the reafferent retinal functionality during the end of the saccade Prablanc et al. (1978) performed two experiments: one in which the peripheral stimulus was cut off at the onset of the orienting saccade and the other one in which the stimulus was cut off during the deceleration phase of the saccade. In the first experiment the probability of having a secondary saccade (partially or fully corrective) turned out to be a function of the primary saccade error. It was compatible with a hypothesis proposed by Shebilske (1976) stating that the error signal between the efference copy and a stored memory of target position could trigger a corrective saccade irrespective of any retinal feedback. The second experiment revealed that when the stimulus was cut off at a velocity lower than $100°/s$ there was a 50% probability of having a corrective saccade although the stimulus had disappeared some hundred milliseconds before. More recently Grealy et al. (1999) and Masson et al. (1999) also reported the existence of retinal processing during the saccade. Thus it seems that some retinal processing occurs before the end of the main saccade, updating the stimulus location, and is able to further trigger a corrective saccade at around 120–150 ms after the end of the main saccade. To sum up with the corrective saccade, its short latency is due to the likelihood of the stimulus retinal error, an absence of decisional processes to trigger it, by contrast with Lünenberger (2003, this volume), and a pre-processing during the deceleration part of the primary saccade.

Coordination between saccadic and limb orientation

When trying to respond optimally (that is to say as quickly and accurately as possible) by a hand pointing toward a peripheral target, there is a natural coupling of eye and hand responses. In order to disentangle the respective roles of the efferent signals, the retinal reafferences from the stimulus and the retinal reafferences from the hand, a paradigm allowing to open the different loops independently (Prablanc et al., 1979a) was developed. The experimental apparatus was inspired by the Held and Gottlieb apparatus (1958) with a mirror allowing to prevent the vision from the hand while maintaining the vision of the stimulus. A half reflecting mirror was used allowing to turn on or off the visual reafferences from the whole limb within a few milliseconds through an electronic shutter controlling a light source in between the plane of the mirror and the plane of pointing. In all conditions subjects were required to point as quickly and accurately as possible to the peripheral target. The observed sequence was always a saccade followed within 50 to 100 ms by a hand movement. In all subsequent experiments (except when mentioned explicitly), vision of the hand was precluded during its whole movement duration, without knowledge of results. When the peripheral stimulus was permanently visible, but the hand was never visible, there was a trend towards undershooting for the eye primary saccade and a corresponding trend toward undershooting for the hand pointing, becoming more pronounced as target eccentricity increased. However, there was no correlation for a given target between the primary saccade amplitude and the corresponding hand pointing accuracy. The same effect was observed when the peripheral stimulus was turned off at saccade onset.

These experiments suggest that there is no correlation for a given target between the oculomotor primary saccade extent or its efference copy and the corresponding amplitude of the hand pointing, indicating independent variabilities, although the two eye and hand responses are synergically initiated.

However, an important factor responsible for the hand pointing accuracy was found to be the vision of the hand prior to the onset of the pointing movement (Prablanc et al., 1979b), a result replicated in many further controlled experiments (Rossetti et al., 1994, 1995; Desmurget et al., 1995b; Vindras et al., 1998). Implementing an accurate response (both in its planning and control components) required the accurate knowledge of the initial hand location, as well as the final target location. This consistent result questioned a theory of motor control: the equilibrium point hypothesis (EPH) put forward by Feldman (1966, 1986) and Bizzi's team (Bizzi et al., 1976, 1978, 1992) stating that a final position irrespective of initial position was encoded for generating a goal-directed movement.

With respect to the coordination between eye and hand, the non-negligible delay between the saccade latency and the hand latency, observed even when subjects are instructed to point as quickly and accurately as possible towards a target (the hand starts near the end of the saccade; Prablanc et al., 1979a; Biguer et al., 1982; Neggers and Bekkering, 2001), drove to an electromyographic (EMG) study (Biguer et al., 1982) to look at the signals at the origin of the upper limb response. This relatively early EMG control signal was nearly synchronous with the saccadic responses, indicating that hand and eye responses were initiated in parallel on the basis of the peripheral retinal signal. When the head was free to move, the same phenomenon of synergic initiation was observed and the increase in the number of degrees of freedom (eye + head for a same gaze direction) induced a better accuracy of the hand pointing, likely because immobilizing the head disrupted a natural mechanism of over-redundant multi-joint synergies involved in visuomotor coordination.

Another experiment performed by Vercher et al. (1994) tested different conditions of eye–head–hand coupling trying to understand the source of accuracy of the pointing. Situations were compared systematically under peripheral vision without gaze orientation, and under synergic or sequential responses of the gaze and hand, with eye, head or trunk free to move. The overall result of this study showed that coupling the eye and hand led to better pointing accuracy than pointing under peripheral vision. However, the sequential organisation of gaze and hand responses had no advantage over the synergic one and the accuracy depended mainly upon the number of degrees of freedom of the motor apparatus allowed by the experimental condition and the amount of visual information available (peripheral versus central). As in this latter experiment all subjects underwent the different conditions with the same initial knowledge, i.e. the hand seen foveally prior to movement onset, it provided a good estimate of the roles of target gaze capture and of synergy of naturally involved joints.

Based on the above observations, the classical hypothesis, according to which the hand motor planning errors should mostly be amended during the end part of the movement based on simultaneous vision of the target and hand pointing movement, was further questioned. The idea that motor error correction does not begin first by retinal error processing between target and hand during its deceleration phase, but rather is based on an early detection of non-visual hand path signal and visual target location, was then proposed.

The unconscious double-step paradigm and the flexibility of motor response

A first paradigm was developed with an initial vision of the hand prior to movement, including always the same instructions (pointing as fast and accurately as possible). The different sessions of this first paradigm included a target turned off at saccade onset, a target turned off 120 ms after saccade end, and a target permanently on. In all sessions the vision of the hand was turned off at movement onset in order to evaluate the effects of initial and final positions coding, but without further visual source of motor modulation of the initially planned movement. A control session was carried out to evaluate the role of an exact knowledge of initial and final conditions prior to movement, by instructing subjects to initiate their movement only after the peripheral target was foveated. Then the target was turned off at hand movement onset in order to disentangle planning and control. The results were in agreement with the notion of an initial planning further modulated by the quality of the updated target location (Prablanc et al., 1986): indeed the poorest planning, based on the peripheral retinal signal followed by updating of the goal through saccadic gaze anchoring during the whole hand movement, produced a higher pointing accuracy than the best planning resulting from a sequential organisation of saccade and hand pointing, despite the lack of visual reafferences from the hand movement and of any final pointing error knowledge.

In order to bring the undoubted evidence that the target-related reafferent retinal signal at the end of the saccade was responsible for the updating of the stimulus and further used for the correction of the unseen hand path, rather than the simultaneous vision of the hand and target, an experiment taking advantage of the inaccuracy of the primary saccade towards a peripheral target, was carried out. The rationale was the following: if a subject is not aware of the natural error at the end of the primary saccade, introducing an artificial error during the saccade when vision is strongly weakened or suppressed should not change anything from a cognitive point of view. The remaining error at the end of the saccade should be corrected when its value stays within some normal biological limits. A paradigm was designed with several peripheral targets both for pointing and orienting, which could be maintained stationary or in a few cases slightly displaced randomly right or left at time of peak velocity of the orienting saccade. The target always moved from a central fixation point along a frontoparallel line towards a peripheral target. The initial fixation point and the target were the same for the eye and the hand so that there was a perfect spatial compatibility between the motion workspaces for the eye and for the hand. Subjects were naive and did not know anything about the possible occurrence of the perturbation. The hypothesis was that the hand planning directed towards the initial target should be amended towards the perturbed one, although no a priori prediction was made on the time necessary to implement the corrections.

The results showed that, although there was some variability in the pointing responses, their mean distribution was shifted by the same amount as the target perturbation, without additional processing time. In addition subjects were totally unaware of the perturbations as well as of any kinaesthetic sensation of correction. The smoothness of the corrections was such that it was not possible to split the kinematics of the trials even on the basis of the acceleration–deceleration profiles (Goodale et al., 1986; Pélisson et al., 1986). When the perturbation shortened the required movement, its duration was reduced, whereas when the perturbation lengthened the required move-

ment, its duration was increased. Moreover, the durations of perturbed movement corresponded to those of normal movements of the same extent. In order to show that subjects did not fail to report the jump, a forced choice control experiment was used, close to the previous one. Perceptual responses were found to be at the level of chance both for perturbed right and left targets.

The previous result was obtained with a perturbation of the amplitude of the required movement, and the next logical step what to test, whether a change in target direction could be handled in such an easy way and still without consciousness. A complementary experiment was thus performed to address this issue (Prablanc and Martin, 1992). The generalisation from amplitude to directional changes was not necessarily expected: indeed many authors have proposed the movement to be encoded through two distinct channels, one specifying the direction, the other one the amplitude (Rosenbaum, 1980; Gordon et al., 1994; Desmurget et al., 1998b, for a review). The experimental paradigm was very similar to the experiment of Goodale et al. (1986) or Pélisson et al. (1986). The starting point of the hand was near the body belly while the fixation and peripheral targets were disposed on a circle centred around the head axis. Two experimental conditions were carried out.

In the first one, the instruction given to the subjects was to point as quickly and accurately as possible to the target. Whereas vision of the static starting position of the hand was available, it was cut off at movement onset preventing the subject from estimating the accuracy of his motor response. At the beginning of each trial, subjects had their hand at the starting location close to the body whereas the eye was fixating the central fixation point. When the target jumped to a peripheral position, the eye and hand initiated their response toward this peripheral target which could either remain stationary or randomly jump to the right or to the left during the early part of the saccade. Subjects were unaware of the jump when it occurred but nonetheless corrected their path direction smoothly with a latency of about 140–170 ms. By contrast with the previous experiment on amplitude perturbation, this experiment exhibited a significant increase of movement duration by about 80 ms despite the fact that movement amplitude remained nearly constant. This increase in movement duration was however not observed in subsequent experiments using a similar paradigm (Desmurget et al., 1999, 2001) but with smaller directional perturbations. As in the previous experiment on amplitude perturbation, subjects were unaware of the perturbation and in a very few cases reported a sensation of inaccuracy they could not explain.

The second experimental condition was identical to the first one except that there was a permanent vision of the hand. This control condition was carried out in order to test if the vision of the hand would bring some additional cues about the perturbations, and to detect a possible earlier correction of the hand path as compared to the first experimental condition without visual reafferences from the hand movement. The results were strikingly similar: the subjects' sensations were the same, without any perception of the jump, corrections of the hand path occurred at the same time as in the first condition, the only difference being the smaller scatter of endpoints under normal vision than under vision cut off at movement onset.

Is the non-conscious percept of the perturbation a pre-requisite for automatic and fast motor corrections?

To answer this question, Komilis et al. (1993) undertook a first experiment in which an amplitude perturbation was triggered exactly as in Goodale et al. (1986), except that the triggering signal producing the random stimulus perturbation was not the saccade but either the hand movement onset or its peak velocity. As subjects were aware of all perturbations (except the very few when saccade and hand movement onset were coincident), the instruction was to point to the second target in the rare cases when a perturbation occurred. Subjects were also instructed not to make a second voluntary corrective hand movement if they felt their response was wrong after touching the stimulus plane, in order to keep the same natural strategy as that used in the experiment of Goodale et al. (1986).

The results clearly showed that the non-conscious aspect of the perturbation was not a prerequisite for the flexibility of the response, as perturbations applied at movement onset were automatically cor-

rected. However, when the perturbation was applied at peak hand movement velocity, no corrections occurred, although theoretically the remaining time (250–300 ms) was long enough to allow for corrections, suggesting the movement was structured in such a way that flexibility of the hand path became more and more difficult after mid-flight, and not only because of the remaining time.

Further experiments of consciously perceived perturbations were carried out to test the flexibility of a reach and grasp behaviour considering that these movements are carried out by distinct anatomic pathways. These experiments also questioned the autonomy of the reach and grasp components (Paulignan et al., 1991; Chieffi et al., 1993). They were conducted with several physical objects, the perturbation consisting in switching the lit object randomly from one to its neighbours like in the pointing experiment by Pélisson et al. (1986). The first object location perturbation experiments involved a substitution (in which the illumination of a target object switched from the initially presented location to a new one at hand movement onset) and showed up an on-line correction of the response, characterized by an early change on the peak and time to peak acceleration profile and a discontinuity on the velocity profile exhibiting frequent double peaks associated with a significant lengthening of the movement duration (Paulignan et al., 1991). Other types of perturbation experiments were carried out with physically displaced objects at hand movement onset either in location (Gréa et al., 2000) or orientation (Desmurget et al., 1995a) and showed up quick on-line hand path corrections with an interesting underlying reorganisation of all joints involved in the movement. The methodological difference between the Paulignan et al. (1991) perturbations and the other related above ones was likely that the object was perceived as a categorical choice between different stationary objects, whereas the second type of perturbation was perceived as a real object displacement. This latter method induced stronger effects, looking like a 'magnetic reaching'.

Thus the non-conscious percept of the perturbation does not appear to be a pre-requisite for automatic and fast motor corrections, whatever the complexity of the task: hand pointing or reaching and grasping an object.

Joints motion in reaching and grasping: which variable may be controlled?

Beyond the demonstration of a large and autonomous motor flexibility, the previous experiments allowed some investigation of the motor variables controlled by the nervous system in such reaching and grasping actions.

In a set of studies involving *orientation perturbation* at movement onset, the existence of a given final posture of the upper limb at object contact was found to be only dependent upon the final tilt of the object, as if the intended posture reached an equilibrium point vector (defined by the set of *n* degrees of freedom) at the different joint angles. Theoretically, the perturbations could have been successfully compensated by changes limited at more distal joints such as wrist pronation or supination, because of a lower inertia in distal than in proximal joints, considering that the required movements were under speed–accuracy constraints. In fact all joints from the more proximal to the more distal were modified to reach the same final posture for a given final orientation of the object (a cylinder). This was far from being trivial, considering the two degrees of freedom in excess between the object and the upper limb joints involved in the task. Thus both the arm and forearm rotations turned out to be equally involved in the corrective process.

A generalisation of this result to even more degrees of freedom in excess, was obtained in an experiment involving a *positional perturbation* at movement onset (Gréa et al., 2000). The object to grasp was a small sphere. In this case, the object to grasp had 3 degrees of freedom whereas the whole hand grip recruited the main 7 degrees of freedom of the upper limb (3 at the shoulder, 2 at the elbow and 2 at wrist). Changing only the location of the sphere at movement onset produced a change in all 7 degrees of freedom of the upper arm, bringing them in the same posture as the one reached for an object directly presented at the final location. A major feature of these corrections was their quick and automatic aspect with little or no training effect, like if the perturbed object seen alone in an otherwise dark environment, acted like a 'magnet' on the upper limb movement and its final posture.

To sum up, the controlled variable in reaching and grasping movements seemed to be the final posture, also proposed by Rosenbaum et al. (1995), as this variable was closely associated with a given object location or orientation, whether it was reached normally or following a perturbation.

Displacement versus positional coding

Based on previous results, Desmurget et al. (1998a) investigated whether the final posture reached by the arm was a real equilibrium point (Feldman, 1966; Bizzi et al., 1992; Feldman et al., 1998) in the 7D joint space, i.e. whether it was independent from the initial arm posture before movement onset. The rationale was the following: if the initial posture was unusual and not properly evaluated, a vector encoding of movement should predict a systematic bias of the final posture as compared to a comfortable initial posture. The EPH on the opposite should predict the same final posture for a given object tilt, whatever the initial posture. Experimentally a consistent and highly significant effect of the starting initial posture on the posture reached at hand contact with the object was found. Despite these posture differences it could still be predicted what the final posture would be, given an initial posture. This last result led to the conclusion that the initial posture of the upper limb had some influence on its final posture hardly compatible with the EPH. Another experiment conducted by Rossetti et al. (1995) led to the same conclusion: a bias was introduced in the perception of the initial hand location (in the sagittal plane 20 cm ahead of the belly) through prisms, but with no bias in the location of the target. As soon as the movement began toward a target lit at the periphery, the hand view was suppressed to keep the planning phase uncontaminated by the visual reafferences from the hand, only the target remaining lit. This experiment was intended to test whether the movement was encoded on the basis of the visual vector joining the seen hand to the seen target, or whether it could be encoded as an equilibrium point corresponding to the final hand location, in a body centred frame of reference, irrespective of the (biased or not) visual knowledge of the initial condition. The result showed that the biased initial visual hand location significantly influenced the hand pointing, despite its limited influence (about 30% only of the visual vector bias being taken into account). On the basis of a purely visual vector coding, a nearly 100% shift should have been expected. This result was hardly compatible with the EPH which predicted the lack of influence of a visual shift of the hand before the onset of movement on the final accuracy of the hand pointing.

A series of experiments on deafferented patients have also been conducted to support or to reject the EPH, which have generally concluded that apart mono-articular movements which support the EPH, most multi-joint movements are severely affected by the lack of proprioception. It is why either visual perturbations or force field perturbations without tactile information, such as Coriolis forces, may be more useful to test theories of motor control, as they do not alter severely proprioception (Coello et al., 1991, 1996; Dizio and Lackner, 1995).

In summary, this series of experiments dealing with either pointing or reaching and grasping objects all indicated that the flexibility of the motor response during the whole response was a general property of visually guided movements. The capability of correcting on-line motor programs was not per se new, as many previous studies had shown the capability of motor responses to be amended continuously throughout the movement (Georgopoulos et al., 1981; Soechting and Lacquaniti, 1983). However, most of these studies had focused on the capability of the CNS to take into account early unexpected on-line events and measured the latency of motor corrections, more than tried to investigate whether these corrections can be smoothly implemented within the frame of the initial programming, or whether they express the capability of the CNS to cancel and reprogram the initial movement. A series of experiments were thus undertaken to show that, although there is some global morphological organisation of the commands undoubtedly reflecting a pre-planning by the prefrontal structures and the premotor cortex (Grafton et al., 1998; Cisek and Kalaska, 2002), these structures are probably no longer involved in the execution of the overall response. And the corrections which occur are under the control of a servo system which takes care of the error signals and convert them into appropriate motor modulations.

Neural substrates of quick automatic guidance of the hand: a clinical hint for the posterior parietal cortex (PPC) involvement

The above series of searches for an automatic process in goal-directed movement has emerged into the association of the visuomotor psychophysics studies with functional visual imaging such as Positron Emission Tomography (PET) and Transcranial Magnetic Stimulation (TMS), which have allowed significant advances in the identification of the main neural substrate responsible for those subtle correction processes, that were difficult to obtain without the psychophysics methodological tool introducing a pseudo-error in the planning process. The clarity of the results obtained are also due to a careful mastering of both the imaging paradigms and its statistical tools. Controlling a single variable at a time, without the subject's awareness was determinant in the extraction of the relevant signals.

The underlying neuroanatomical correlates of the functional properties described above are shortly considered by Johnson and Grafton (2003, this volume) with exactly the same psychophysical experiments of eye–hand pointing to unconsciously displaced targets during the orienting saccade as in Prablanc and Martin (1992). These experiments were carried out under simultaneous PET, oculomotor and arm movement recordings, which allowed quantification of spatio-temporal characteristics of eye and hand kinematics together with contrast brain activity. The sharp contrast between images of perturbed and unperturbed visuomotor responses (which were perceived as being exactly the same by the subjects) revealed the activity of a network including isolated patches in the contralateral PPC and the upper arm related motor cortex and in the ipsilateral anterior cerebellum (Desmurget et al., 2001). Another identical type of experiment with TMS stimulation alone showed that when a pulse inhibited the contralateral PPC to the used arm in exact synchrony with hand movement onset, the fast automatic corrections were cancelled (Desmurget et al., 1999), whereas when the hand ipsilateral to the stimulated PPC was tested, there was no impairment in the automatic correction, thus showing that the motor impairment observed with the controlateral pointing hand was not related to a visual impairment. These two converging results, reported by Johnson and Grafton (2003, this volume), demonstrate how sharp psychophysical experiments may become powerful tools combined with neuroimaging investigation techniques, as well as transcranial magnetic stimulation used as a transient functional inhibition of given cortical structures.

Along this chapter an indirect clinical evidence will be presented showing that the lack of PPC may be responsible for the absence of smooth on-line corrections to the movement. Although the role of PPC in sensorimotor processes has been generally considered as essential for movement planning (Andersen et al., 1998; Snyder et al., 2000), the above-mentioned functional neuroanatomical studies in Johnson and Grafton (2003, this volume), indicate that the PPC participates to on-line regulation of movement. However, there was no clinical evidence that it did. Many previous experimental paradigms that have investigated goal-directed movements have not been able to differentiate between the two components of planning and control. To further assess with a clinical approach the involvement of PPC not only in planning but in on-line motor control, the kinematics of hand movements was studied in a patient with a bilateral PPC lesion who had no clinical deficit in planning her grasping movements in central vision and whose characteristics were close to normal subjects (see Figs. 1 and 2). Although this patient had recovered from her lesion, she still presented an ataxic pointing behaviour in her far peripheral visual field, characteristic of the optic ataxia described by Perenin and Vighetto (1988). This case of a bilateral PPC lesion was chosen rather than an ipsilateral one, because the behavioural recovery could not be related to a functional substitution by the ipsilateral PPC of the lacking contralateral one. The patient was instructed to reach and grasp a small cylinder presented at different locations within an apparent angle of about 10 degrees and her motor performance was compared to that of four healthy control subjects. To address on-line control specifically, the cylinder quickly and unexpectedly jumped, on a few trials at movement onset, to a new location some 10 degrees (of apparent visual angle) apart. Despite her optic ataxia, the patient could easily grasp stationary objects seen in foveal vision, exhibiting the same kinematical pattern as controls. Therefore she could plan movements accurately. In response to the object

jump, healthy control subjects produced smooth and fast corrections. However, unlike the controls, the patient was unable to amend her ongoing movement when the target suddenly jumped. In this situation, she completed two distinct movements, a first one toward the initial object location, followed by a second one toward the final object location. These results, in agreement with those emphasized by Johnson and Grafton (2003, this volume), support the idea that beyond a role in movement planning, PPC plays a major role in the on-line control of reach-to-grasp movements and that quick amendments to the motor program cannot be embedded within the ongoing response in patients with a parietal lesion.

A functional schema for eye–hand coordination of rapid movements

This schema is mainly based upon the existence of both a general planning and of a fast feedback control derived from the comparison between the target representation and the current hand signal (Fig. 2). This latter signal has two potential sources: the first one is efferent and is the output of the controller acting upon the upper limb apparatus, also referred to as the efference copy, available without sensory transmission delays. The action of such outflow signals has received some support from an experiment reporting an unconscious correction in a deafferented patient submitted to the unconscious double-step paradigm, a correction (Bard et al., 1999) suggesting that part of movement corrections could be mediated without proprioception. The second source of correction is afferent and comes from the different receptors among which the muscle spindles transmitting the essential proprioceptive signals (Gandevia and Burke, 1988; Prochazka and Hulliger, 1998). However, many authors have argued that such signals had a non-negligible delay, too long to enter within a servo-loop, knowing that there are also delays on the efferent side where conduction and contraction increase the total delay. Such systems with non-negligible time delays with respect to the duration of fast movements are known to be unstable and to induce oscillations (Hollerbach, 1982; Gerdes et al., 1994). Nonetheless, this stability problem has been tackled by several researchers who basically have shown that the combination of an efferent signal and of a delayed afferent signal could

164

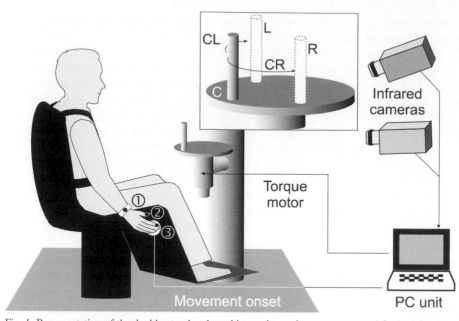

Fig. 1. Representation of the double-step hand reaching and grasping apparatus used for both healthy subjects and a young patient having a bilateral PPC lesion. The object to grasp was a cylinder which the subjects took with all fingers. After a beep instruction the object could either remain stationary or move towards another random location a few degrees away at movement onset, without delay within a duration less than 80 ms. To prevent any strategy the perturbations represented no more than 80% of the total trials.

be used to predict through an internal model the actual signal (Hoff and Arbib, 1992; Miall et al., 1993; Wolpert et al., 1995; Miall, 1998; Schweighofer et al., 1998a,b; Scarchilli et al., 1999; Desmurget and Grafton, 2000; Spoelstra, 2000) and then to allow an efficient non-delayed feedback action.

The simplified diagram of Fig. 3 illustrates the operating mode of the eye–hand coordination and both its fast and slow processing modes. A description of the fast processing mode is presented when both time and accuracy constraints are required: if a target appears at the periphery, the difference between the eye position and the target position produces a retinal error which triggers after a detection/decision delay, a saccade planning and a hand pointing planning, based on a poor spatial resolution. At the end of the saccade, the target is updated through the addition of the oculomotor efference copy and of the residual retinal error, to give a sharp target central representation. Due to inertia, the hand starts near the saccade end. During the initial phase of the hand movement, together with the delayed (Pd) signal from hand position, the efference copy of the hand movement is sent to the internal model (see Vercher

et al., 2003, this volume; Kawato et al., 2003, this volume), which in turn predicts the current hand position. The error processing between the updated target central representation and the current hand position, i.e. the instantaneous motor error (presumably located within the PCC) drives fast corrections if necessary.

The slow corrections are processed by a retinal signal comparing directly the target and the hand, which is delayed by Vd, without involving the internal model thus without prediction.

This schema explains how a given error may be processed and quickly amended when the target suddenly jumps a few degrees apart. Because such a situation mimics a slightly erroneous initial planning, the error processing is speeded up by an internal model which predicts, from the hand efferent signals and from its delayed (Pd) afferent signal, the current hand position. Thus the hand motor error acts upon the fast corrections.

If we now consider another condition with a full vision of the hand, with a prism viewing corresponding to the same dynamic error as the previous jump, the hand motor planning will be aimed at the vir-

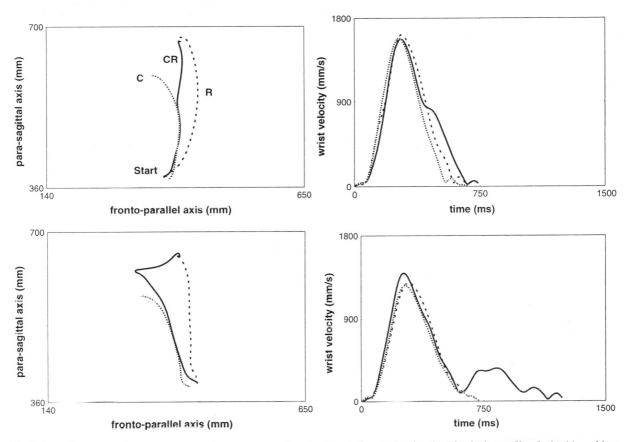

Fig. 2. It can be seen on the more representative responses to jumping targets that the hand path and velocity profile of a healthy subject exhibited an early and smooth correction without increase in movement time. Conversely the patient had nearly the same behaviour with stationary targets whereas in response to jumping targets she made two successive non-overlapping movements towards the two target locations, showing clearly the lack of online correction.

tual image, but as the hand is seen displaced by the prisms, the output of the internal model will be inappropriate and useless to be compared to the target central representation. In that case the only efficient and reliable signal will be the retinal target-to-hand signal transmitted and processed with a visual delay Vd. Then the movement will have to be much more slowed down than under the unconscious double-step condition, in order to be correctly amended, a phenomenon everybody can experience under the first prism displaced attempt to reach an object.

Conclusion

The above psychophysical data, both in healthy subjects and in a young patient with bilateral lesion of

the PPC have demonstrated a remarkable capability of the CNS to modulate on-line an already planned action, and have shown the dramatic effect of PPC lesion on the production of these corrections. First the healthy subjects' behaviour has shown that these corrective signals were embedded within the overall motor response without conscious awareness and that they were likely to modulate an already present error even when no perturbation was applied. When the perturbation of the goal to be reached was applied with a conscious perception at movement onset, the corrective behaviour did not change significantly. In addition other similar studies have shown that the self-perception of the corrective action arises much latter than the action itself (Castiello et al., 1991), indicating that the corrections are under the con-

166

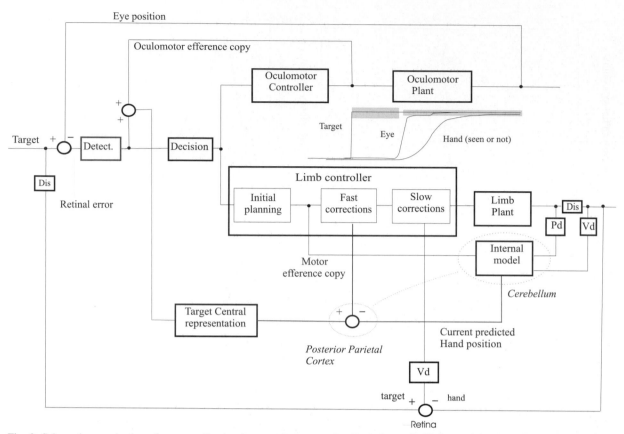

Fig. 3. Schematic organization of eye coordination in an optimum eye–hand pointing task. Under straight ahead, the onset of a target on the peripheral retina elicits after a detection and decision stage a parallel initiation of saccade and limb movement, based on the fuzzy localization of the target (large hatched bar). Due to the higher inertia of the upper limb the hand begins to start near the end of the saccade. By the end of the saccade, the efference copy of eye position is added to the residual retinal error to update the central representation of the target (thin hatched bar), a process which occurs during the very early part of hand movement, when a subject is required to point optimally to the target. Meanwhile a limb efferent signal from the hand is sent towards an internal model together with the delayed (Pd) proprioceptive and visual (Vd) information whose output predicts the current hand location. The posterior parietal cortex which receives the target- and hand-related signals, is supposed to compute the dynamic error between the central target representation and the current hand location given by the internal model presumably in the cerebellum and to send, through a cortico-ponto-cerebello-thalamo-cortical loop, the fast corrective modulations. The outer loop is represented by the delayed processed (Vd) retinal error between target and hand, which only acts slowly on the fine errors during the last part of the deceleration phase of the upper limb movement. Dis represents a possible distortion of visual signals introduced by goggles for instance displacing the whole visual image. If Dis = 0, the internal model is fed with coherent signals and its output is an accurate representation of the current limb position. If Dis equals for instance 10 degrees, the internal model is fed with a correct proprioceptive signal and a wrong visual signal which prevents it from doing its predictor operation.

trol of an automatic process. This type of automatic control that could hardly be cancelled in normal subjects, was further investigated by Pisella et al. (2000) and was found to depend upon the integrity of the PPC. The interpretation of these latter authors was based upon the knowledge of two distinct visuomotor pathways.This simplified dichotomy of two ventral and dorsal streams has been established

by Ungerleider and Mishkin (1982) in monkey, and then in man by neuropsychological lesion studies of either the ventral occipito-temporal pathway or of the dorsal occipito-parietal pathway (Goodale et al., 1991; Goodale and Milner, 1992). These studies showed a distinction between perception for identification and perception for action, and recently a study from Pisella et al. (2000) led to the conclusion that in normal subjects, the fast dorso-occipito-parietal pathway acting like an 'automatic pilot' could not be overcome by the slower occipito-temporo-frontal pathway.

However, the implication of the PPC in on-line control does not allow by itself to choose between feedforward or feedback processes. Alternative explanations have been proposed which do not consider the corrective processes described above as relying upon feedback processes but rather on feedforward processes, either as a cancellation of the initial motor program and its substitution by a new one (Gielen et al., 1984; Flash and Henis, 1991), or as a superposition of a second step corresponding to the amplitude of the perturbation (Flanagan et al., 1991, 1993). A strong argument for a feedback process is probably the reaction time to the perturbation, being much smaller than the initial reaction time, although it is not fully decisive, because some stages such as the decision to move have already been processed. But the most compelling argument for a feedback processing is probably the very small or absent increase of movement duration together with the smoothness of the corrections observed under the unconscious double-step paradigm. If the corrective process is under feedback control it may result from a comparison with the updated target location or orientation and the ongoing 3D hand movement kinematics signals (velocity and position and orientation).

In addition although the target perturbation induced a corrective saccade with short reaction times as for normal stimuli, the experiments carried out so far do not allow to conclude that the efference copy of the corrective saccade is responsible for the early path correction of the hand, as the association of the efference copy of the primary saccade together with the retinal error at the end of this saccade may be sufficient to yield a correct updating of the target. On the other hand, psychophysical experiments of eye–hand coordination with a simultaneous saccade associated with the unseen hand pointing have led Van Donkelaar (1997) to conclude that there was some correlation between the hand pointing accuracy and the initial fixation point for the eye, which would indicate some coupling between the planning of both responses. More recently he found that TMS applied on the PPC during the saccade disrupted the weak but significant link between saccadic ampli-

tude and hand pointing amplitude (Van Donkelaar et al., 2000), suggesting that planning of both saccade and hand pointing could have some common origin within PPC. However, there is no clear agreement between investigators on that last point. For instance, Blouin et al. (1995) showed that the efference copy per se was not accurate enough and needed some additional retinal signal (even null) to sharpen the efference copy signal. These authors showed that pointing towards a briefly presented target, flashed again after the orienting saccade, was more accurate than pointing towards the same target without further flash on the fovea, despite the delay between target presentation and hand pointing response.

If the role of the PPC in the eye–hand coordination is now clearly established, it is likely not an exclusive one, and other researches are pursued on saccade and reach cells (Lünenburger et al., 2000) within the deep layers of the superior colliculus structure (i.e. at a very low level) with population cells coding not only for gaze saccade but also for hand reaching. It is also important to mention that some double-step hand reaching experiments, similar to those mentioned above in man, have been carried out in cats (Alstermak et al., 1990). They showed that very fast corrections of about 80 ms latency to double-step target were observed, and explained this behaviour by the hypothetical action of feedforward tecto-spinal pathways. In addition the observed very short reaction time may have been related to the little spatial uncertainty, as the animal's paw response had only a two-choice situation.

There remains to be determined whether the different fast loops evoked above are coupled together or whether they correspond to specific circuitries. In Johnson and Grafton (2003, this volume) the contribution of a fast parieto-cerebello-frontal network has been evoked in the unconscious process of error correction (Desmurget et al., 1999, 2001), without additional time, perhaps facilitated by the quick triggering of the corrective saccade bringing the gaze onto the target. It has to be mentioned that a recent paper from Neggers et al. (2000) investigating the saccade to hand pointing coupling has suggested that secondary saccades were nearly prevented as long as the hand pointing toward the target where the gaze was anchored, had not reached its goal. This could appear in contradiction with the description of the oculomotor behaviour in this paper during the unconscious double-step target paradigm. In fact the two experimental conditions are at odd. In our paradigm there was a single purpose: to capture both by gaze and hand the target perceived as unique. In Bekkering et al.'s paradigm the subject was faced with a dual competitive task: look and point at the target and then look at another target. From both their results and ours we suggest that gaze and hand are so strongly associated that they are overriding the second instruction when a dual task is required.

Although the fast corrective processes seem to involve the contribution of a higher-level structure such as the posterior parietal cortex controlling indirectly cerebellar activation as mentioned by Johnson and Grafton (2003, this volume), it does not exclude their direct coupling to other lower structures such as the superior colliculus.

Acknowledgements

We wish to thank Yann Coello for critically reading the manuscript.

References

Alstermak, B., Gorska, T., Lundberg, A. and Petterson, L.G. (1990) Integration in descending motor pathways controlling the forelimb in the cat, 16. Visually guided switching of target-reaching. *Exp. Brain Res.*, 80: 1–11.

Andersen, R.A., Snyder, L.H., Batista, A.P., Buneo, C.A. and Cohen, Y.E. (1998) Posterior parietal areas specialized for eye movements (LIP) and reach (PRR) using a common coordinate frame. *Novartis Found. Symp.*, 218: 109–122.

Bahill, A.T., Bahill, K.A., Clark, M.R. and Stark, L. (1975) Closely spaced saccades. *Invest. Ophthalmol.*, 14: 317–321.

Bard, C., Turrell, Y., Fleury, M., Teasdale, N., Lamarre, Y. and Martin, O. (1999) Deafferentation and pointing with visual double-step perturbations. *Exp. Brain Res.*, 125: 410–416.

Becker, W. (1976) Do correction saccades depend exclusively on retinal feedback? A note on the possible role of non-retinal feedback. *Vis. Res.*, 16: 425–427.

Becker, W. and Fuchs, A.F. (1969) Further properties of the human saccadic system: eye movements and correction saccades with and without visual fixation points. *Vis. Res.*, 9: 1247–1258.

Biguer, B., Jeannerod, M. and Prablanc, C. (1982) The coordination of eye, head, and arm movements during reaching at a single visual target. *Exp. Brain. Res.*, 46: 301–304.

Bizzi, E., Polit, A. and Morasso, P. (1976) Mechanisms underlying achievement of final head position. *J. Neurophysiol*, 39: 435–443.

Bizzi, E., Morasso, P. and Polit, A. (1978) Effect of load disturbances during centrally initiated movements. *J. Neurophysiol.*, 41: 542–556.

Bizzi, E., Hogan, N., Mussa-Ivaldi, F.A. and Giszter, S. (1992) Does the nervous system use the equilibrium point control to guide single and multiple joint movements. *Behav. Brain Sci.*, 15: 603–613.

Blouin, J., Gauthier, G.M. and Vercher, J.L. (1995) Internal representation of gaze direction with and without retinal inputs in man. *Neurosci. Lett.*, 183: 187–189.

Campbell, F.W. and Wurtz, R.H. (1978) Saccadic omission: why we do not see a gray-out during a saccadic eye movement. *Vis. Res.*, 18: 1297–1303.

Castiello, U., Paulignan, Y. and Jeannerod, M. (1991) Temporal dissociation of motor responses and subjective awareness: a study in normal subjects. *Brain*, 114: 2639–2655.

Chieffi, S., Gentilucci, M., Allport, A., Sasso, E. and Rizzolatti, G. (1993) Study of selective reaching and grasping in a patient with unilateral parietal lesion. Dissociated effects of residual spatial neglect. *Brain*, 116: 1119–1137.

Cisek, P. and Kalaska, J.F. (2002) Simultaneous encoding of multiple potential reach directions in dorsal premotor cortex. *J. Neurophysiol.*, 87: 1149–1154.

Coello, Y., Orliaguet, J.P., Ohlman, C. and Marendaz, C. (1991) Spatial adaptation for a fast pointing disturbed in distance and in direction. *Innov. Technol. Biol. Med.*, 2: 30–38.

Coello, Y., Orliaguet, J.P. and Prablanc, C. (1996) Pointing movement in an artificial perturbing inertial field: a prospective paradigm for motor control study. *Neuropsychologia*, 34: 879–892.

Desmurget, M. and Grafton, S. (2000) Forward modeling allows feedback control for fast reaching movements. *Trends Cogn. Sci.*, 4: 423–431.

Desmurget, M., Prablanc, C., Rossetti, Y., Arzi, M., Paulignan, Y., Urquizar, C. and Mignot, J.C. (1995a) Postural and synergic control for three-dimensional movements of reaching and grasping. *J. Neurophysiol.*, 74: 905–910.

Desmurget, M., Rossetti, Y., Prablanc, C., Stelmach, G.E. and Jeannerod, M. (1995b) Representation of hand position prior to movement and motor variability. *Can. J. Physiol. Pharmacol.*, 73: 262–272.

Desmurget, M., Gréa, H. and Prablanc, C. (1998a) Final posture of the upper limb depends on the initial position of the hand during prehension movements. *Exp. Brain Res.*, 119: 511–516.

Desmurget, M., Pélisson, D., Rossetti, Y. and Prablanc, C. (1998b) From eye to hand: planning goal directed movements. *Neurosci. Biobehav. Rev.*, 22: 761–788.

Desmurget, M., Epstein, C.M., Turner, R.S., Prablanc, C., Alexander, G.E. and Grafton, S.T. (1999) Role of the posterior parietal cortex in updating reaching movements to a visual target. *Nat. Neurosci.*, 2: 563–567.

Desmurget, M., Gréa, H., Grethe, J.S., Prablanc, C., Alexander, G.E. and Grafton, S.T. (2001) Functional anatomy of non-visual feedback loops during reaching: a positron emission tomography study. *J. Neurosci.*, 21: 2919–2928.

Deubel, H., Wolf, W. and Hauske, G. (1982) Corrective saccades: effect of shifting the saccade goal. *Vis. Res.*, 22: 353–364.

Deubel, H., Wolf, W. and Hauske, G. (1986) Adaptive gain control of saccadic eye movements. *Hum. Neurobiol.*, 5: 245–253.

Dizio, P. and Lackner, J.R. (1995) Motor adaptation to Coriolis force perturbations of reaching movements: endpoint but not trajectory adaptation transfers to the nonexposed arm. *J. Neurophysiol.*, 74: 1787–1792.

Eggert, T., Ditterich, J. and Straube, A. (1999) Intrasaccadic target steps during the deceleration of primary saccades affect the latency of corrective saccades. *Exp. Brain Res.*, 129: 161–166.

Feldman, A.G. (1966) Functional tuning of the nervous system during control of movement or maintenance of a steady posture, II. Controllable parameters of the muscle. *Biophysics*, 11: 565–578.

Feldman, A.G. (1986) Once more on the equilibrium-point hypothesis (L model) for motor control. *J. Mot. Behav.*, 18: 17–54.

Feldman, A.G., Ostry, D.J., Levin, M.F., Gribble, P.L. and Mitnitski, A.B. (1998) Recent tests of the equilibrium-point hypothesis (lambda model). *Motor Control*, 2: 189–205.

Fischer, B. and Ramsperger, E. (1984) Human express saccades: extremely short reaction times of goal directed eye movements. *Exp. Brain Res.*, 57: 191–195.

Flanagan, J.R., Feldman, A.G. and Ostry, D.J. (1991) Equilibrium control vectors subserving rapid goal-directed arm movements. In: J. Requin and G.E. Stelmach (Eds.), *Tutorials in Motor Neuroscience*. Kluwer, Dordrecht, pp. 357–367.

Flanagan, J.R., Ostry, D.J. and Feldman, A.G. (1993) Control of trajectory modifications in target-directed reaching. *J. Motor Behav.*, 25: 140–152.

Flash, T. and Henis, E.A. (1991) Arm trajectory modifications during reaching toward visual targets. *J. Cogn. Neurosci.*, 3: 220–230.

Gandevia, S.C. and Burke, D. (1988) Projection to the cerebral cortex from proximal and distal muscles in the human upper limb. *Brain*, 111(Pt 2): 389–403.

Gerdes, V.G. and Happee, R. (1994) The use of internal representation in fast gold-directed movements: a modeling approach. *Biol. Cybern.*, 70: 513–524.

Georgopoulos, A.P., Kalaska, J.F. and Massey, J.T. (1981) Spatial trajectories and reaction times of aimed movements: effects of practice, uncertainty, and changes in target location. *J. Neurophysiol*, 46: 725–743.

Gielen, C.C.A.M., Van den Heuvel, P.J.M. and Van Gisbergen, J.A.M. (1984) Coordination of fast eye and arm movements in a tracking task. *Exp. Brain Res.*, 56: 154–161.

Goodale, M.A. and Milner, A.D. (1992) Separate visual pathways for perception and action. *Trends Neurosci.*, 15: 20–25.

Goodale, M.A., Pélisson, D. and Prablanc, C. (1986) Large adjustments in visually guided reaching do not depend on vision of the hand or perception of target displacement. *Nature*, 320: 748–750.

Goodale, M.A., Milner, A.D., Jacobson, L.S. and Carey, D.P. (1991) A neurological dissociation between perceiving objects and grasping them. *Nature*, 349: 154–156.

Gordon, J., Ghilardi, M.F. and Ghez, C. (1994) Accuracy of planar reaching movements, 1. Independence of direction and extent variability. *Exp. Brain Res.*, 99: 97–111.

Grafton, S.T., Fagg, A.H. and Arbib, M.A. (1998) Dorsal premotor cortex and conditional movement selection: a PET functional mapping study. *J. Neurophysiol.*, 79: 1092–1097.

Gréa, H., Desmurget, M. and Prablanc, C. (2000) Postural invariance in three-dimensional reaching and grasping movements. *Exp. Brain Res.*, 134: 155–162.

Grealy, M.A., Craig, C.M. and Lee, D.N. (1999) Evidence for on-line visual guidance during saccadic gaze shifts. *Proc. R. Soc. Lond., B Biol. Sci.*, 266: 1799–1804.

Harris, C.M. (1995) Does saccadic undershoot minimize saccadic flight-time? A Monte-Carlo study. *Vis. Res.*, 35: 691–701.

Henson, D.B. (1979) Investigation into corrective saccadic eye movements for refixation amplitudes of 10 degrees and below. *Vis. Res.*, 19: 57–61.

Hoff, B. and Arbib, M.A. (1992) A model of the effects of speed, accuracy, and perturbation on visually guided reaching. *Exp. Brain Res.*, 22: 285–306.

Hollerbach, J.M. (1982) Computers, brains and the control of movement. *Trends Neurosci.*, 5: 189–192.

Johnson, S.H. and Grafton, S.T. (2003) From 'acting on' to 'acting with': the functional anatomy of object-oriented action schemata. In: C. Prablanc, D. Pélisson and Y. Rossetti (Eds.), *Neural Control of Space Coding and Action Production. Progress in Brain Research*, Vol. 142. Elsevier, Amsterdam, pp. 127–139 (this volume).

Komilis, E., Pelisson, D. and Prablanc, C. (1993) Error processing in pointing at randomly feedback-induced double-step stimuli. *J. Motor Behav.*, 25: 229–308.

Kawato, M., Kuroda, T., Imamizu, H., Nakano, E., Miyauchi, S. and Yoshioka, T. (2003) Internal forward models in the cerebellum: fMRI study on grip force and load force coupling. In: C. Prablanc, D. Pélisson and Y. Rossetti (Eds.), *Neural Control of Space Coding and Action Production. Progress in Brain Research*, Vol. 142. Elsevier, Amsterdam, pp. 171–188 (this volume).

Li, W. and Matin, L. (1997) Saccadic suppression of displacement: separate influences of saccade size and of target retinal eccentricity. *Vis. Res.*, 37: 1779–1797.

Lünenburger, L., Kutz, D.F. and Hoffmann, K.P. (2000) Influence of arm movements on saccades in humans. *Eur. J. Neurosci.*, 12: 4107–4116.

Lünenburger, L., Lindner, W. and Hoffmann, K.-P. (2003) Neural activity in the primate superior colliculus and saccadic reaction times in double-step experiments. In: C. Prablanc, D. Pélisson and Y. Rossetti (Eds.), *Neural Control of Space Coding and Action Production. Progress in Brain Research*, Vol. 142. Elsevier, Amsterdam, pp. 91–107 (this volume).

Masson, G.S., Mestre, D.R. and Stone, L.S. (1999) Speed tuning of motion segmentation and discrimination. *Vis. Res.*, 39: 4297–4308.

Miall, R.C. (1998) The cerebellum, predictive control and motor coordination. *Novartis Found. Symp.*, 218: 272–284.

Miall, R.C., Weir, D.J., Wolpert, D.M. and Stein, J.F. (1993) Is the cerebellum a Smith predictor. *J. Mot. Behav.*, 25: 203–216.

Neggers, S.F. and Bekkering, H. (2001) Gaze anchoring to a pointing target is present during the entire pointing movement and is driven by a non-visual signal. *J. Neurophysiol.*, 86: 961–970.

Neggers, S.F. and Bekkering, H. (2000) Ocular gaze is anchored to the target of an ongoing pointing movement. *J. Neurophysiol.*, 83: 639–651.

Paulignan, Y., MacKenzie, C.L., Marteniuk, R.G. and Jeannerod, M. (1991) Selective perturbation of visual input during prehension movements, 1. The effects of changing object position. *Exp. Brain Res.*, 83: 502–512.

Pélisson, D., Prablanc, C., Goodale, M.A. and Jeannerod, M. (1986) Visual control of reaching movements without vision of the limb, II. Evidence of fast unconscious processes correcting the trajectory of the hand to the final position of a double-step stimulus. *Exp. Brain Res.*, 62: 303–311.

Perenin, M.T. and Vighetto, A. (1988) Optic ataxia: a specific disruption in visuomotor mechanisms, I. Different aspects of the deficit in reaching for objects. *Brain*, 111: 643–674.

Pisella, L., Gréa, H., Tilikete, C., Vighetto, A., Desmurget, M., Rode, G., Boisson, D. and Rossetti, Y. (2000) An 'automatic pilot' for the hand in human posterior parietal cortex: toward reinterpreting optic ataxia. *Nat. Neurosci.*, 3: 729–736.

Prablanc, C. and Jeannerod, M. (1975) Corrective saccades: dependence on retinal reafferent signals. *Vis. Res.*, 15: 465–469.

Prablanc, C. and Martin, O. (1992) Automatic control during hand reaching at undetected two-dimensional target displacements. *J. Neurophysiol.*, 67: 455–469.

Prablanc, C., Massé, D. and Echallier, J.F. (1978) Error correcting mechanisms in large saccades. *Vis. Res.*, 18: 557–560.

Prablanc, C., Echallier, J.E., Jeannerod, M. and Komilis, E. (1979a) Optimal response of eye and hand motor systems in pointing at a visual target, II. Static and dynamic visual cues in the control of hand movement. *Biol. Cybern.*, 35: 183–187.

Prablanc, C., Echallier, J.F., Komilis, E. and Jeannerod, M. (1979b) Optimal response of eye and hand motor systems in pointing at a visual target, I. Spatio-temporal characteristics of eye and hand movements and their relationships when varying the amount of visual information. *Biol. Cybern.*, 35: 113–124.

Prablanc, C., Pélisson, D. and Goodale, M.A. (1986) Visual control of reaching movements without vision of the limb, I. Role of retinal feedback of target position in guiding the hand. *Exp. Brain Res.*, 62: 293–302.

Prochazka, A. and Hulliger, M. (1998) The continuing debate about CNS control of proprioception. *J. Physiol.*, 513(Pt 2): 315.

Rosenbaum, D.A. (1980) Human movement initiation: specification of arm direction and extent. *J. Exp. Psychol. Gen.*, 109: 444–474.

Rosenbaum, D.A., Loukopoulos, L.D., Meulenbroek, R.G.J., Vaughan, J. and Engelbrecht, S.E. (1995) Planning reaches by evaluating stored postures. *Psychol. Rev.*, 102: 28–67.

Rossetti, Y., Stelmach, G., Desmurget, M., Prablanc, C. and Jeannerod, M. (1994) The effect of viewing the static hand prior to movement onset on pointing kinematics and variability. *Exp. Brain Res.*, 10: 323–330.

Rossetti, Y., Desmurget, M. and Prablanc, C. (1995) Vectorial coding of movement: vision proprioception or both?. *J. Neurophysiol.*, 74(1): 457–463.

Scarchilli, K., Vercher, J.L., Gauthier, G.M. and Cole, J. (1999) Does the oculo-manual co-ordination control system use an internal model of the arm dynamics? *Neurosci. Lett.*, 265: 139–142.

Schweighofer, N., Arbib, M.A. and Kawato, M. (1998a) Role of the cerebellum in reaching movements in humans, I. Distributed inverse dynamics control. *Eur. J. Neurosci.*, 10: 86–94.

Schweighofer, N., Spoelstra, J., Arbib, M.A. and Kawato, M. (1998b) Role of the cerebellum in reaching movements in humans, II. A neural model of the intermediate cerebellum. *Eur. J. Neurosci.*, 10: 95–105.

Shebilske, W.L. (1976) Extraretinal information in corrective saccades and inflow vs outflow theories of visual direction constancy. *Vis. Res.*, 16: 621–628.

Snyder, L.H., Batista, A.P. and Andersen, R.A. (2000) Saccade-related activity in the parietal reach region. *J. Neurophysiol.*, 83: 1099–1102.

Soechting, J.F. and Lacquaniti, F. (1983) Modification of trajectory of a pointing movement in response to a change in target location. *J. Neurophysiol.*, 49: 548–564.

Spoelstra, J., Schweighofer, N. and Arbib, M.A. (2000) Cerebellar learning of accurate predictive control for fast-reaching movements. *Biol. Cybern.*, 82: 321–333.

Ungerleider, L.G. and Mishkin, M. (1982) Two cortical visual systems. In: D.J. Ingle, M.A. Goodale and R.J.W. Mansfield (Eds.), *Analysis of Visual Behavior*. MIT Press, Cambridge, MA, pp. 549–586.

Van Donkelaar, P. (1997) Eye–hand interactions during goal-directed pointing movements. *Neuroreport*, 8: 2139–2142.

Van Donkelaar, P., Lee, J.H. and Drew, A.S. (2000) Transcranial magnetic stimulation disrupts eye–hand interactions in the posterior parietal cortex. *J. Neurophysiol.*, 84: 1677–1680.

Vercher, J.L., Magenes, G., Prablanc, C. and Gauthier, G.M. (1994) Eye–head–hand coordination in pointing at visual targets: spatial and temporal analysis. *Exp. Brain Res.*, 99: 507–523.

Vercher, J.-L., Sarès, F., Blouin, J., Bourdin C. and Gauthier, G. (2003) Role of sensory information in updating internal models of the effector during arm tracking. In: C. Prablanc, D. Pélisson and Y. Rossetti (Eds.), *Neural Control of Space Coding and Action Production*. *Progress in Brain Research*, Vol. 142. Elsevier, Amsterdam, pp. 203–222 (this volume).

Vindras, P., Desmurget, M., Prablanc, C. and Viviani, P. (1998) Pointing errors reflect biases in the perception of the initial hand position. *J. Neurophysiol.*, 79: 3290–3294.

Wolpert, D.M., Ghahramani, Z. and Jordan, M.I. (1995) An internal model for sensorimotor integration. *Science*, 269: 1880–1882.

C. Prablanc, D. Pélisson and Y. Rossetti (Eds.)
Progress in Brain Research, Vol. 142
© 2003 Elsevier Science B.V. All rights reserved

CHAPTER 11

Internal forward models in the cerebellum: fMRI study on grip force and load force coupling

Mitsuo Kawato [1,*], Tomoe Kuroda [2], Hiroshi Imamizu [1], Eri Nakano [1], Satoru Miyauchi [3] and Toshinori Yoshioka [1]

[1] *ATR Human Information Science Laboratories, 2-2-2, Hikaridai, Seika-cho, Soraku-gun, Kyoto 619-0288, Japan*
[2] *JST/ERATO Kawato Dynamic Brain Project, 2-2-2, Hikaridai, Seika-cho, Soraku-gun, Kyoto 619-0288, Japan*
[3] *Communications Research Laboratory, 588-2, Iwaoka, Iwaoka-cho, Nishi-ku, Kobe, Hyogo 651-2492, Japan*

Abstract: Internal models are neural mechanisms that can mimic the input–output or output–input properties of the motor apparatus and external objects. Forward internal models predict sensory consequences from efference copies of motor commands. There is growing acceptance of the idea that forward models are important in sensorimotor integration as well as in higher cognitive function, but their anatomical loci and neural mechanisms are still largely unknown. Some of the most convincing evidence that the central nervous system (CNS) makes use of forward models in sensory motor control comes from studies on grip force–load force coupling. We first present a brief review of recent computational and behavioral studies that provide decisive evidence for the utilization of forward models in grip force–load force coupling tasks. Then, we used functional magnetic resonance imaging (fMRI) to measure the brain activity related to this coupling and demonstrate that the cerebellum is the most likely site for forward models to be stored.

Introduction

Internal models are neural mechanisms located inside the brain that can mimic the input–output properties of the motor apparatus and external objects (located outside the brain), or their inverse transformations. Forward internal models predict sensory consequences of executed movements from information on efference copies of motor commands, whereas inverse internal models determine the appropriate motor commands from information on the desired motor consequences. Several computational theories have proposed that forward and/or inverse models are learned in the cerebellum (Kawato et al., 1987; Kawato and Gomi, 1992; Miall et al., 1993; Wolpert et al., 1998; Kawato, 1999).

We have accumulated quite convincing data from both electrophysiological studies (Shidara et al., 1993; Gomi et al., 1998; Kitazawa et al., 1998; Kobayashi et al., 1998; Takemura et al., 2001; Yamamoto et al., 2002) and human imaging studies (Imamizu et al., 2000) demonstrating that inverse models are acquired through motor learning based on Purkinje cell synaptic plasticity and stored in the cerebellum. Even though many behavioral (Miall et al., 1993; Wolpert et al., 1995; Flanagan and Wing, 1997; Scarchilli and Vercher, 1999; Mehta and Schaal, 2002) and theoretical studies (Kawato et al., 1987; Jordan and Rumelhert, 1992; Miall et

* Correspondence to: Mitsuo Kawato, ATR Human Information Science Laboratories, 2-2-2, Hikaridai, Seika-cho, Soraku-gun, Kyoto 619-0288, Japan. Tel.: +81-774-95-1058; Fax: +81-774-95-2647;
E-mail: kawato@atr.co.jp

al., 1993; Wolpert and Kawato, 1998; Kawato, 1999) have suggested that forward models are functionally and computationally critical for a broad repertoire of behaviors ranging from sensorimotor integration to higher cognitive function, the anatomical loci and neural mechanisms of forward models are still largely unknown. In addition to their use in sensory–motor control, Blakemore et al. (1998, 1999, 2001)) demonstrated that forward models are used for cancellation of sensory inputs generated by one's own movements; in this series of elegant perceptual studies, they suggested that the forward models are located in the cerebellum (see also Vercher et al., 2003, this volume).

Some of the most convincing evidence showing that the CNS makes use of forward models in sensory–motor control comes from studies on grip force–load force coupling. Grip force–load force coupling is a common phenomenon that has been observed in the following situation. When an object is held in a precision grip (e.g. a grasp between the tips of the thumb and forefinger) and moved by voluntary movements (e.g. arm movements), the grip force perpendicular to the contact surfaces changes in phase with, and in a similar temporal waveform to, the load force induced by the movements (Johansson and Westling, 1984; Flanagan and Tresilian, 1994; Johansson, 1996). The coupling between the two forces prevents the object from slipping while using the minimal grip force. This grip force modulation is anticipatory in the sense that changes in the grip force occur at the same time as, or even prior to, changes in the load force.

Previously we proposed computational models that explain grip force–load force coupling with forward models (Kawato, 1999), and their predictions have been confirmed by recent behavioral studies (Flanagan and Wing, 1996; Flanagan et al., 2003). Here, we summarize these previous computational and behavioral studies that demonstrate the utilization of forward models in grip force–load force coupling. Then, we present a functional magnetic resonance imaging (fMRI) experiment that investigates the possible brain loci of the forward models used for the coupling and suggest that the cerebellum is the likeliest site.

Computational models and behavioral experiments that support the use of forward models in grip force–load force coupling

We first briefly explain a simple example of grip force–load force coupling to facilitate clear understanding of the phenomenon. In preparation for the fMRI experiment, we measured grip force and load force outside the MRI scanner to confirm that the two forces were coupled in the current task paradigm (Fig. 1). A subject lay down in a supine position and made cyclic up-and-down arm movements paced by beep sounds (2 Hz) while holding a ping-pong ball between the tips of the thumb and forefinger. At each beep, the subject made a set of up and down strokes above the abdomen. The LED marker of a position recording system (OPTOTRAK, Northern Digital, Inc., Canada) was mounted on top of the object. The marker's vertical position was sampled at 500 Hz. We obtained the object's acceleration due to arm movement by twice differentiating the time series of the position data. Load force was then calculated as the absolute value of the product of the object's acceleration and mass (0.015 kg), where acceleration was the sum of the acceleration due to movement and gravitational acceleration. Grip force was measured by small and light pressure gauges (PS-10KA, Kyowa Electronic Instruments Co., Japan) attached to the contact surfaces. The amplitude of the arm movements was 30–40 cm. Because grip force is coupled with the absolute value of load force, it had two peaks coinciding with the acceleration and deceleration peaks of the arm movement within one cycle. Thus with a 2 Hz movement, the primary frequency of the grip force (solid line in Fig. 1B) and load force modulation was 4 Hz (dotted line in Fig. 1B). As has been reported in numerous studies (Johansson and Westling, 1984; Flanagan and Tresilian, 1994; Johansson, 1996), the grip force was temporally coupled with the load force during movement, and a cross-correlation analysis indicated that the phase of the grip force preceded that of the load force by approximately 15 ms with a correlation coefficient of 0.88. These values are in close agreement with previously reported values for cyclic movement (Flanagan and Wing, 1995).

Previous studies on grip force–load force coupling have suggested that both feedback (Johansson

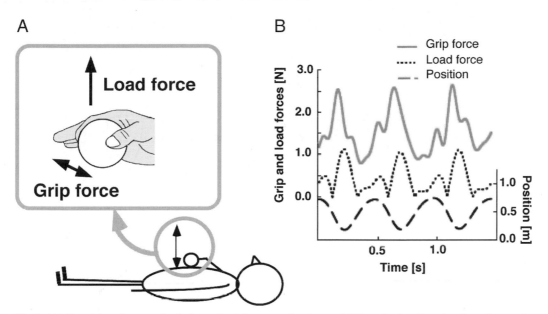

Fig. 1. (A) Experimental setup of grip force–load force coupling in our fMRI study. A subject lay down in a supine position and made cyclic up-and-down arm movements above the abdomen while holding a ping-pong ball between the tips of the thumb and forefinger. (B) A subject's sample record of the temporal pattern of grip force (solid line), load force (dotted line) and vertical position (broken line) of the grasped object. Grip force and load force coupling were observed while transporting a ping-pong ball.

and Westling, 1984) and feedforward (Flanagan and Tresilian, 1994) components are necessary for controlling grip force. Feedback control is important for establishing a stable grip force/load force ratio and for responding to unexpected disturbances, while feedforward control is important for rapid, predictive and accurate coupling of grip force to load force during movement. The fact that the change in grip force precedes the change in load force suggests that pure sensory feedback, which has large (70 ms) time delays, cannot be the sole source of grip force modulation. Therefore the CNS predicts changes in load force to modulate grip force.

There may be a number of computational and neural models that can explain the observed grip force–load force coupling. However, because of the above mentioned predictive nature of grip force modulation, we can assume that either forward or inverse models, or a combination of the two, are utilized in grip–load coupling. Accordingly, there are three models that can potentially explain the observed grip force–load force coupling (Fig. 2). The first model (Fig. 2A) consists of a single inverse dynamics model (IDM) of the combined arm, hand and object dynamics. The combined IDM generates

the arm motor command as well as the hand motor command. For generation of hand motor commands, this model is not computationally attractive since the entire IDM must be relearned every time a different hand grasping posture is taken and a different object is manipulated. In other words, this model has the least structural and functional modularity with respect to separation of object manipulation, hand posture control and arm movement control. This model is the least economically compatible in terms of the number of modules required when it is combined with the MOSAIC structure, that contains multiple models (Wolpert and Kawato, 1998). The second model shown in Fig. 2B has modularity between arm and hand control. The IDM of the arm and object generates the motor command for the arm while receiving the desired trajectory information. The object's IDM predicts the load force necessary to transport the object along the desired trajectory. This load force information is fed to the grip force controller, which generates the hand motor commands required for the grip force that is proportional to the predicted load force. Specifically, the future load force is computed by the object's IDM, which is divided by a friction coefficient and multiplied by

174

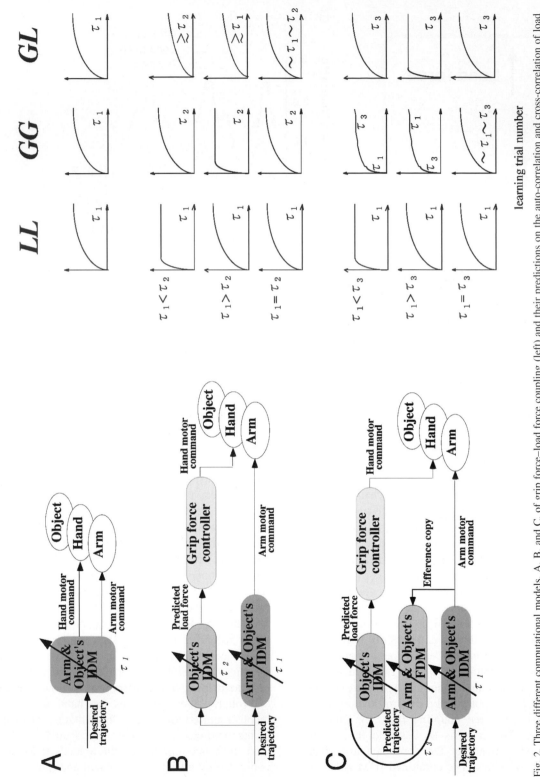

Fig. 2. Three different computational models, A, B, and C, of grip force–load force coupling (left) and their predictions on the auto-correlation and cross-correlation of load (L) and grip (G) forces (right). Only the third model shown in C utilizes the forward model.

a safety factor to derive an appropriate future grip force. Finally, this necessary force is realized in a predictive manner by the grip force controller.

Kawato (1999) proposed the computational model of grip force–load force coupling shown in Fig. 2C. In this framework, the IDM of the combined dynamics of the arm, hand, and object calculates the appropriate arm motor commands from the desired trajectory of the arm. This command is sent to the arm muscles as well as to the forward model of the combined dynamics of the arm, hand, and object as an efference copy (see also Flanagan and Wing, 1997). The forward model predicts the arm trajectory 50 to 100 ms in the future. From this predicted arm trajectory, a hand motor command is generated in the same way as for the model shown in B. The third model has the largest modularity and utilizes both forward and inverse models of the arm and object. Its extension to multiple models in the framework of MOSAIC (Wolpert and Kawato, 1998) was also proposed by Kawato (1999) so that multiple-object manipulation could be easily switched. Even in the models of B and C, the IDM of the combined arm and object should be relearned or switched every time when a new object is grasped. However, this combined IDM is used for only arm control in B and C, and arm motor commands are less influenced by different object characteristics than hand motor commands, while hand motor command should be drastically altered for different objects. The MOSAIC architecture is best suited for the computational model C, because both the forward and inverse models are utilized, and the learning of object IDM for hand motor command generation is decoupled from learning of arm dynamics.

From the viewpoint of grasp control, the essential difference between models B and C is that the former uses the desired arm trajectory in computing the necessary grip force while the latter uses the arm trajectory estimated by the forward model. If the environment is a well-learned one, the desired arm trajectory is accurately realized and should be similar to the estimated trajectory. Therefore, the behaviors of the two kinds of models are similar and cannot be discriminated between. However, for novel environments that are not well controlled, the desired trajectory and the predicted trajectory could be very different, allowing us to discriminate between the

three models. In particular, if one assumes that the forward model is learned more rapidly than the inverse model, an idea consistent with the MOSAIC model, then one would expect good coupling between grip force and load force before good control over the movement trajectory is established.

The right side of Fig. 2 shows predictions of the three models in terms of how three different correlations — involving grip and load forces — will change when learning to manipulate an object with novel dynamics. These correlations are the correlation between load force in a given trial with load force after adaptation (LL), the correlation between grip force in a given trial and grip force after adaptation (GG), and the correlation between the grip force and load force in a given trial. By definition, both LL and GG start from a low value and increase to 1 as learning progresses. From previous studies on grip force–load force coupling, we know that GL takes a high value in the late stages of learning when subjects are well experienced at manipulating the objects (Flanagan and Wing, 1997).

For the single IDM of model A, LL, GG and GL, as shown in the right side of Fig. 2A, should all have a similar rate of increase because a single common neural network generates both hand and arm motor commands as a single unit. If the load dynamics are highly altered, compared with objects subjects are familiar with, the novel dynamics alter the realized trajectory, and induce different acceleration patterns, thus altering the load-force time course while the grip-force time course is inappropriate for the new object and starts from the old pattern for a familiar object. Therefore, at the early stage of learning, GL is low, but as learning progresses both the arm and hand motor commands become appropriate for the new object dynamics, and GL approaches a high value.

Quantitative details of predictions made by model B depend on the relative lengths of the learning time constants of the combined object and arm IDM and the object IDM. The LL-increase time course is determined solely by the learning rate of the combined IDM of arm and object (τ_1), while the GG-increase time course is determined solely by the learning rate of the object IDM (τ_2). At the early phase of learning, after a new object dynamic is imposed, GL is low because the load-force time course is altered, as in A. As learning progresses, both the combined IDM and object IDM become better models of the controlled objects, and GL increases for two reasons. First, due to combined IDM learning, the desired arm trajectory is better realized and the load force approaches that predicted from the desired trajectory. Secondly, the predicted grip force becomes closer to that required with the new dynamics for the actual arm trajectory because the object IDM improves, and the final realized trajectory approaches the desired trajectory. Consequently, the time course of GL-increase is governed by both of the two time constants of the two IDM learning rates (τ_1 and τ_2). This can also be seen from the block diagram of model B, since GL is the correlation computed through the cascade of the two IDMs (Fig. 2B).

For the third model, C, GL is determined by the third time constant (τ_3) of the forward model of the arm and object as well as the object IDM because the predicted arm trajectory can be close to the actual trajectory even if it is greatly distorted only if the forward model is good. On the other hand, GG is governed by both the third time constant (τ_3) and the first time constant (τ_1), because the grip-force time course is determined by the cascade of all four elements in C (combined IDM and FDM, object IDM, and grip controller). Quantitative details of the time courses of LL, GG and GL differ depending on relative lengths of the learning time constants of each of the different elements within these models. However, regardless of this we can make some qualitative predictions. For the model A, the GL rise rate is exactly the same as those of GG and LL. For the model B, the GL rise rate is not larger than that of either LL or GG. Only model C can have a GL rise rate higher than that of LL. This will occur if the learning rate of the combined IDM (τ_1) is slower than that of the forward model (τ_3). As described below, recent experimental data unequivocally support model C's predictions, and the utilization of forward models is strongly supported.

Behavioral studies done by Flanagan and Wing (1996, 1997) supported model C. In their experiments, they changed the dynamics of manipulated objects by using a one-degree-of-freedom robotic manipulator. This alternation of the object's dynamics significantly disrupted both the hand trajectory and the grip force–load force coupling. Even in

these novel situations generated by inertia, viscous, or spring force, grip and load forces became closely coupled after a relatively small number of learning trials, whereas the learning of the hand trajectory was much slower. In other words, during early learning trials, good grip force–load force coupling was quickly acquired even though the arm velocity profile was irregular and poorly controlled. One of the limitations of these studies is that grip–load correlations were examined across learning trials where the load force waveform was changing. Recently, Flanagan et al. (2003) dealt with this potential confound by having subjects produce trajectories — after having adapted to the novel load — that were similar to those observed in early learning. They found that after some four learning trials, subjects generated grip–load coupling that was similar to that observed after adaptation and for similar movements (and hence load force waveforms). Consequently, utilization of forward models in grip force–load force coupling is well established. Based on this, we have explored the possible sites of forward models through fMRI experiments.

Materials and methods

Subjects

Three females (ranging in age from 25 to 31) and three males (from 27 to 43) participated in the experiment after giving written informed consent. The protocol was approved by the ethics committee of CRL. All subjects were right-handed.

Task and procedure

The transporting task shown in Fig. 1A includes three components: arm movement control, grip force modulation, and coordination of arm movement and grip force. Therefore, if we remove the first two components, we can extract the brain activity exclusively related to coordination or, more specifically, to forward models. We used a 2 by 2 factorial design of tasks to compare neural activity under conditions with and without arm movement and with and without grip force modulation (Fig. 3). Accordingly, the experimental tasks were (A) transporting an object, (B) loaded arm movement, (C) grip force modula-

Grip Force Modulation

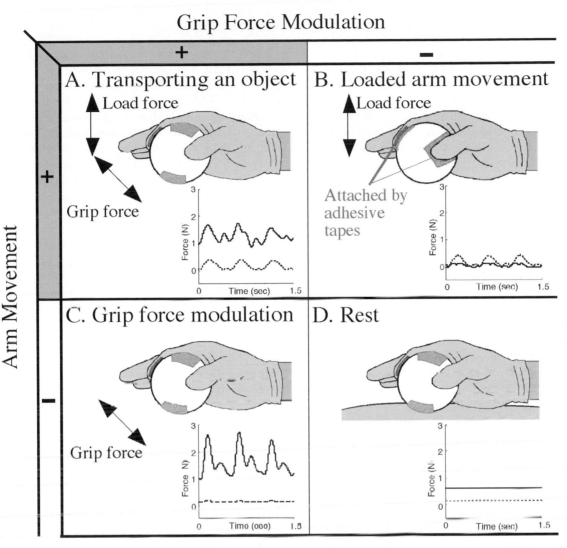

Fig. 3. A 2 × 2 factorial design (with/without arm movement/grip force modulation) of four tasks in the fMRI experiment. The solid lines in the inset boxes depict temporal patterns of grip force, and the dotted lines depict temporal patterns of load force. These measurements were made during behavioral experiments performed outside of the MRI scanner under similar experimental conditions (see section 'Materials and methods').

tion, and (D) rest. In all four tasks, the subjects wore a glove. In the transport and loaded arm movement tasks, movement amplitude was 20–25 cm because of the limited workspace in the gantry. The glove did not alter the basic coupling between grip force and load force (compare Fig. 1 and the inset of Fig. 3A). The loaded arm movement task was similar to the transport task except that the object was attached at the tips of the thumb and forefinger by removable adhesive tape. In this case, grip force modulation is not necessary, and the actual grip force modulation was very small as shown by the solid line in the inset of Fig. 3B. In retrospective inquiries, subjects reported that they were not conscious about the absence of grip force modulation in the loaded arm movement task. Thus, it is unlikely that some kinds of voluntary suppression of grip force in the loaded arm movement condition took place, and this factor influenced brain imaging data. The pressure gauges were attached to the glove underneath the adhesive tape rather than on the ping-pong ball to avoid any artifact caused by the adhesive tape. During the grip force modulation condition, the subjects held the object in the same grip as in the transport task and periodically changed the grip force voluntarily at 4 Hz (see the inset of Fig. 3C). They were instructed to produce a larger grip force than in the transport task. In the rest period, they made no overt movements. For brevity, the three task conditions A, B and C will be called transport, arm and grasp movements, respectively.

The dynamics of both arm movement and hand configuration were similar in the two arm-movement tasks (A and B) because the object was attached to the fingers during loaded arm movement. Thus, arm motor commands, hand motor commands for hand and finger postural maintenance, and the proprioceptive feedback would also be expected to be similar in these two tasks. Furthermore, the preliminary measurement outside the scanner confirmed that grip force changes that occurred during the grip force modulation task were as large as, or larger than, changes during the transport task (compare the insets of Fig. 3A and 3C). Consequently, finger tactile feedbacks due to modulation of grip forces perpendicular to contact surfaces would be expected to be similar in these two tasks (A and C). Because volitional control of grip force in the grip force modulation task (C) may be more demanding than automatic adjustment of the force in the transport task (A), the subtraction of the signal values in the grasping task from those in the transport task could cause an underestimation of the brain activity related to components other than the grasping component in the transport. However, more importantly it is unlikely that such activation was overestimated.

Each subject performed the tasks with her or his dominant, right arm and hand. Their heads were fixed by using individually molded bite bars. An experimental session consisted of four blocks; in each block, and for all subjects, each of the four task periods occurred for 35.2 s in the fixed order of A, B, C and D as shown in Fig. 3. The subjects prepared for the task during the first 4.4 s of each task period, and performed the task for the successive 30.8 s. Eight functional image volumes of the whole brain were acquired in each task period. Thus, total 128 volumes were acquired in each session.

Brain imaging

A 1.5 T Magnetom Vision system (Siemens, Erlangen) was used to acquire both sixteen axial gradient-echo, echo-planar $T2^*$ weighted image volumes [TR = 4.4 s, TE = 66 ms, flip angle = 90°, thickness = 7 mm, slice gap = 2.8 mm, in-plane resolution = 2 mm × 2 mm] and T1 weighted structural image volumes for anatomical co-registration [TR = 560 ms, TE = 6 ms, flip angle = 90°, thickness = 7 mm, slice gap = 2.8 mm, in-plane resolution = 1 mm × 1 mm]. Each session began with two 'dummy' scans, the data of which were discarded to allow for T1 equilibration effects. Each subject participated in six separate sessions of functional imaging. All the multiple session data were analyzed at once in the following two methods. Session-specific effects were modeled and removed as confounding effects in the general linear model explained below.

Analyses

We used SPM99 [http://www.fil.ion.ucl.ac.uk/spm] for all of the preprocessing and statistical inference procedures except motion correction. To remove motion artifacts, all volumes of each functional imaging session were realigned to the reference, the 65th volume, by using AIR3.08 [http://bishopw. loni.ucla.edu/AIR3]. After that, they were stereotactically normalized using affine and nonlinear transformation and then resampled using sinc interpolation into the space of a standard brain. The volumes were then smoothed with a Gaussian kernel of 4 mm full-width half-maximum (FWHM). The first two image volumes of each task period were regarded as a preparation phase and discarded in order to avoid the effects of task transition, and six other volumes were regarded as a test phase. High-frequency noises were removed with a Gaussian filter (FWHM = 4 s).

Condition and session effects were estimated according to the general linear model at each and every voxel with delayed boxcar waveforms. To investigate regionally specific condition effects of interest, the estimated coefficients were compared using appropriately weighted linear contrasts (Friston et al., 1995). In the first half of the analyses to obtain transport > rest, grasp > rest, and arm > rest con-

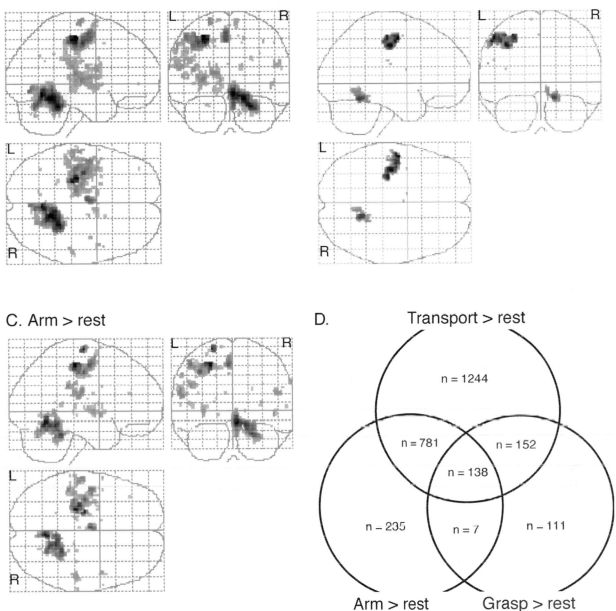

A. Transport > rest

B. Grasp > rest

C. Arm > rest

D.

Transport > rest

n = 1244

n = 781   n = 152

n = 138

n – 235   n = 7   n – 111

Arm > rest   Grasp > rest

Fig. 4. Statistical parametrical maps (SPM*t*) illustrating activation loci of transport > rest (A), grasp > rest (B) and arm > rest (C). Topography of brain regions related to transport movements (A), grasp movements (B) and loaded arm movements (C) are expected to be revealed by these contrasts. (D) The numbers of voxels.

trasts (Fig. 4) and transport > arm and transport > grasp contrasts (Figs. 5 and 6), a conjunction analysis across subjects (Friston et al., 1999) was applied to find common activation to the subjects at

the threshold of 5% corrected for multiple comparisons.

In the latter half of the analysis, the so-called factorial analysis was carried out to identify co-

A. Transport > Arm

B. Transport > Grasp

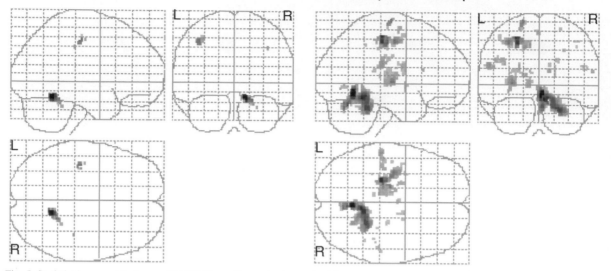

Fig. 5. Statistical parametrical maps (SPM*t*) illustrating activation loci of the transport > arm (A) and transport > grasp (B).

ordination-related brain regions (Fig. 8A). Namely, coordination-related areas were investigated in terms of the interaction between arm movement and grip force modulation effects: (a-b)–(c-d) (a, transport; b, loaded arm; c, grip force modulation; and d, rest). The resulting set of voxel values for each contrast constitutes a statistical parametric map of the *t* statistic, SPM*t*. Here, conjunction analysis was not utilized, and SPM99b was used.

Results

Fig. 4A–C shows the topography of brain regions related to object transport, grip force modulation and loaded arm movement, respectively. More specifically, they show statistical parametric maps (SPM*t*) illustrating the activation loci of transport > rest (A), grasp > rest (B), and arm > rest (C). The main effect of transport movement (Fig. 4A) was observed in many cerebral cortical areas including the bilateral sensory–motor cortices, bilateral premotor cortices, bilateral SMA, bilateral inferior frontal gyri, left middle frontal gyrus, bilateral cingulate gyri, bilateral inferior parietal lobules, right intraparietal sulcus, and bilateral insula (Table 1). The activity was also observed in the bilateral thalamus, basal ganglia, and cerebellum. In cerebral cortical areas, the thalamus and in the basal ganglia, activity was

stronger in the contralateral (left) hemispheres to the using hand. This was not the case in the parietal cortex. However, the cerebellum had much stronger ipsilateral activation (Table 1). The main effect of grip force modulation (Fig. 4B) revealed activity in the left primary sensorimotor cortex, left premotor cortex, left SMA, left insula, and right anterior cerebellum, which are mainly small subsets of brain loci activated during transport movements. The primary effect of loaded arm movement (Fig. 4C) revealed activity in a wide range of regions including the left primary motor cortex, left premotor cortex, left SMA, bilateral postcentral gyri, inferior and middle frontal gyri, left cingulate gyrus, bilateral inferior parietal lobules, bilateral insula, bilateral thalamus, left basal ganglia, and the right anterior cerebellum, which are mainly large subsets of brain loci activated during transport movements.

Fig. 4D shows the numbers of activated voxels examined in the above three SPM contrasts in the format of the Venn diagram. One might first note that the number of activated voxels for transport movement was by far the largest, that for the loaded arm movement was medium, and that for the grasp was the smallest. A large portion (79%) of the arm-activated voxels was also activated in transport movement. Similarly, a large portion (71%) of the grasp-activated voxels was also activated in transport

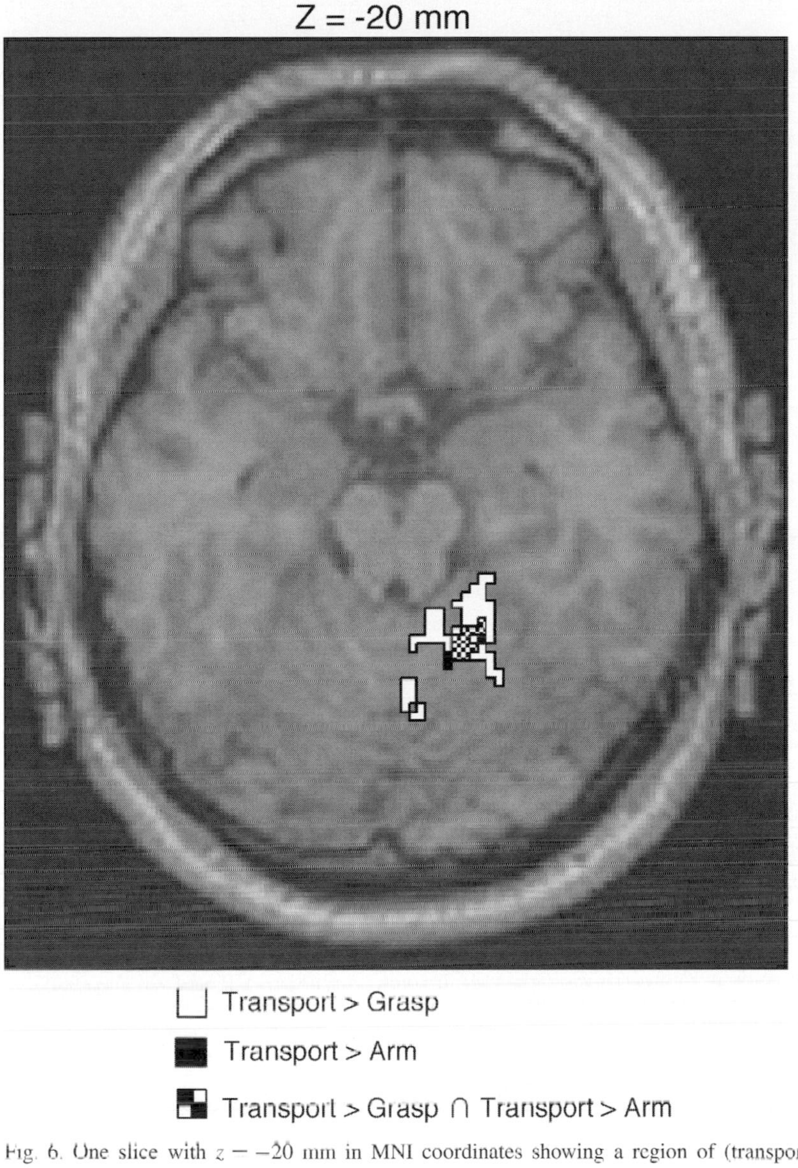

Z = -20 mm

⬜ Transport > Grasp

⬛ Transport > Arm

▨ Transport > Grasp ∩ Transport > Arm

Fig. 6. One slice with $z = -20$ mm in MNI coordinates showing a region of (transport > grasp) and (transport > arm) in the right anterior cerebellum. The open area shows the voxels that were more activated in transport than in grasp. The filled area shows the voxels that were more activated in transport than in arm. The mosaic area shows the conjunction of these two areas.

movement. On the other hand, a large portion (54%) of the transport-activated voxels was not activated in either arm or grasp movement.

Fig. 5 shows voxels that were more activated in transport than in loaded arm movement and those that were more activated in transport than in grasp movement, respectively. As expected from the results of Fig. 4, only the left primary motor cortex, right postcentral gyrus, and right anterior cerebellum were more activated in transport movements than in arm movements (Fig. 5A and Table 2). On the other hand, many brain loci, including the left primary motor cortex, left premotor cortex, left SMA, bilateral postcentral gyri, right inferior frontal gyrus, left cingulate gyrus, bilateral inferior parietal lobules, left thalamus, bilateral basal ganglia, and right anterior cerebellum, were more activated in transport than in grasp movements (Fig. 5B and Table 2).

TABLE 1

Principal areas of activation related to three movement tasks compared with the rest condition

	Transport > rest				Grasp > rest				Arm > rest			
	MNI coordinates			t value	MNI coordinates			t value	MNI coordinates			t value
L. BA4	−28	−22	54	10.24	−38	−18	44	5.00	−24	−26	52	9.03
R. BA4	38	−6	48	2.13								
L. BA6	−22	−16	72	4.06	−10	0	72	1.59	−22	−16	70	7.03
R. BA6	8	2	72	2.68								
L. SMA	−4	−8	56	6.00	−2	−4	54	1.64	−4	−10	52	5.17
R. SMA	10	−2	54	1.54								
L. postcentral gyrus	−54	−24	18	3.41	−58	−18	22	1.78	−58	−18	24	3.60
R. postcentral gyrus	58	−24	16	1.80					48	−26	22	3.21
L. inferior frontal gyrus	−52	−2	8	2.73					−60	4	28	2.04
R. inferior frontal gyrus									60	4	4	1.66
L. middle frontal gyrus	−40	48	0	1.96					−38	34	20	1.73
L. cingulate gyrus	−22	−10	42	1.64					−18	−10	40	1.68
R. cingulate gyrus	14	10	46	1.61								
L. inferior parietal lobule	−52	−34	48	2.40					−46	−34	28	3.59
R. inferior parietal lobule	52	−28	20	2.79					56	−26	26	1.60
R. intraparietal sulcus	26	−56	26	1.56								
L. insula	−40	2	16	3.25	−38	0	16	1.63	−44	−4	4	1.77
R. insula	46	4	−2	2.61					46	2	−4	2.72
L. thalamus	−18	−22	12	4.18					−18	−12	14	1.56
R. thalamus	14	−8	20	2.16					14	−28	0	1.57
L. basal ganglia	−28	−14	6	3.84					−32	−6	−2	3.06
R. basal ganglia	14	0	16	1.63								
R. cerebellum	14	−50	−16	10.35	16	−54	−18	3.76	6	−58	−12	7.85
L. cerebellum	−24	−42	−24	1.98								

$p < 0.05$, corrected. Activation peaks are reported in MNI coordinates. The MNI coordinates and t scores (degrees of freedom = 4481) for maxima of activations are presented. R and L indicate the right hemisphere and left hemisphere, respectively.

TABLE 2

Principal activations related to the transport task compared with two other movement tasks

	Transport > arm				Transport > grasp			
	MNI coordinates			t value	MNI coordinates			t value
L. BA4	−40	−20	48	2.24	−26	−26	54	6.32
L. BA6					−18	−16	72	3.65
L. SMA					−2	−8	60	1.98
L. postcentral gyrus					−56	−26	20	2.59
R. postcentral gyrus	38	−28	40	1.86	50	−28	22	2.00
R. inferior frontal gyrus					60	20	16	1.91
L. cingulate gyrus					−16	−24	44	2.54
L. inferior parietal lobule					−40	−26	28	2.26
R. inferior parietal lobule					44	−32	50	1.76
L. thalamus					−22	−4	20	2.43
L. basal ganglia					−30	−14	2	3.59
R. basal ganglia					12	0	18	2.04
R. cerebellum	12	−54	−16	3.44	2	−58	−12	7.84

$p < 0.05$, corrected. Activation peaks are reported in MNI coordinates.

When we consider the conjunction of Fig. 5, then activated voxels were found only in the right anterior and superior cerebellum. That is, voxels that were simultaneously more activated in transport than in grasp movements, and more activated in transport than in arm movements were only found to exist in the cerebellum. Fig. 6 shows these activated voxels in the cerebellum at the slice of $z = -20$ mm of MNI coordinates. Here, the open areas show the voxels that were more activated in transport than in grasp. The filled areas show the voxels that were more activated in transport than in arm movement. The mosaic areas show the conjunction of these two areas and indicate the voxels that were simultaneously more activated in transport than in grasp and more activated in transport than in arm movement. The number of these conjointly activated voxels was 37.

The region of interest was defined as the above conjointly activated areas (mosaic, 37 voxels), and the relative blood oxygen level dependent (BOLD) signal increase compared with the rest condition was averaged over all voxels across all subjects. Fig. 7 shows that the BOLD signal increase was the largest for transport movements, slightly smaller for arm movements, and the smallest for grasp movements.

Finally, the coordination-related area was identified by the factorial analysis, which was explained in the latter half of the method. As shown in Fig. 8, the left biventer in the cerebellum was the only region identified as having a statistically significant relation to coordination (uncorrected $p < 10^{-4}$ for each voxel, larger than 62 voxels for cluster, corrected $p < 0.05$).

Fig. 8B shows the relative BOLD signal in this region of interest (ROI). As shown in Fig. 8B, the mean BOLD signal in the ROI was higher under the rest condition (d) than under the other three conditions (a, b, and c); i.e. this region was deactivated by all movement tasks. The amount of deactivation by transporting task (a from d) was much smaller than the combined amount of deactivation by arm movement (b from d) and grip force modulation (c from d) tasks.

Discussion

Most regions related to arm movement and grip force modulation corresponded to those that were reported in many previous studies on simple hand or arm movement tasks (e.g. Fink et al., 1997). In particular, the coordinate of the peak t-score in grip force modulation (x, y, z in MNI coordinates: $-38, -18, 44$) in the primary sensorimotor cortex was located inferiorly and laterally to that found with arm movements ($-24, -26, 52$). This different location of peaks is congruent with the somatotopic organization of the hand and arm (Penfield and Rasmussen, 1950). Furthermore, in the anterior cerebellum the peak in grip force modulation ($16, -54, -18$) was located laterally to that found with arm movements ($6, -58, -12$). This difference in peak location is also congruent with previous findings that distal parts of the body are represented more laterally in the anterior cerebellum than more proximal parts of the body (Snider and Eldred, 1952; Grodd et al., 2001).

According to the computational model of grip force–load force coupling shown in Fig. 2C, the four different task conditions of Fig. 3 are expected to activate the three computational elements, the inverse model, the forward model and the grip force controller differently. None of the three elements is utilized in the rest condition. Only the grip force controller is activated for grip force modulation (grasp), and only the inverse model is activated for loaded arm movements (arm). On the other hand, all three

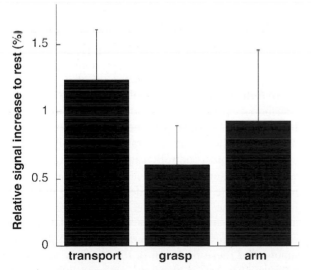

Fig. 7. Relative signal increase averaged across subjects in common regions of transport > grasp and transport > arm. Error bars show standard deviations between subjects.

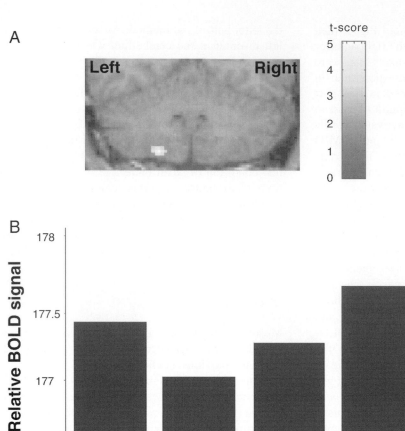

Fig. 8. Coordination-related activation superimposed on an anatomical coronal slice of a subject normalized to the MNI space. Only voxels with *t*-scores above 3.09 ($p < 10^{-4}$, uncorrected) were analyzed. We only found an active cluster of voxels in the left biventer of the cerebellum ($p < 0.05$, corrected on the basis of the random field theory). The MNI coordinates and *t*-score (df = 4481) for maxima of activations were −17, −58, −54 and 5.01. Adjusted BOLD contrast signals relative to the fitted mean in the cerebellar ROI related to coordination.

elements are utilized simultaneously for transport of the object. Consequently, with the transport > rest contrast shown in Fig. 4A, we expected to observe union of the activities of the three elements. For the grasp > rest contrast of Fig. 4B, activated voxels were assumed to contain activity of the grip force controller of Fig. 2C. Similarly, for the arm > rest contrast of Fig. 4C, we expected to observe activity related to the inverse model for arm. As Fig. 4D demonstrated, more than half of the activated voxels for the transport > rest contrast were not significantly more activated during either arm or grasp compared with the rest. Therefore, these voxels may contain activity of the forward model.

To further explore this possibility, the two contrasts transport > arm and transport > grasp were examined in Fig. 5. According to the computational model of Fig. 2C, the former contrast may reveal activity of the grip force controller and the forward model, while the latter may show activity of the inverse model and the forward model. Logically, the conjunction of the grip controller or the forward model and the inverse model or the forward model should reveal the locus of the forward model, and the conjunction of these is shown in Fig. 6. Only the small number of voxels in the right, anterior and superior cerebellum showed statistical significance, and may correspond to the forward model locus. The BOLD signal increase for this ROI (Fig. 7) is compatible with the hypothesis that the ROI contains the forward model used for grip force–load force coupling.

If one simply assumes that the BOLD signal increases induced by activation in the three elements of Fig. 2C are linearly added to each other, the transport signal increase would have to be larger than the summation of the grasp increase and the arm increase because the forward model increase must also be added. However, this simple expectation was apparently not met, as shown by the BOLD signal of the right anterior cerebellum in Fig. 7. Consequently, in parallel to the above conjunction analysis, we further explored the possible forward model locus by the factorial analysis (a-b)–(c-d), based on this linear addition assumption (a = transport; b = loaded arm; c = grip force modulation; and d = rest). With the linear addition assumption, (a-b)–(c-d) should reveal only the forward model activation. Using these assumptions, multiple regression analysis showed that the left biventer in the cerebellum could be the only statistically significantly activated region involved in arm movement–grip force coordination. The previous conjunction analysis did not show this second ROI because it was deactivated by all movement tasks. This deactivation is consistent with the results of previous research that reported that hand movement could deactivate the cerebellum contralateral to the employed hand (Allison et al., 2000). The amount of deactivation by the transporting task was much smaller than the amount of summation of deactivation by the two simple movement tasks. Furthermore, the second ROI was more activated in the transporting task than in the arm movement or grip force modulation task. Therefore, according to the linear addition assumption, this ROI can be regarded as a potential coordination related region.

The finding that the second ROI was in the left, i.e. contralateral, cerebellum strengthens the argument that this increased activation is related to coordination per se and not to grip force or arm movement control itself, since simple movements of a motor effector activate the anterior cerebellum ipsilaterally (Nitschke et al., 1996). Because most corticopontine projections and almost all cerebellar projections to the cerebral cortex are contralateral (Middleton and Strick, 1998), this activity in the left cerebellum during transport with the right hand is congruent with previous findings that lesions of the right cerebral cortex are often associated with ipsilateral impairments of complex sensorimotor tasks (Winstein and Pohl, 1995). More recently, Ehrsson et al. (2000) conducted an fMRI study with normal human subjects and found that the right cerebral cortex was engaged in a precision grip task performed with the right hand, although muscles of the left hand did not show reliable electromyogram (EMG) activity. Furthermore, Ehrsson et al. (2001) found that the right intraparietal cortex was more activated when subjects generate small grip forces than when they employ large grip forces. The small grip forces were representative of the forces that are typically used when manipulating small objects with precision grips in everyday situations. Thus, the left cerebellum together with the right cerebral cortex may be recruited in tasks more demanding than simple movement, in this case, coordination between the right arm and hand. Independently to the current work, Ehrsson et al. (2003) conducted a closely related fMRI experiment to examine cortical representations of coordinated grip and lift force control. Although their motivation was very similar to ours, the actual experimental paradigm was different. Their task was purely isometric and did not involve arm movement. The caudal two thirds of the cerebellum were not covered ($z > -22$ in the MNI standard space). They did not find any cerebellar activity in the coordination task compared with the other two tasks. They instead found that the coordination was specifically associated with activation of a posterior section of the right intraparietal cortex. The left biventar lobule activation, which we found, was outside their coverage, and might have anatomical connection with their right intraparietal cortex. Different experimental paradigms or different scanning coverage may explain the different results on right anterior cerebellum activity.

In summary, the same data were analyzed twice, in ways that are both expected to detect the additional activation due to coupled arm and grip action compared to either alone. The two analyses give different results, most spectacularly in that the cerebellar activation site shifts from right anterior cerebellum to left posterior. The different results obtained are due to different assumptions made in the two different analyses. In the first analysis, simple overlap between arm and grasp conditions was assumed small, which was quantitatively supported by Fig. 4D. In the second analysis, linear summation assumption of BOLD signals corresponding to different brain functions was made, which should be wrong in general. However, as Fig. 8B shows, the left biventar activation was certainly larger during transport than arm or grip, thus the analysis was validated. Consequently, our data and the two analysis methods suggested that the right, anterior and superior cerebellum and/or biventer in the left cerebellum were the only regions related to grip force–load force coupling.

We hypothesized that the coordination-related regions include the neural substrate of the internal forward model. The present results suggest that the right anterior and superior cerebellum and/or the left biventer may contain such forward models. This supports the prediction by previous computational theories (Kawato et al., 1987; Kawato and Gomi, 1992; Miall et al., 1993; Wolpert et al., 1998; Kawato, 1999) that forward models are located in the cerebellum.

Finally, we compared the locations of the first and the second ROIs revealed in our study with the cerebellar locations of interests, which are related to forward models (Blakemore et al., 2001; Miall et al., 2001). The first ROI in the right, anterior and superior cerebellum is located approximately 25 mm medial and 20 mm superior to the right superior cerebellar locus, which was found to be significantly correlated with the delay in the self-tickling task of Blakemore et al. (2001). Both studies involved right arm and hand movement, but ours involved grip force modulation while theirs involved perceptual modulation due to forward model prediction. Since cancellation of tactile sensation due to self-movement is thought to be more cognitive than grip force–load force coupling as motor coordination, the more lateral and inferior location of more cognitive forward models is not surprising. The second ROI, in the left biventar location in our study is about 15 mm medial and 20 mm inferior to the locus that was found to be correlated with asynchrony and independence of eye–hand coordination by Miall et al. (2001). Both studies involved right hand movements, but ours dealt with arm–hand coordination while theirs dealt with eye–hand coordination. Physically, the arm and hand are coupled more closely, and the

grip force–load force coupling tasks may be interpreted as a more basic form of motor coordination. Thus, it was not surprising to find the more sophisticated eye–hand coordination induced more lateral and more superior activation near the bottom of the left cerebellum.

In the current behavioral paradigm, the forward model predicts future arm movement and load force from the efference copy of the arm motor command. Recent studies have rigorously demonstrated that the cerebellum plays an essential role in the coordination of movements with multiple degrees of freedom (Bastian et al., 1996). In this study, we supported a specific computational model of coordination as shown in Fig. 2C. That is, we explained the coupling of grip force and load force by the mechanism where the forward model in the cerebellum predicts a trajectory of one motor effector (arm) and this prediction is used to control another motor effector (hand). Apparently, this computational framework can be generalized to arbitrary pairs of motor effectors such as eye and hand (Scarchilli and Vercher, 1999; Miall et al., 2000, 2001) and right and left hands; moreover, the framework might be considered a general principle of coordination.

Conclusions

The present experiment adopted a factorial deconvolution of the transporting task when subjects transported an object with a precision grip using the right arm and hand. The obtained imaging data suggested that the right, anterior and superior cerebellum and/or biventer in the left cerebellum were the only regions related to grip force–load force coupling. This agrees with previous findings that the right cerebral cortex is involved in more complex precision grip tasks than simple motor control while using the right hand. Furthermore, from a computational viewpoint, these cerebellar regions might contain forward models of arm movements.

References

Allison, J.D., Meador, K.J., Loring, D.W., Figueroa, R.E. and Wright, J.C. (2000) Functional MRI cerebral activation and deactivation during finger movement. *Neurology*, 54: 135–142.

Bastian, A.J., Martin, T.A., Keating, J.G. and Thach, W.T. (1996) Cerebellar ataxia: abnormal control of interaction torques across multiple joints. *J. Neurophysiol.*, 76: 492–509.

Blakemore, S.J., Wolpert, D.M. and Frith, C.D. (1998) Central cancellation of self-produced tickle sensation. *Nat. Neurosci.*, 1: 635–640.

Blakemore, S.J., Wolpert, D.M. and Frith, C.D. (1999) The cerebellum contributes to somatosensory cortical activity during self-produced tactile stimulation. *Neuroimage*, 10: 448–459.

Blakemore, S.J., Frith, C.D. and Wolpert, D.M. (2001) The cerebellum is involved in predicting the sensory consequences of action. *Neuroreport*, 12: 1879–1884.

Ehrsson, H.H., Fagergren, A., Jonsson, T., Westling, G., Johansson, R.S. and Forssberg, H. (2000) Cortical activity in precision versus power-grip tasks: an fMRI study. *J. Neurophysiol.*, 83: 528–536.

Ehrsson, H.H., Fagergren, A. and Forssberg, H. (2001) Differential fronto-parietal activation depending on force used in a precision grip task: an fMRI study. *J. Neurophysiol.*, 85: 2613–2623.

Ehrsson, H.H., Fagergren, A., Jonsson, T., Johansson, R.S. and Forssberg, H. (2003) Cortical representation of fingertip forces used in human manipulation: grip force, lift force and coordinated grip and lift forces. *J. Neurophysiol.*, submitted.

Fink, G.R., Frackowiak, R.S.J., Pietrzyk, U. and Passingham, R.E. (1997) Multiple nonprimary motor areas in the human cortex. *J. Neurophysiol.*, 77: 2164–2174.

Flanagan, J.R. and Tresilian, J.R. (1994) Grip–load force coupling: a general control strategy for transporting objects. *Exp. Psychol. Hum. Percept. Perform.*, 20: 944–957.

Flanagan, J.R. and Wing, A.M. (1995) The stability of precision grip force during cyclic arm movements with a hand-held load. *Exp. Brain Res.*, 105: 455–464.

Flanagan, J.R. and Wing, A.M. (1996) Internal models of dynamics in motor learning and control. *Soc. Neurosci. Abstr.*, 22(2): 897.

Flanagan, J.R. and Wing, A.M. (1997) The role of internal models in motion planning and control: evidence from grip force adjustments during movements of hand-held loads. *J. Neurosci.*, 17: 1519–1528.

Flanagan, J.R., Vetter, P., Johansson, R.S. and Wolpert, D.M. (2003) *Curr. Biol.*, in press.

Friston, K.J., Holmes, A.P., Worsley, K.J., Poline, J.P., Frith, C.D. and Frackowiak, R.S.J. (1995) Statistical parametric maps in functional imaging: A general linear approach. *Hum. Brain Mapp.*, 2: 189–210.

Friston, K.J., Holmes, A.P., Price, C.J., Buchel, C. and Worsley, K.J. (1999) Multisubject fMRI studies and conjunction analyses. *NeuroImage*, 10: 385–396.

Gomi, H. and Kawato, M. (1996) Equilibrium-point control hypothesis examined by measured arm-stiffness during multi--joint movement. *Science*, 272: 117–120.

Gomi, H., Shidara, M., Takemura, A., Inoue, Y., Kawano, K. and Kawato, M. (1998) Temporal firing patterns of Purkinje cells in the cerebellar ventral paraflocculus during ocular following responses in monkeys I. Simple spikes. *J. Neurophysiol.*, 80: 818–831.

Grodd, W., Hulsmann, E., Lotze, M., Wildgruber, D. and Erb, M. (2001) Sensorimotor mapping of the human cerebellum: fMRI evidence of somatotopic organization. *Hum. Brain Mapp.*, 13: 55–73.

Imamizu, H., Miyauchi, S., Tamada, T., Sasaki, Y., Takino, R., Putz, B., Yoshioka, T. and Kawato, M. (2000) Human cerebellar activity reflecting an acquired internal model of a new tool. *Nature*, 403: 192–195.

Johansson, R.S. (1996) Sensory control of dexterous manipulation in humans. In: A.M. Wing, P. Haggard and J.R. Flanagan (Eds.), *Hand and Brain: The Neurophysiology and Psychology of Hand Movements*. Academic, New York, pp. 381–414.

Johansson, R.S. and Westling, G. (1984) Roles of glabrous skin receptors and sensorimotor memory in automatic control of precision grip when lifting rougher or more slippery objects. *Exp. Brain Res.*, 56: 550–564.

Jordan, M.I. and Rumelhert, D.E. (1992) Forward models: Supervised learning with a distal teacher. *Cogn. Sci.*, 16: 307–354.

Kawato, M. (1999) Internal models for motor control and trajectory planning. *Curr. Opin. Neurobiol.*, 9: 718–727.

Kawato, M. and Gomi, H. (1992) The cerebellum and VOR/OKR learning models. *Trends Neurosci.*, 15: 445–453.

Kawato, M., Furukawa, K. and Suzuki, R. (1987) A hierarchical neural-network model for control and learning of voluntary movement. *Biol. Cybern.*, 57: 169–185.

Kitazawa, S., Kimura, T. and Yin, P.B. (1998) Cerebellar complex spikes encode both destinations and errors in arm movements. *Nature*, 392: 494–497.

Kobayashi, Y., Kawano, K., Takemura, A., Inoue, Y., Kitama, T., Gomi, H. and Kawato, M. (1998) Temporal firing patterns of Purkinje cells in the cerebellar ventral paraflocculus during ocular following responses in monkeys. II. Complex spikes. *J. Neurophysiol.*, 80: 832–848.

Mehta, B. and Schaal, S. (2002) Forward models in visuomotor control. *J. Neurophysiol.*, 88: 942–953.

Miall, R.C., Weir, D.J., Wolpert, D.M. and Stein, J.F. (1993) Is the cerebellum a Smith predictor? *J. Mot. Behav.*, 25: 203–216.

Miall, R.C., Imamizu, H. and Miyauchi, S. (2000) Activation of the cerebellum in co-ordinated eye and hand tracking movements: an fMRI study. *Exp Brain Res.*, 135: 22–33.

Miall, R.C., Reckess, G.Z. and Imamizu, H. (2001) The cerebellum coordinates eye and hand tracking movements. *Nat. Neurosci.*, 4: 638–644.

Middleton, F.A. and Strick, P.L. (1998) The cerebellum: an overview. *Trends Cogn. Sci.*, 2: 348–354.

Nitschke, M.F., Kleinschmidt, A., Wessel, K. and Frahm, J. (1996) Somatotopic motor representation in the human anterior cerebellum. A high-resolution functional MRI study. *Brain*, 119: 1023–1029.

Penfield, W. and Rasmussen, T. (1950) *The Cerebral Cortex of Man: A Clinical Study of Localization of Function*. Macmillan, New York.

Scarchilli, K. and Vercher, J.L. (1999) The oculomanual coordination control center takes into account the mechanical properties of the arm. *Exp. Brain Res.*, 124: 42–52.

Shidara, M., Kawano, K., Gomi, H. and Kawato, M. (1993) Inverse-dynamics model eye movement control by Purkinje cells in the cerebellum. *Nature*, 365: 50–52.

Snider, R.S. and Eldred, E. (1952) Cerebro-cerebellar relationships in the monkey. *J. Neurophysiol.*, 15: 27–40.

Takemura, A., Inoue, Y., Gomi, H., Kawato, M. and Kawano, K. (2001) Change in neuronal firing patterns in the process of motor command generation for the ocular following response. *J. Neurophysiol.*, 86: 1750–1763.

Vercher, J.-L., Sarès, F., Blouin, J., Bourdin, C. and Gauthier, G. (2003) Role of sensory information in updating internal models of the effector during arm tracking. In: C. Prablanc, D. Pélisson and Y. Rossetti (Eds.), *Neural Control of Space Coding and Action Production. Progress in Brain Research*, Vol. 142. Elsevier, Amsterdam, pp. 203–222 (this volume).

Winstein, C.J. and Pohl, P.S. (1995) Effects of unilateral brain damage on the control of goal-directed hand movements. *Exp. Brain Res.*, 105: 163–174.

Wolpert, D.M. and Kawato, M. (1998) Multiple paired forward and inverse models for motor control. *Neural Networks*, 11: 1317–1329.

Wolpert, D.M., Ghahramani, Z. and Jordan, M.I. (1995) An internal model for sensorimotor integration. *Science*, 269: 1880–1882.

Wolpert, D.M., Miall, C. and Kawato, M. (1998) Internal models in the cerebellum. *Trends Cogn. Sci.*, 2: 338–347.

Yamamoto, K., Kobayashi, Y., Takemura, A., Kawano, K. and Kawato, M. (2002) Computational studies on the acquisition and adaptation of ocular following responses based on the synaptic plasticity in the cerebellar cortex. *J. Neurophysiol.*, 87: 1554–1571.

C. Prablanc, D. Pélisson and Y. Rossetti (Eds.)
Progress in Brain Research, Vol. 142
© 2003 Elsevier Science B.V. All rights reserved

CHAPTER 12

A multisensory posture control model of human upright stance

T. Mergner [1,*], C. Maurer [1] and R.J. Peterka [2]

[1] *Neurological University Clinic, Freiburg, Germany*
[2] *Neurological Sciences Institute, Oregon Health and Science University, Portland, OR, USA*

Abstract: We present a multisensory postural control model based on experiments where the balance in normal subjects and vestibular loss patients was perturbed by application of external torque produced by force-controlled pull stimuli. The stimuli were applied while subjects stood on a stationary or body-sway-referenced motion platform with eyes closed and auditory cues masked. Excursions of the center of mass (COM) and the center of pressure (COP) were analyzed using a systems analysis approach. The results were compared to an 'inverted pendulum' model of posture control. The model receives input from four sensors: ankle proprioceptors, semicircular canals, otoliths, and plantar pressure sensors (somatosensory graviceptors). Sensor fusion mechanisms are used to yield separate internal representations of foot support motion, gravity, and external torque (pull). These representations are fed as global set point signals into a local control loop based on ankle proprioceptive negative feedback. This set point control upgrades the proprioceptive body-on-foot (support) stabilization into a body-in-space control which compensates for support tilt, gravity, and contact forces. This compensation occurs even when the stimuli are combined or a voluntary lean is superimposed. Model simulations paralleled our experimental findings.

Introduction

It is still not understood how humans control their upright stance and how they embed their voluntary actions into postural mechanisms. Research in this field faces the problem of a high complexity of the mechanisms involved (multi-segment dynamics, biomechanics of the human body, multisensory integration, volition, cognition, etc.). The complexity of the system requires that researchers develop conceptual hypotheses concerning the involved sensors, the internal 'reconstruction' and representation of the external stimuli by means of sensor fusion mecha-

nisms (multisensory integration), and the implementation of these internal stimulus representations into the postural control mechanism (for the clinical approach to multisensory integration of space see also Kerkhoff, 2003, this volume, and Rode et al., 2003, this volume). Conceivably, such an approach has to build upon a number of simplifications, such as the assumption that the control is based to a large extent on a sensory negative feedback mechanism (e.g. Johansson and Magnusson, 1991; Fitzpatrick et al., 1996).

We conceptualized the *physical stimuli*, which challenge body equilibrium of an upright standing human, as consisting of the following.

(1) Force field due to gravity.
(2) Motion of the body's support surface. We consider here only support surface tilt about an axis through the ankle joints of both feet, i.e. tilt in the anterior–posterior (a–p) direction.

* Correspondence to: T. Mergner, Neurozentrum, Breisacher Str. 64, 79106 Freiburg, Germany. Tel.: +49-761-270-5313; Fax: +49-761-270-5310;
E-mail: mergner@uni-freiburg.de

(3) External contact forces, such as a pull on, or a push against the body.

Humans use several sensors to obtain internal estimates of these stimuli. The most relevant sensory cues are derived from visual input (Berthoz et al., 1979; Amblard et al., 1985; Bronstein, 1986; Van Asten et al., 1988; Peterka and Benolken, 1995), proprioceptive input (Kavounoudias et al., 2001), the vestibular system (Hajos and Kirchner, 1984; Britton et al., 1993), and the somatosensory system (Mittelstaedt, 1996; Jeka et al., 1998).

To simplify, we consider here subjects who have no visual or auditory spatial orientation cues (i.e. eyes are closed and no relevant sound source). In this situation, we assume that the aforementioned three physical stimuli are perceived predominantly with the help of the following four *sensory signals*.

(1) *An otolith-derived signal of the body lean in space*. It is known from clinical and experimental work that imbalance between the vestibular sensors in the two labyrinths, resulting from unilateral lesion or stimulation, give rise to postural reactions (see Massion, 1994; Horak and Macpherson, 1996; Massion and Woollacott, 1996). It is generally believed that a relevant part of the vestibular information stems from the otolith system. This is thought to provide a signal related to the body orientation with respect to the earth vertical. After shaping it according to current body geometry, it yields an appropriate 'antigravity' extensor muscle tone, such that the gravitational reaction forces are neutralized.

(2) *A canal-derived signal of support surface motion in space*. There is experimental evidence that humans perceive rotation of the body support with the help of vestibular semicircular canal signals, and it has been suggested that the corresponding internal signals are also used for postural control (Mergner et al., 1997).

(3) *A somatosensory graviception from deep plantar mechanoreceptors*. There is clinical evidence that posture control is impaired following loss of plantar somatosensory afferents as well as experimental evidence that stimulation of these afferents evokes postural reactions (see Maurer et al., 2000, 2001).

(4) *A proprioceptive signal of body angular posi-tion with respect to the foot*. Normally, postural reactions take place at several joints along the body axis. However, here we assume for simplification that the proprioceptive signal stems from one joint only (in this view the body is conceptualized as an 'inverted pendulum' with a single head–trunk–leg segment rotating about the ankle joint).

It is still an enigma how these four sensors interact and what their functional relevance is during posture control. For an analytical approach (such as a systems analysis approach), it would be desirable to further reduce the number of sensors and to compare the system's behavior in the absence versus the presence of a given sensor. We conceived of two possibilities. One would be to compare the postural responses to external perturbations of patients with bilateral loss of vestibular function with those of normal controls. In the above adopted view, the patients would have only the ankle proprioceptive cue and the somatosensory graviceptive cue for postural control, while normal subjects would have all four sensors.

The second possibility would be to 'freeze' the proprioceptive signal by a procedure called 'body-sway referencing of the platform' (BSRP). BSRP is performed by making a motion-controlled platform rotate 1:1 (i.e. in fixed register) with the body sway angle. This procedure has been commonly used in posture control studies to 'open' the ankle joint proprioceptive feedback loop by keeping the ankle angle constant during body sway while the subject is still able to apply torque about the ankle joint. In the envisaged comparison between patients and normal subjects, the patients now would have to maintain balance relying solely on somatosensory graviception, while the normal subjects would have, in addition, the otolith and canal signals.

In the present study we performed these comparisons using a contact force as an external perturbation. The stimulus was created by applying a force-controlled pull on a subject's body around the ankle joints in the a–p direction. We measured center of mass (COM) and center of pressure (COP) excursions to sinusoidal pull stimuli at different frequencies and with various force magnitudes. Gain and phase curves obtained from the responses were compared to simulated data using a dynamic postural control model into which we implemented the four sensors, sensor fusion mechanisms, a sensorimotor transformation, and the corresponding physics and biomechanics.

Methods

Subjects

Experiments were performed in six normal subjects (age 34–53 years) and four patients with loss of vestibular function (age 33–42 years). Loss of vestibular function in patients was assumed on the basis of routine clinical examinations (e.g. balancing problems when standing on foam rubber with eyes closed) and electronystagmographic criteria (absence of caloric nystagmus and of rotation-evoked VOR) as well as on case histories (meningitis and oto-toxic medication in childhood). Apart from hearing problems and slight vertigo during rapid head movements, patients showed no neurological symptoms. In compliance with the Helsinki declaration (1964) all subjects gave their informed consent to the study which was approved by the local Ethics Committee of the Freiburg University Clinics.

Experimental setup and procedures

The experiments were conducted with a setup which allowed us to apply a pull on the subjects' body in the sagittal plane and thereby to exert a defined torque about their ankle joints. The stimuli were applied via a body harness by means of two force-controlled cable winches (servo motors) under computer control, as shown schematically in Fig. 1. Sinusoidal stimulus profiles were applied at five different frequencies (0.05, 0.1, 0.2, 0.4, and 0.8 Hz) and three different amplitudes of torque about the ankle joint (± 1, ± 4, and ± 16 N m). During these stimuli subjects were standing upright, heels 5 cm apart, on a custom-built motion platform. The platform rested on six 'legs', each incorporating a motor capable of producing a change in the length of the leg (hexapod with Stuart principle). The motors were controlled by a computer to generate platform tilts in the sagittal plane with the axis through subjects' ankle joints during some of the stimuli.

Mounted on the motion platform was a force-transducing platform (Kistler®, platform type 9286, Winterthur, Switzerland) that registered subjects' COP shift in the a–p direction. We also measured subjects' hip-to-ankle and shoulder-to-hip angular excursions in the sagittal plane by means of an optoelectronic device with active markers (Optotrack 3020®, Waterloo, Canada). These measures were used to obtain estimates of subjects' COM angular excursion in the sagittal plane.

Two experiments were performed. In one experiment, the pull stimuli were applied while the platform was kept stationary ('pull alone' experiment). In the other, the pull stimuli were applied while platform position was coupled 1 : 1 to subjects' COM angular position, by which their ankle angle essentially was held constant ('pull with BSRP' experiment). In the BSRP condition, any spontaneous, actively produced, or stimulus-evoked angular excursion of the body off its primary position causes the platform to rotate with the body with a small time delay (<40 ms) and error (<2%).

Subjects were instructed to always remain upright and to maintain balance. The stimuli with the longest duration (0.05 and 0.1 Hz) were presented as two separate trials with 4 stimulus cycles each, while those with shorter duration were presented within one trial which comprised either 8 stimulus cycles (0.2 and 0.4 Hz) or 16 cycles (0.8 Hz). The order of these presentations was varied, starting always with a stimulus in the mid-frequency range with 4 N m, but varying the remaining ones in random order. The pull stimuli on stable support were always performed prior to those in the BSRP condition, in order to allow subjects to become accustomed to the stimuli. No attempt was made to hide from the subjects which of the two conditions was applied. The patients and three of the normal subjects were completely naive as concerns the postural tests used, the remaining three normal subjects were naive as to the stimulus frequency and amplitude presented. During the stimulus presentations, we instructed the subjects to perform simple mental arithmetic, in order to draw their attention away from the postural stimuli.

Data analysis

Optotrak and Kistler output signals as well as platform rotation and pull stimulus signals were recorded

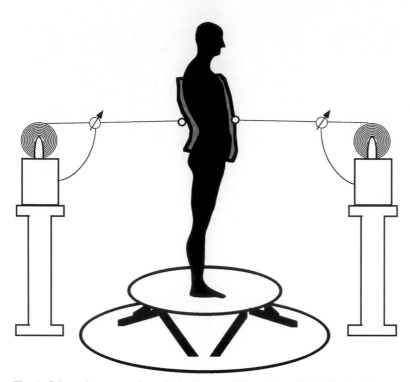

Fig. 1. Schematic presentation of stimulus conditions. Sinusoidal pull stimuli were applied by means of two force-controlled cable winches via a padded body harness to exert defined torques about the subject's ankle joints in the a–p direction. The subject stood on a motion platform which was either stationary or was tilted in fixed register with spontaneous and stimulus-evoked body excursions (body-sway-referenced platform, BSRP).

on a computer system (IBM compatible Pentium®) via analog-digital converter with a 100 Hz sampling rate. The data were recorded with software programmed in LabView® (National Instruments, Austin, TX, USA) and analyzed off-line with custom-made software programmed in MATLAB® (The MathWorks Inc., Natick, MA, USA). COM angular displacement was calculated from the shoulder-to-hip and hip-to-ankle angular displacements according to anthropometric data of Winter (1990). Within-subject averages were obtained for six cycles of each stimulus. Further analysis was performed using a spread sheet program (Microsoft Excel®) and a statistics program (StatView®, SAS Inc., Cary, NC, USA).

A spectral analysis was performed on the pull stimulus and response (COP and COM) waveforms using a discrete Fourier transformation. Fourier coefficients at the frequency corresponding to the stimulus frequency were used to calculate gain (peak response amplitude divided by peak stimulus amplitude) and phase (relative timing of the response

compared to the stimulus). Gain measures have units of cm/N m for measures related to COP displacements caused by the pull stimulus, and °/N m for COM angular displacements caused by the pull stimulus. Gain values of zero indicate that the pull stimulus had no effect on the subject's COM angle or COP displacement. Gain and phase change patterns as a function of stimulus frequency characterize the dynamic behavior of the postural control system.

By developing models of postural control that explain these patterns, we hope to understand how sensorimotor integration is achieved in the postural control system. The model was implemented in Simulink/MATLAB®.

Results

Pull alone

Fig. 2A shows the results of normal subjects to pull stimuli on a stationary support for the different stim-

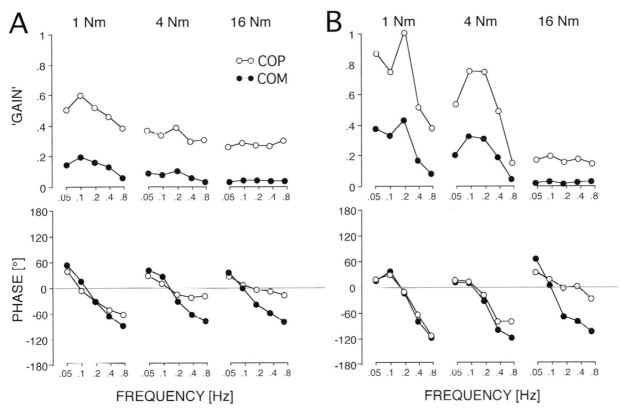

Fig. 2. Responses of normal subjects (A) and vestibular loss patients (B) to sinusoidal pull stimuli on a stationary platform. The angular excursion of COM and the linear shift of COP are given in terms of mean gain (in °/N m and cm/N m, respectively) and phase values as a function of peak ankle torque (1, 4, 16 N m) and of stimulus frequency, as indicated. COM and COP gains show a clear dependency on stimulus amplitude (reflecting that excursions were relatively larger, the smaller the stimulus was), unlike the corresponding phase values. Furthermore, gain and phase of COM and COP change as a function of stimulus frequency (exception: gains with the 16 N m stimulus). The responses of patients in (B) are similar to those of normal subjects, apart from larger gain values in the mid- to low-frequency range with the 1 N m and 4 N m stimuli.

ulus frequencies and the three peak ankle torques. In the upper panel we give the gain measures for the COM (in °/N m) and the COP (in cm/N m). In the lower panel the corresponding phase values are given.

Peak COM excursion by the pull stimulus in normal subjects did not exceed 1° in absolute values, even with the largest stimulus magnitude (16 N m). This is reflected in the rather low COM gain values. Noticeably, the gain values decrease with increasing stimulus magnitude (thus, the small stimuli were counteracted relatively less than the large ones). For instance, gain was about 0.2 with the 1 N m/0.1 Hz stimulus and decreased to 0.02 with the 16 N m/0.1 Hz stimulus. In contrast to this clear gain

nonlinearity, COM phase is essentially independent of stimulus magnitude.

COM gain also depends on stimulus frequency. With the smallest stimulus magnitude (1 N m), increase of frequency leads to an increase in COM excursion, with a peak at 0.1 to 0.2 Hz, after which it decreases at higher frequencies. This frequency-dependent modulation levels off when gain becomes small with the larger stimuli. COM phase is approximately in phase with the stimulus at 0.1 and 0.2 Hz and develops some lead at 0.05 Hz and some lag at 0.4 and 0.8 Hz.

Normal subjects' COP shows qualitatively a very similar gain behavior in terms of both the nonlinearity related to stimulus magnitude and the modulation in relation to stimulus frequency. Also COP phase is similar to COM phase, especially with the smallest stimulus magnitude (±1 N m). At higher magnitudes, however, the COP phase tended to level off at about 0°, losing the frequency modulation almost completely with the 16 N m stimulus, similar to the COP gain curve.

The results of vestibular loss patients are shown in Fig. 2B. Patients exhibit qualitatively similar COM and COP responses as normals during the pull stimuli on the stationary platform. This applies to the gain nonlinearity, the gain modulation with frequency, and the phase modulation with frequency. A clear difference, however, concerns the gain of COM and COP at low frequencies and small stimulus magnitudes. Gain is then almost double compared to that in normal subjects. At the higher frequencies and the highest stimulus magnitude (16 N m), gain is essentially in the normal range (thus, patients behave like normal subjects and limit their COM and COP excursions to values <1° and <3 cm, respectively).

Pull with body-sway-referenced platform

Normal subjects have no difficulty maintaining stance on a sway-referenced platform with their eyes closed. However, stance in this condition is associated with a relatively large and irregular body sway. The effect of this variability was largely removed, however, from the experimental data by the averaging process. Subjectively the platform is experienced as unstable in this situation, since any body lean is associated with a corresponding tilt of the platform. Subjects tend to avoid this and normally try to keep the body orientation vertical.

Fig. 3 shows the COM and COP gain and phase curves of normal subjects obtained with the pull stimuli in the sway-referenced condition. The COM gain curves are qualitatively similar to those obtained with the stationary platform, showing again the nonlinearity related to stimulus magnitude and the modulation in relation to frequency. However, overall gain is higher by a factor of approximately 2 (i.e. pull-evoked body excursions were essentially doubled). Also COM phase is qualitatively similar as before (lead at low and lag at high frequency, no major change related to stimulus magnitude). But

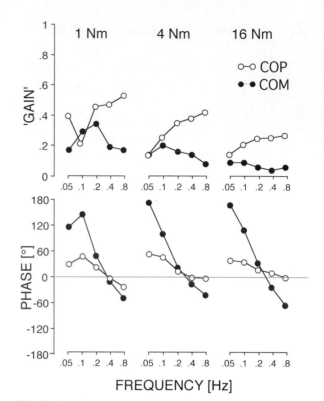

Fig. 3. Responses of normal subjects to sinusoidal pull stimuli on body-sway-referenced platform (BSRP). Presentation as in Fig. 2. Compared to the normals' responses on the stationary platform (Fig. 2A) the gain and phase curves of COM are similar, apart from slightly higher gain values and a shift of the phase towards lead. The latter also applies to COP phase. In contrast, the COP gain curves now start with relatively small values at low frequency and increase with increasing frequency, unlike on the stationary platform. Vestibular loss patients were unable to maintain balance in the BSRP condition (not shown).

overall there is a shift towards lead as compared to the stationary condition; already at 0.2 Hz the phase shows a lead, which further increases at the lower frequencies and reaches approximately counter-phase (180°) at 0.05 Hz. Thus it appears that normal subjects produce a counter-leaning body position when compensating for the pull at this low frequency. This counter-leaning position allows gravity to act on the body to counteract the pull.

COP gain in the sway-referenced condition shows a nonlinearity related to stimulus magnitude as before, while its modulation by frequency is clearly different compared to the stable-platform experiment. The largest gain is reached at the highest frequency, and shows a monotonic decrease with decreasing frequency. COP phase is slightly shifted towards a lead as compared to the platform stationary condition, but otherwise it remains very similar.

Patients are not able to maintain balance on the sway-referenced surface with eyes closed. When standing on the body-sway-referenced platform with eyes open, they can maintain balance even with the pull stimulus. However, as soon as they close their eyes, they fall, even without the pull stimulus.

Discussion

To reduce the high complexity of the human postural control system during upright stance, we restricted access to visual and auditory orientation sources, thus limiting the postural control system to information from mainly four sensors (otolith, canal, ankle proprioceptive, and somatosensory graviceptive sources). The external physical events, which may endanger body equilibrium, consist mainly of three stimuli (gravitational pull on the body, external pull produced by a contact force, and tilt of the body support surface). The interactions of these physical factors were investigated in normal and vestibular loss subjects using a system analysis approach by measuring COM and COP excursions during force-controlled pull stimuli. In vestibular loss subjects, it was assumed that equilibrium control is achieved only by means of ankle proprioceptive and plantar somatosensory cues. We further challenged the postural control system by introducing tilts of the platform that tracked COM body sway (the BSRP condition). This 'opened the proprioceptive loop' and limited sensory information solely to somatosensory cues in vestibular loss subjects, and to somatosensory and vestibular (otolith and canal) cues in normals. To better understand the interactions of sensory information required for postural control, we developed a computer model that allowed us to compare experimental results with model predictions based on plausible sensory integration schemes.

We found that the pull-evoked COM and COP excursions on stable support are very small in normal subjects, indicating a very efficient control mechanism for the effects of this stimulus. At 0.1–0.2 Hz (approximately the *eigen*-frequency of body sway) the pull-evoked excursions are maximal and in phase with the stimulus (with a phase lead/lag when frequency was decreased/increased). The responses showed a clear nonlinearity in that the gain was largest (the pull-evoked excursions became relatively larger) with the smallest stimulus magnitudes. Since this nonlinearity was also observed in patients and was a consistent finding in normal subjects in the BSRP condition, it appears to represent a property of the postural sensorimotor control mechanism.

Patients' pull responses on stable support were similar to those of normals, apart from a higher gain in the mid- to low-frequency range (larger body excursions). In terms of our concept, the gain difference would be explained mainly by the absence of the otolith signal in patients. This requires patients to produce responses solely using ankle proprioceptive and somatosensory graviceptive cues. Admittedly, one could conceive, as an alternative, that patients used solely a proprioceptive negative feedback loop. However, our previous work showed that patients have at least some sensory information on gravity from plantar pressure receptors during platform tilt (Maurer et al., 2000), and we postulate that they use this cue to control balance during the pull stimulus. But we assume that somatosensory graviceptive cues cannot be used to distinguish between the pull evoked by an external contact force and the pull arising from gravity during body leans away from a vertical orientation. In contrast, normal subjects, using the 'force field meter' provided by the otolith system in addition to the 'contact force meter' in the plantar sole, should be able to make this distinction. Patients indeed failed to keep balance with the pull stimuli in the BSRP condition, while normal subjects were able to do so.

Normal subjects' COM response to the pull stimuli in the BSRP condition showed a pronounced phase lead at low frequency. Extrapolating from this observation to a static situation, this is consistent with subjects producing a counter lean of the body in space such that the gravitational pull almost counterbalances the stimulus pull, with some control error remaining, as indicated by the small COP shift in the direction of the stimulus. In the dynamic situation with increasing stimulus frequency, body inertia resists more and more the force that evokes body excursion, and responses become more and more similar to the stable-platform condition where subjects produced an appropriate counter force scaled to the stimulus.

Since there is platform tilt associated with the pull-evoked body lean in the BSRP condition, canal-derived estimates of platform tilt can contribute to postural responses. Because the responses in the BSRP condition became similar to those in the stable-platform condition at high frequency and with large stimulus magnitude, one can conclude that normal subjects were able to use canal information to compensate for the platform tilt to a large degree (as they do for body tilt produced by their spontaneous sway in the BSRP condition; see the section Results).

When implementing our assumptions into a postural control model for comparison with the experimental data, we proceeded from the concept (Mergner et al., 1997; Mergner and Rosemeier, 1998) that the control is built around an ankle proprioceptive negative feedback loop, which stabilizes the body with respect to the foot and its support base. During support tilt, a canal-derived internal estimate of the tilt is fed into this 'local' loop as a set point signal, by which the body-on-support control becomes upgraded into a body-on-support-*in-space* control. This concept originally was based on psychophysical data obtained in the earth-horizontal rotational plane (i.e. perpendicular to the gravity vector). Since body sway occurs in the vertical planes, we have to consider additional mechanisms that can also cope with the effects of gravity. Furthermore, postural control mechanisms also need to cope with external contact forces, such as the pull stimuli we used in our experiments.

We developed a model, shown in Fig. 4, based on the concepts described above. The model includes a 'physics' part and a 'subject' part. The physics part includes a body composed of two mutually coupled pendulums, one being the body segment, the other the foot-platform segment. Both segments are interconnected by a joint (see inset), an actuator produces torque at this joint, and only rotations around this joint are considered. We assume that the body is always oriented approximately upward and the foot-platform segment downwards, so that gravity presses the foot firmly on the support, as long as only small angular excursions about the upright

position occur. With the foot-platform segment held stationary in space (foot-in-space angle, FS $= 0°$), the body-to-foot angle (BF; i.e. the reverse of the foot-to-body angle, FB; FB $= -$BF) is coupled 1 : 1 to the body-in-space angle (BS). This coupling is eliminated (FB $= -$BF $= 0$) when FS is made to exactly follow BS (mimicked by opening the switch BSRP). Our subjects' anthropometric data were implemented in the box 'body inertia, gravity'. The input signals to the physics part consist of an external torque (the pull stimulus), a muscle torque produced by the subject in the ankle joint, and FS (platform tilt). As outputs of this part and as inputs into the 'subject', BF is sensed by ankle proprioception (PROP), BS by the vestibular system (VEST), and a shift of COP by plantar somatosensory receptors (SOMAT; determined by the shift of the COM's gravitational vector, the actively produced muscle torque, and the external torque evoked by the contact force, i.e. the pull stimulus).

The PROP sensor is considered to have essentially ideal transfer characteristics (broad band pass filter characteristics) and a gain of about unity. The PROP sensor combined with a neural controller in the form of a PID controller (P, proportional; D, differential; I, integrative) yields the local proprioceptive negative feedback loop in the ankle joint. The PID controller was set such that BS follows rather accurately a voluntary lean signal (input VOLUNT. LEAN) in the absence of all external stimuli including gravity. The VEST sensor was considered to contain two parts, one representing the canal system, the other the otolith system. We assumed that by way of a canal–otolith interaction (not shown; see Merfeld, 1995; Mergner and Glasauer, 1999; Zupan et al., 2002) the canal transfer characteristics are improved in the vertical rotational planes such that an essentially veridical internal representation of BS rotation results (signal bs). A combination of canal and proprioceptive cues in terms of a sensor fusion (Mergner et al., 1997; Mergner and Rosemeier, 1998) is taken to yield an internal estimate of foot-in-space motion (fs; fs $=$ bs $-$ bf), which is fed into the local loop as a set point signal. A detection threshold, T$'$, is included in the canal-derived fs signal pathway (T$'$ is about 0.1°/s and is expressed as a velocity threshold because the canal signal at early stages of processing codes angular velocity). This threshold, combined

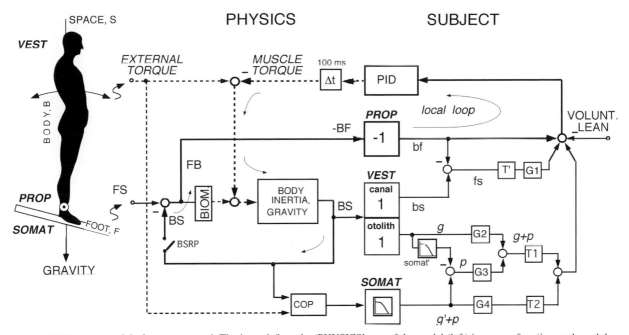

Fig. 4. Multisensory model of posture control. The inset defines the 'PHYSICS' part of the model (left) in terms of an 'inverted pendulum body' (one segment for head, trunk, and legs) that pivots about the ankle joint on a potentially rotating platform (axis through the ankle joint). Pull on the body yields an 'external torque' stimulus acting on the body, together with the 'muscle torque'. FS, foot-in-space angle (resulting from platform tilt); FB, foot-to-body angle (equal to −BF); BS, body-in-space angle; BSRP, body-sway-referenced platform (open switch mimics the BSRP condition). Box BIOM (for biomechanics) represents the transformation of FB into ankle torque (in the present case passive viscous–elastic properties are assumed to be zero, since these would be small as compared to external and muscle torques). Subjects' anthropometric parameters are contained in the box 'BODY INERTIA, GRAVITY'. Dashed lines represent torque and solid lines angles. All delays in the system are represented as one dead time (Δt). BS excursion leads to a shift of the COP (box COP; also affected by the external torque stimulus). The 'SUBJECT' part of the model (on the right) establishes internal representations of the external stimuli (torque, stemming from gravitational and external pull on the body, and FS angle), which are fed as set point signals, together with a voluntary signal (VOLUNT. LEAN), into a local proprioceptive negative feedback loop for body-on-support control (loop indicated by thin arrows). PROP, proprioceptive sensor; VEST, vestibular sensors; SOMAT, plantar pressure cue ('somatosensory graviceptor'; it is assumed to have low-pass frequency characteristics with a corner frequency of 0.8 Hz); somat', internal model of SOMAT; bf, bs, and fs, internal representations of BF, BS and FS, respectively; g, otolith derived internal estimate of gravitational pull (g', somatosensory derived version of g); p, internal estimate of external pull; T1, T2, and T', detection thresholds; G1–G4, gain of set point signals (on the order of 0.7–0.9; held constant for all simulations of the results of normals).

with other thresholds discussed below, accounts for the observed amplitude nonlinearity of the system.[1]

The presumed canal–otolith interaction in the box VEST, in addition, is thought to extract from the

otolith signal the gravitational component (assumed to show essentially ideal transfer characteristics as well). This yields an internal representation of the body's orientation with respect to the gravitational vertical, g, and thereby a measure of the 'gravitational pull' on the COM (zero with upright orientation of the inverted pendulum). The somatosensory plantar cue (SOMAT) is assumed to show low-pass frequency characteristics, and to yield an internal representation of the sum of (1) the COM's gravitational vector with respect to the foot support base (signal g'), and (2) the additional shift of the COP induced by the pull stimulus (p). (The acceleration

---

[1] Note that the thresholds here are thought to represent central mechanisms, in contradistinction to the thresholds of the sensors in classical sensory physiology. In our previous psychophysical studies, the central thresholds were related to mechanims that minimise noise in the system and thereby help to achieve perceptual stability (Mergner et al., 2001). The presumed central thresholds in the present context, however, are considerably lower than those in the psychophysical studies. Their functional significance and underlying processes remain to be elucidated.

components contained in COP, that are mainly due to active changes in ankle torque, are assumed to be removed by way of an interaction with acceleration signals from shear force receptors in the feet or by an efference-copy-like signal.)

Fusion of an otolith-derived signal (a sign-reversed version of the otolith signal is given the low-pass characteristics of the plantar signal by feeding it through an internal model of the SOMAT cue; somat') with the plantar cues is thought to yield an internal representation of the effect of pull, $p = (g' + p) - g'$. This then yields, in combination with the original otolith-derived signal, a set point signal for the local loop to compensate for the external forces in any adopted body position $(g + p)$.[2] The set point signal is given a detection threshold, T1, on the order of 0.1°.

This form of the model was used for simulation of the results of our normal subjects obtained with the pull stimulus on stationary support (note that the model contains, in addition, a direct set point signal from SOMAT, $g' + p$, which was disabled here; see below). The simulation results, given in Fig. 5A, are consistent with the essential features of the experimental data. Preliminary testing showed that the model also yields similar successful simulations of our previous data obtained with tilt stimuli (Maurer et al., 2000).

In order to describe the data obtained from the patients, we first considered a model that included only the local proprioceptive loop. The simulation results described the experimental results rather well for the 1 N m pull stimulus if the PID values in the neural controller were slightly increased. However, the experimental results obtained with 4 and 16 N m stimuli were clearly better than the predicted ones (gain was smaller, reflecting smaller body excursions than expected from model simulations). This led us to assume that patients use, in addition to the proprioceptive loop, a set point signal derived from the

SOMAT sensor (the $g' + p$ signal). This signal includes a threshold, T2, whose value is about 0.6° (which corresponds to a COP displacement of about 1 cm). The simulations described rather accurately the experimental findings (Fig. 5B). This modeling result suggests that the patients control small body-on-support excursions entirely with the proprioceptive loop, while larger excursions require the help of the plantar somatosensory cues to prevent the center of ground reaction force from shifting beyond the base of support given by the foot. This extended model for patients is also able to describe their tilt responses from the earlier experiments (Maurer et al., 2000). In addition, the model correctly predicts the experimental finding that patients cannot maintain stance in the BSRP condition.

We conceive furthermore that normal subjects also make use of the somatosensory signal, but use it with a wider threshold, so that there is only a small somatosensory contribution for the pull stimulus on stationary support. In fact, for the simulation of the experiment in Fig. 2A (Fig. 5A) the somatosensory derived signal was not included in the model. In contrast, when simulating the results of normals for pull in the BSRP condition, we used the somatosensory signal with a low threshold (and disabled the $g + p$ signal by raising its threshold). This allowed us to simulate the normals' results with the 1 N m stimulus where COP phase and gain curves became clearly dissociated from those of COM (Figs. 3 and 6). The results obtained with the 4 N m and 16 N m stimuli were also well simulated. Therefore, we postulate that normal subjects can make use of two internal estimates of $g + p$, one that is primarily derived from the otolith signal and the other that is based primarily on the somatosensory cue alone. We speculate that normal subjects can shift the weighting to emphasize the use of one or the other (in the extreme, this weighting of the two thresholds, T1 and T2, can be considered to represent a 'switch' between the use of vestibular and somatosensory graviceptive control). From the simulation of the data, we determined that normal subjects balanced the pull stimulus in the BSRP condition mainly by using the COP-like somatosensory cue.

Using sinusoidal stimuli we cannot exclude that our subjects used predictive mechanisms to some extent for their postural responses (this despite the

---

[2] Note that during a voluntary body lean, for instance, these signals are used to compensate the external forces that arise with the lean, such as the gravitational pull, by providing the appropriate ankle torque (in the sense of a force or load compensation). They are not used to bring the body to an upright position and therefore do not interfere with the kinematic control (which in the model is provided by the internal signals bf, fs, and the voluntary signal VOLUNT. LEAN).

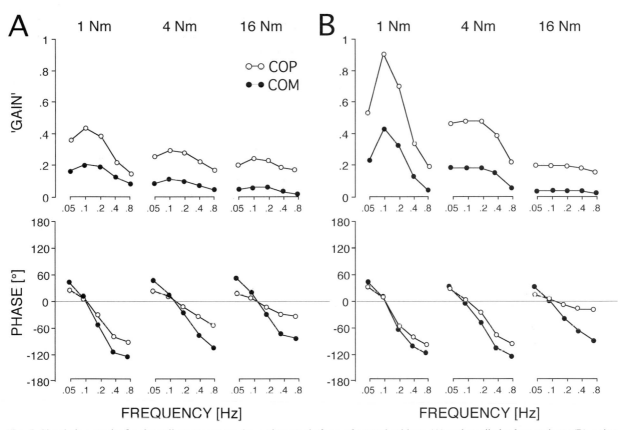

Fig. 5. Simulation results for the pull responses on the stationary platform of normal subjects (A) and vestibular loss patients (B), using the model shown in Fig. 4. Presentation as in Fig. 2 which shows the corresponding experimental results.

fact that they performed mental arithmetic during the trials and often did not perceive consciously the stimuli, especially the 1 N m stimuli). The possibility exists that prediction may have led to a reduction of the effective feedback time delay. Therefore, the choice of the time delay in the model might already be accounting for predictive effects. But this idea still has to be tested in future work. Future models may include a more complete representation of prediction, possibly including feed-forward pathways.

One major aim in our modeling was to establish a parsimonious description of postural control mechanisms which can cope simultaneously with all three external physical stimuli (tilt, pull, gravity) and with voluntary lean, while at the same time minimizing the need for a task-dependent adjustment of parameters (i.e. without explicit sensory reweighting). We were successful for conditions of pull and tilt stimuli on stationary support. In this case, the necessary

'sensory weighting' occurred implicitly because the external stimuli are internally implemented in an appropriate way. However, successful simulation of the condition of the pull stimulus with BSRP required additional parameter adjustments.

Another aim of the modeling was to establish a mechanism which successfully predicts changes that occur with a reduction of sensory information. We were successful at predicting the results for vestibular loss patients by disabling the VEST sensor in the model and the related sensor fusion mechanisms, and making a simple threshold adjustment. This model was also able to predict that vestibular loss patients are able to maintain stability during low-frequency tilt of the support surface (see Maurer et al., 2000). A future experiment is motivated by the prediction that loss of the SOMAT sensor should have a limited effect on stability (e.g. by evaluating patients with distal neuropathy of the legs).

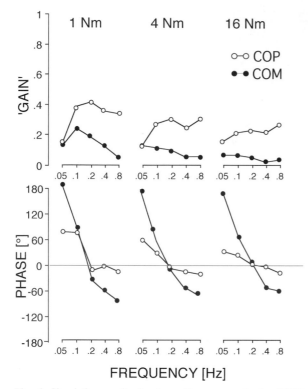

Fig. 6. Simulation results for the pull responses in the BSRP condition of normal subjects. The corresponding experimental results are shown in Fig. 3.

We are aware of the fact that many more receptor systems are involved in postural control, but consider the four sensors considered here as the essential minimum. We also learned from the modeling that many different model topologies yield essentially equivalent results, as long as they are implemented within the same basic framework (internal representations of the external stimuli, their use as set point signals of the local proprioceptive loop). We consider our modeling as a first and preliminary step in a novel approach whose aim is to understand the reasons for the high flexibility and robustness of the human postural control system. This approach clearly distinguishes it from otherwise similar work in the literature (e.g. Nashner, 1972; Johansson and Magnusson, 1991; Van der Kooij et al., 1999; Jeka et al., 2000; Peterka, 2002).

Acknowledgements

DFG Me 715/5-1, NIH AG17960.

References

Amblard, B., Cremieux, J., Marchard, A.R. and Carblanc, A. (1985) Lateral orientation and stabilization of human stance: static versus dynamic visual cues. *Exp. Brain Res.*, 61: 21–37.

Berthoz, A., Lacour, M., Soechting, J.F. and Vidal, P.P. (1979) The role of vision in the control of posture during linear motion. *Prog. Brain Res.*, 50: 197–210.

Britton, T.C., Day, B.L., Brown, P., Rothwell, J.C., Thompson, P.D. and Marsden, C.D. (1993) Postural electromyographic responses in the arm and leg following galvanic vestibular stimulation in man. *Exp. Brain Res.*, 94: 143–151.

Bronstein, A.M. (1986) Suppression of visually evoked postural responses. *Exp. Brain Res.*, 63: 655–658.

Fitzpatrick, R., Burke, D. and Gandevia, S.C. (1996) Loop gain of reflexes controlling human standing measured with the use of postural and vestibular disturbances. *J. Neurophysiol.*, 76: 3994–4008.

Hajos, A. and Kirchner, W. (1984) Körperlageregelung des Menschen bei elektrischer Reizung des Vestibularsystems. In: L. Spillmann and B.R. Wooten (Eds.), *Sensory Experience, Adaptation, and Perception*. Lawrence Erlbaum, London, pp. 255–280.

Horak, F.B. and Macpherson, J.M. (1996) Postural orientation and equilibrium. In: L. Rowell and J. Shepherd (Eds.), *Handbook of Physiology, 1. Exercise: Regulation and Integration of Multiple Systems*. Oxford University Press, New York, NY, pp. 255–292.

Jeka, J., Oie, K., Schöner, G., Dijkstra, T. and Henson, E. (1998) Position and velocity coupling of postural sway to somatosensory drive. *J. Neurophysiol.*, 79: 1661–1674.

Jeka, J., Oie, K.S. and Kiemel, T. (2000) Multisensory information for human postural control: integrating touch and vision. *Exp. Brain Res.*, 134: 107–125.

Johansson, R. and Magnusson, M. (1991) Human postural dynamics. *Biomed. Eng.*, 18: 413–437.

Kavounoudias, A., Rool, R. and Roll, J.-P. (2001) Foot sole and ankle muscle inputs contribute jointly to human erect posture regulation. *J. Physiol. (Lond.)*, 5532: 869–878.

Kerkhoff, G. (2003) Modulation and rehabilitation of spatial neglect by sensory stimulation. In: C. Prablanc, D. Pélisson and Y. Rossetti (Eds.), *Neural Control of Space Coding and Action Production. Progress in Brain Research*, Vol. 142. Elsevier, Amsterdam, pp. 257–271 (this volume).

Massion, J. (1994) Postural control system. *Curr. Opin. Neurobiol.*, 4: 877–887.

Massion, J. and Woollacott, M.H. (1996) Posture and equilibrium. In: A.M. Bronstein, T. Brandt and M.H. Woollacott (Eds.), *Clinical Disorders of Balance, Posture and Gait*. Arnold, London, pp. 1–18.

Maurer, C., Mergner, T., Bolha, B. and Hlavacka, F. (2000) Vestibular, visual, and somatosensory contributions to human control of upright stance. *Neurosci. Lett.*, 281: 99–102.

Maurer, C., Mergner, T., Bolha, B. and Hlavacka, F. (2001) Human balance control during cutaneous stimulation of the plantar soles. *Neurosci. Lett.*, 302: 45–48.

Merfeld, D.M. (1995) Modeling the vestibulo-ocular reflex of the squirrel monkey during eccentric rotation and roll tilt. *Exp. Brain Res.*, 106: 123–134.

Mergner, T. and Glasauer, S. (1999) A simple model of vestibular canal–otolith signal fusion. *Ann. N.Y. Acad. Sci.*, 871: 430–434.

Mergner, T. and Rosemeier, T. (1998) Interaction of vestibular, somatosensory and visual signals for posture control and motion perception under terrestrial and microgravity conditions. *Brain Res. Rev.*, 28: 118–135.

Mergner, T., Huber, W. and Becker, W. (1997) Vestibular–neck interaction and transformations of sensory coordinates. *J. Vestib. Res.*, 7: 119–135.

Mergner, T., Nasios, G., Maurer, C. and Becker, W. (2001) Visual object localisation in space. Interaction of retinal, eye position, vestibular and neck proprioceptive information. *Exp. Brain. Res.*, 141: 33–51.

Mittelstaedt, H. (1996) Somatic graviception. *Biol. Psychol.*, 42: 53–74.

Nashner, L.M. (1972) Vestibular postural control model. *Kybernetik*, 10: 106–110.

Peterka, R.J. and Benolken, M.S. (1995) Role of somatosensory and vestibular cues in attenuating visually induced human postural sway. *Exp. Brain Res.*, 105: 101–110.

Peterka, R.J. (2002) Sensorimotor integration in human postural control. *J. Neurophysiol.*, 88: 1097–1118.

Rode, G., Pisella, L., Rossetti, Y., Farnè, A. and Boisson, D. (2003) Bottom-up transfer of sensory-motor plasticity to recovery of spatial cognition: visuomotor adaptation and spatial neglect. In: C. Prablanc, D. Pélisson and Y. Rossetti (Eds.), *Neural Control of Space Coding and Action Production. Progress in Brain Research*, Vol. 142. Elsevier, Amsterdam, pp. 273–287 (this volume).

Van Asten, W.N.J.C., Gielen, C.C.A.M. and Van der Gron, J.J. (1988) Postural movements induced by rotations of visual scenes. *J. Opt. Soc. Am.*, 5: 1781–1789.

Van der Kooij, H., Jacobs, R., Koopman, B. and Grootenboer, H. (1999) A multisensory integration model of human stance control. *Biol. Cybern.*, 80: 299–308.

Winter, D.A. (1990) *Biomechanics and Motor Control of Human Movement*. 2nd ed., Wiley, New York, NY.

Zupan, L., Merfeld, D.M. and Darlot, C. (2002) Using sensory weighting to model the influence of canal, otolith and visual cues on spatial orientation and eye movements. *Biol. Cybern.*, 86: 209–230.

C. Prablanc, D. Pélisson and Y. Rossetti (Eds.)
Progress in Brain Research, Vol. 142
© 2003 Elsevier Science B.V. All rights reserved

CHAPTER 13

Role of sensory information in updating internal models of the effector during arm tracking

Jean-Louis Vercher *, Frédéric Sarès, Jean Blouin, Christophe Bourdin and
Gabriel Gauthier

*UMR 6152 'Mouvement et Perception', CNRS and Université de la Méditerranée, Campus scientifique de Luminy, F-13288 Marseille
cedex 9, France*

Abstract: This chapter is divided into three main parts. Firstly, on the basis of the literature, we will shortly discuss how the recent introduction of the concept of internal models by Daniel Wolpert and Mitsuo Kawato contributes to a better understanding of what is motor learning and what is motor adaptation. Then, we will present a model of eye–hand co-ordination during self-moved target tracking, which we used as a way to specifically address these topics. Finally, we will show some evidence about the use of proprioceptive information for updating the internal models, in the context of eye–hand co-ordination. Motor and afferent information appears to contribute to the parametric adjustment (adaptation) between arm motor command and visual information about arm motion. The study reported here was aimed at assessing the contribution of arm proprioception in building (learning) and updating (adaptation) these representations. The subjects (including a deafferented subject) had to make back and forth movements with their forearm in the horizontal plane, over learned amplitude and at constant frequency, and to track an arm-driven target with their eyes. The dynamical conditions of arm movement were altered (unexpectedly or systematically) during the movement by changing the mechanical properties of the manipulandum. The results showed a significant change of the latency and the gain of the smooth pursuit system, before and after the perturbation for the control subjects, but not for the deafferented subject. Moreover, in control subjects, vibrations of the arm muscles prevented adaptation to the mechanical perturbation. These results suggest that in a self-moved target tracking task, the arm motor system shares with the smooth pursuit system an internal representation of the arm dynamical properties, and that arm proprioception is necessary to build this internal model. As suggested by Ghez et al. (1990) (Cold Spring Harbor Symp. Quant. Biol., 55: 837–8471), proprioception would allow control subjects to learn the inertial properties of the limb.

Motor control schemes should have an element of control and an element of co-ordination. The former is a source of initiative and a product of the brain's work (mind, intelligence, or 'homunculus') while the latter can be viewed as a process with *constraints emerging at a hierarchically lower, autonomous level. Limiting scientific analysis to an object smaller than the universe necessarily leads to a hierarchical (cybernetic) approach.*

Mark Latash (1997)

Do we need an internal model to control our actions?

* Correspondence to: J.-L. Vercher, UMR 6152 'Mouvement et Perception', CNRS and Université de la Méditerranée, Campus scientifique de Luminy, F-13288 Marseille cedex 9, France. Tel.: +33-491-17-22-62; Fax: +33-491-17-22-52; E-mail: vercher@laps.univ-mrs.fr

Prior to any action, the central nervous system (CNS) must solve a series of problems, which Jean Massion (1997) clearly identified as mainly related to me-

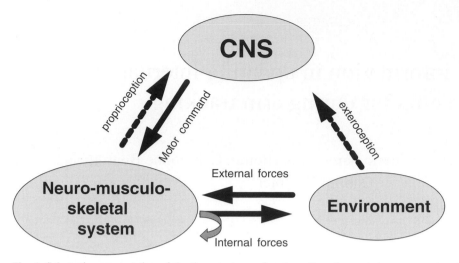

Fig. 1. Schematic representation of the three partners of motor action: the central nervous system (CNS), the musculo-skeletal system, and the external world. Adapted from Massion (1997).

chanics (see Fig. 1). A movement is the result of the interaction of at least three actors, the CNS, the body and the environment. Information and force flows are continuously exchanged between these actors. For this reason, obviously a movement is not only the result of a motor command. In other words, the dynamical constraints put by the external world have an influence on the trajectory. On the other side, a motor command cannot result in an appropriate action if the properties of the effector and the environment are not taken into account. Among these properties, the ones pertaining to the CNS itself are not the least, for instance the delays.

The concept of internal model, of robotic inspiration, has been recently introduced in motor control theories as a way to explain how a motor system can overcome its own delays and how it may take into account the physical properties of the effector (Wolpert et al., 1995; Wolpert and Kawato, 1998; Kawato, 1999; Kawato et al., 2003, this volume). Many authors now consider that in order to perform complex motor actions involving motor segments with distinct geometrical, mechanical and neural properties (e.g. the arm and the eyes), the CNS must build and update internal models of the motor systems. In this framework, motor skill acquisition can be seen as resulting from the elaboration of an internal model of a sensory–motor system, and motor adaptation may be a long-term change of this internal model,

driven by changes in the environment or the motor system itself, and mediated by sensory signals. The existence of an internal model of arm properties, shared by both the eye and arm motor systems, could explain the synchrony between the eye and the arm in a self-moved target tracking task (Gauthier and Hofferer, 1976). This point will be extensively discussed further in this chapter.

What is meant by the term 'internal model'? Chris Miall and Daniel Wolpert proposed the following definition (see Fig. 2): an internal model is a causal representation of the motor apparatus, which mimics its behavior. It allows to predict what the effector will do when it receives a given motor command. It delivers an estimate of the sensory feedback, with no delay (Fig. 2B).

There is another form of internal model, called 'inverse'. In an inverse internal model (Fig. 2A) the informational flow is reversed: it allows to predict the command to be applied to the effector in order to get a given state. In other words, the inverse internal models receives as an input the intended movement and delivers, as an output, a set of motor commands, to be applied to the effector. The general idea is that if the inverse model mirrors the dynamical properties of the effector, then the transfer function of the combination of inverse model and effector is equal to unity (the intended movement is transformed into a real movement). For instance, Kawato (1999) proposed that an

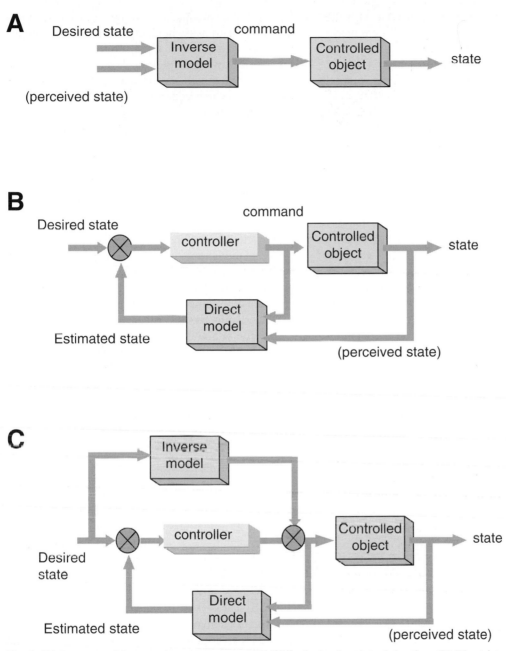

Fig. 2. (A) Inverse model, generating a motor command on the basis of an intended action. (B) Direct internal model, generating a prediction of the sensory inflow, on the basis of a copy of the motor command. (C) Integrated model, combining inverse and direct internal model. Adapted from Miall et al. (1993) and Wolpert et al. (1998).

internal model allows to determine the torques to be applied to the joint in order to reach a position.

Wolpert et al. (1998) combined the two types of internal models in a classical feedback control system: the forward internal model is inserted in the feedback loop while the inverse internal model is in parallel with the forward branch (Fig. 2C). It appears that in order to be kept operative, the internal models must maintain themselves in tune with the real controlled system. This is what the engineers call adaptive control.

As judiciously pointed out by Normand Teasdale (personal communication) the concept of internal model was announced more than a quarter of a century ago by Schmidt's (1975) theory of motor program (or schema). Indeed, Schmidt proposed that when performing movement, the subject stored the *initial conditions*, the *response specifications*, the *sensory consequences of the movement*, and the *response outcome*. After learning, when a movement is intended, the schema receives two inputs: the desired outcome and the initial conditions. Then the schema generates the commands which result in the movement. The schema also generates a set of expected sensory inflows (Schmidt distinguished between the proprioceptive and the exteroceptive feedbacks). After movement, the expected sensory consequences are compared with the actual inflow, in order to identify the errors, which drive the necessary changes of the motor schema. Conceptually, the major difference between the two concepts (motor schema and internal model) is that for Schmidt (1975) the motor program works on an iterative (discrete) way, while the internal model is described as a continuous (on-line) mechanism. There is now a large amount of evidence (starting from the study of Prablanc and Martin, 1992; see also Prablanc et al., 2003, this volume) that error correction is a continuous, early starting process during movement execution itself.

Internal models play a role in motor co-ordination and adaptation

To understand how these models build up, how they stay in tune with the effectors, in spite of some physical changes, is an open door for studying motor learning and sensorimotor adaptation. For instance, Shadmehr and Mussa-Ivaldi (1994) used a robotic manipulator to simulate an artificial force field, which perturbed the pointing movement. After some trials, the subject could compensate for the perturbation and produced a straight trajectory. When the force field was suddenly turn off, the subject produced again distorted trajectories, mirroring the trajectories before adaptation. The authors concluded that the subject built an internal representation of the force field, which could even be extrapolated to the non-visited space.

Internal models may also be used to control the co-ordination between two motor systems, as evidenced by Flanagan and Wing (1997), who used a grip-and-push task. When the impedance (inertia, viscosity, elasticity) of the manipulandum was changed, the grip force was modulated in a parallel way with push forces, and thus anticipated the changes in manipulandum load. This means that the CNS can predict the load force and the kinematics of hand movement on which the load depends. Flanagan and Wing proposed that this was achieved by updating an internal model of both the motor system and external loads.

Guédon et al. (1998) showed another type of motor adaptation, involving bi-dimensional arm movements, and specifically addressed the role of proprioception. The task was to move the stretched out arm, to move a cursor in pace with a target on a screen. Unexpectedly, the gain between the arm motion and the cursor motion could be changed, along the vertical, horizontal or both directions. The subjects were then allowed to practice and to learn this new relationship. Finally, after adaptation, the subjects produced in visual open loop an ellipse with the arm to achieve a circle on the screen (Fig. 3A). In contrast, a deafferented subject (a patient suffering a complete loss of proprioception below neck level) tested in the same conditions failed to achieve a similar adaptation, as evidenced by his tracking performance, in terms of error, delay and curvature (Fig. 3B). Paradoxically, when unexpectedly exposed to the gain change, the deafferented subject was less affected than control subjects. It has to be noted that the tested patient has certainly developed along time a repertoire of 'cognitive strategies' which he may be using to perform the task while control subjects are

Fig. 3. Adaptation of 2D tracking to a change of gain. The task was to track a target moving along a circular path at constant radial velocity. During the adaptation block (50 trials), the gain was increased by 2.5 times along the horizontal axis. VCL, visual closed loop; VOL, visual open loop. (A) Control subjects. (B) Deafferented subject. (C) Model. Adapted from Guédon et al. (1998).

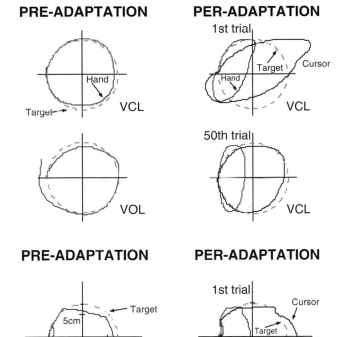

A   PRE-ADAPTATION   PER-ADAPTATION   POST-ADAPTATION

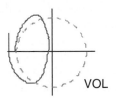
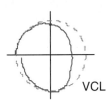
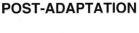

B   PRE-ADAPTATION   PER-ADAPTATION   POST-ADAPTATION

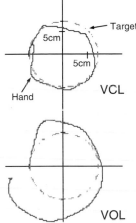
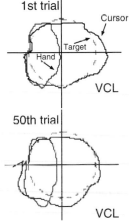
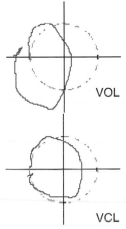

C

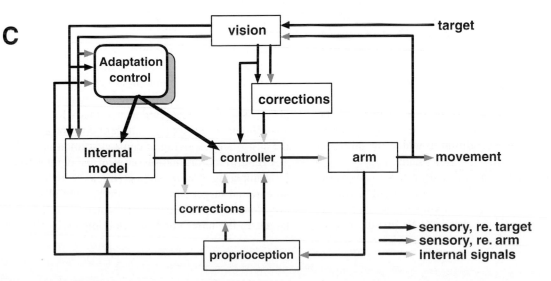

certainly using more low-level, sensorimotor mechanisms (Ingram et al., 2000).

Guédon (1998) proposed a model (Fig. 3C), to explain how visual and proprioceptive signals were used to adapt the motor system to a new condition. According to this model, vision and proprioception are used simultaneously to correct errors during the execution of the movement (in-line control) and to update the arm controller, included the internal model (adaptive control). Guédon and co-workers also focused on the fact that adaptation control may be understood as *performance control*, as opposed to *execution control*. The role of the adaptation control is to maintain a fairly stable level of performance in spite of changes in the motor plant or the external world. It is usually difficult to distinguish between those two control modes, because most of the time they are studied on the same motor apparatus, and because it is practically impossible to suppress all sources of feedback. One way to overcome the difficulty is to examine what happens when two motor systems, as different and mechanically uncoupled as possible, are involved in a common task. Eye–hand co-ordination during tracking is a good candidate.

How are the eyes and the arm co-ordinated in a tracking task?

At this point, it may be necessary to define the term 'co-ordination', because we may be using it in a singular way. We call *co-ordination control* the process by which when two sensorimotor systems (for instance the eyes and the arm, or the head and the eyes) are involved in the execution of a motor task, the accuracy and the characteristics of each system improve, as compared to the performance observed separately in each system when used alone (see also Engel and Soechting, 2003, this volume). As opposed to most of the studies dealing with eye–hand co-ordination, which show that the arm takes advantage of vision and eye motion to increase its accuracy, we consider how the eye motor system takes advantage of a condition in which the target is directly attached to the observer's hand.

The term 'smooth pursuit' (SP) refers to a type of eye movements observed when an animal is tracking with the eyes a target moving in front of it. It has long been believed that smooth pursuit is not under voluntary control: slow eye movements are not possible without a visual target (Westheimer and Conover, 1954) and are directly driven by signals related to target velocity, e.g. an internal reconstruction of target motion in space, since retinal signals are not sufficient to code target motion as soon as the eyes and/or the head are moving (Rashbass, 1961). Usually, smooth pursuit starts between 100 and 120 ms after target onset. It has to be noted that this time is much longer than the sum of all the conduction times in the path between the retina and the extra-ocular muscles (Fuchs, 1967). The extra time needed to start smooth pursuit could be a sign that some central process (reconstruction, representation?) is underlying. More recently, Duhamel et al. (1992) proposed that parietal neurons are taking into account the retinal consequences of eye movements in order to update target representation in space coordinates.

However, Gauthier and Hofferer showed in 1976 that if a subject tracks a LED attached to his moving finger, smooth pursuit is not discontinued when the LED is turned off, providing that the subject continues moving the finger. If the subject stops moving the finger when the target is off, smooth pursuit disappears. Thus vision is not the only source of information able to trigger and control smooth pursuit.

Let us consider what happens when a subject fixates a visual target with the eyes. The target suddenly starts moving. The pattern of eye motion in response to such a stimulus is well known: after a latency of 90–120 ms, the eyes start moving slowly and smoothly. Because of the delay, the eyes are not on the target. 250 ms after target onset, a saccade is triggered to catch-up the target, allowing the visual image of the target to be on the fovea, after which the pursuit will continue by a combination of smooth pursuit segments and small saccades. The velocity of the smooth pursuit segments is generally very close to target velocity, except when the latter exceeds 40–50°/s, which is considered as a velocity limit for the smooth pursuit system. A similar behavior applies if the target is not moving at constant velocity.

eye–arm co-ordination control is demonstrated by comparing how a subject tracks with the eyes an external target (this condition is generally called *eye-alone tracking*) to how he tracks a self-moved target. In the latter condition, a completely different eye movement pattern develops. The smooth pursuit movement starts earlier than in the former: the latency is close to 0 instead of 100 to 130 ms. The maximum smooth pursuit velocity is much higher than in eye-alone tracking ($\sim 100°/s$, Gauthier et al., 1988). As a consequence there is generally no catch-up saccade and the contribution of smooth pursuit to the overall tracking is higher. At this point, let us remember that the synchrony between the arm and the eyes could not be explained only by a common command addressed to the oculomotor system and the arm motor system. Indeed, since the mechanical properties of the eyes and the arm are obviously completely different (the viscous–elastic forces have much more influence on the eye than the inertia), in transient situations a common command would result in the eyes leading the arm.

Role of proprioception in eye–arm co-ordination

Although a major part of co-ordination between the eye and the arm is based on vision, we may suggest that some part of this control relies on arm inflow and outflow information. Arm proprioception may be responsible for smooth pursuit during tracking of the hand in darkness. These signals may also account for the higher velocity of smooth pursuit eye movements and the shorter tracking delay when the hand is used as a target. In order to determine the role played by arm proprioception in the arm–eye co-ordination, we tested eye–arm co-ordination during passive movements of the arm (Vercher et al., 1996). In this study, we showed that the latency distributions observed in the active condition are significantly different from the two others (eye-alone and passive condition). There was no difference between the latencies observed in eye-alone and passive arm movement conditions (the passively moved arm is 'considered' by the smooth pursuit system as if it were an externally driven target), which is an argument to say that:

- active control of the arm motion is necessary to synchronize eye and arm motions;
- in passive condition smooth pursuit is initiated by the same process as in eye-alone condition.

In the same study, the participation of two subjects suffering complete loss of proprioception allowed us to assess the contribution of arm motor command signals operating alone. Though both deafferented subjects are almost unable to produce accurate goal-directed motor behavior in complete darkness, they can produce, with visual control, almost all the movements required for a normal life: they can move by themselves, feed themselves and write. The difference between them is that one subject has neck proprioception whereas the other does not. If we consider the latency criterion, the deafferented subjects did not differ from controls: in eye-alone tracking the latency is 150 ms in average while in self-moved target tracking, it is exactly 0 ms. However, the variability is significantly higher in deafferented subjects (Vercher et al., 1997a,b). We thus may say that active control of the arm is sufficient to trigger short-latency smooth pursuit. Comparing the performance of controls tracking with the eye their passively moved arm and deafferented tracking the actively moved arm showed that the will to move is necessary to synchronize arm and eye movements. Thus, we may say that:

- non-visual signals coding arm movements are responsible for the short latency;
- active control of arm movement is necessary and sufficient to produce short-latency eye tracking;
- arm inflow is necessary to increase the dynamic performance and the accuracy of the smooth pursuit system.

Finally, arm–eye co-ordination results in an improvement of smooth pursuit performance. Arm command is necessary for the eye-to-arm motion onset synchronization, while afferent information does not seem to contribute to timing. However, afferent information appears to contribute to the adjustment between arm command and visual information about arm motion.

It is amazing how far we can go in perturbing the system and how it is able to compensate for the perturbation. For instance, if the target path is reversed relative to the arm path without informing the subject, during the first 200 ms of ocular tracking, smooth pursuit movement is produced in the direction of the arm motion, thus opposed to the visual stimulus (Vercher et al., 1995). After that initial interval, the eye velocity decays, and a saccade is issued in the direction of the visual target motion, and for the rest of the trial, the eyes remain in pace with the visual target. Exposure to reversal during a long period resulted in an adaptation to the constraint: on average, less than ten trials were sufficient to induce a reversal of the gain of the initial smooth pursuit. When returning to a normal hand-to-target relationship, a reversal on the initial smooth pursuit was taken as the sign for an after-effect. Again, deafferented subjects behaved almost like control subjects when the target path was randomly reversed to the arm, but they did not adapt at all to the perturbation (Vercher et al., 1996).

The model

On the basis of previous studies, we proposed in 1997 a model for co-ordination control between the arm motor system and the smooth pursuit system as observed in human subjects during eye tracking of a self-moved target (Lazzari et al., 1997). The model is based on an exchange of information between the two sensorimotor systems, mediated by sensory (vision, arm muscle proprioception) and arm motor signals. Both motor systems are completely independent from each other. The interaction is mediated by the lateral cerebellum (Vercher and Gauthier, 1988): monkeys were trained to perform a self-moved target tracking; the performance was quantified before and after lesion of the dentate nucleus. Before lesion, the monkeys behaved almost as human subjects: eye tracking of the hand was more accurate that tracking of an external target. The only difference was that monkeys had to see a LED attached to their real hand to show the eye–arm coupling while vision of target projected on a screen was sufficient for humans (direct and complete vision of the real hand does not improve the performance on humans). After lesion, monkeys tracked the self-moved target as if it was an external target. Experiments on patients (Van Donkelaar and Lee, 1994) or using functional neuroimaging techniques (Miall et al., 2001) confirmed the involvement of the lateral cerebellum in arm–eye coordination. The model implies that the properties of the arm are stored, and taken into account by the eye motor system (see Fig. 4).

Computer simulation of the model yielded results which both qualitatively and quantitatively fit the behavior of human subjects (Vercher et al., 1996, 1997a,b). The model is based on the following rules.

- Co-ordination control is based on an exchange of non-visual signals (proprioception, efferent copy) between the arm motor system and the oculomotor system. As a corollary, co-ordination is not based on a common command simultaneously addressed to the two motor systems.
- Co-ordination control is mediated by a structure of the CNS (the lateral cerebellum) receiving signals from both sensory–motor systems.
- Efferent copy from the moving arm plays a crucial role in timing aspects, while arm proprioception is needed for spatial accuracy.

The model developed, implemented and simulated on the basis of empirical research, has been designed as a prototype in order to test the veracity of hypotheses addressing the way information about movement is used to co-ordinate different motor systems. We tried to maintain a high level of parallelism between the model and what is known about neurophysiology of motor control. We also tried to make sure that the same model will behave in the appropriate way in the different tracking conditions.

The model presented in Fig. 4 features three main parts: (1) the eye motor control (including a smooth pursuit branch and a saccadic branch) inspired from the models proposed by Larry Young and by David Robinson; (2) the arm motor control; and (3) the co-ordination control in between. The co-ordination control is carried out via an exchange of information between the arm and the eye sensorimotor systems, mediated by sensory signals (vision, proprioception) and motor command copy. This cross-talk results in improved smooth pursuit system performance.

Role of proprioception in eye–arm co-ordination adaptation

So far the model is absolutely static (adaptation control has not been included), meaning that if some parameter is changed somewhere (for instance the properties of the arm, or a change in the environment), then there is no way to maintain the performance of the task. Due to the mechanical differences between the eye plant and the arm, to maintain the synchrony between the hand and the eyes, the co-ordination system must be aware of these changes and take them into account.

With a model, it is easy to change inertia, stiffness or viscosity and play around with the parameters.

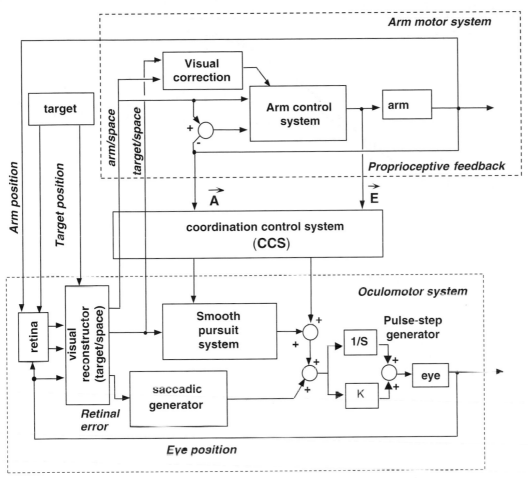

Fig. 4. Model of eye–arm co-ordination. See text for details. Adapted from Lazzari et al. (1997).

Still, a major problem appears at this point: what happens if some part of the model, or the real system, is changed, for instance the mechanical properties of the arm? How could the oculomotor system stay in tune with the arm in order to maintain synchrony? Let us see what results if the friction is increased at arm level.

Fig. 5A shows a simulation of the model, in which a dry friction was added to the dynamics of the manipulandum. When the system generates a command, the produced force may not be enough to compensate for the friction. The simulation shows that in this case, smooth pursuit starts long before the arm, and a saccade is triggered back to the arm position. This is due to the fact that when the arm motor command is issued, friction delays the initiation of the arm motion. At the same time, the arm motor command has

been addressed to the oculomotor system through the co-ordination control system, and has triggered the non-visual smooth pursuit which results in an anticipation of the eyes on the arm. We tested these predictions with control subjects, to test the ability of the oculomotor system to remain adapted with the properties of the arm. A variable friction system was attached to the manipulandum, and we recorded eye movements and arm muscles EMG during self-induced arm-movements. The EMG signal was used to date the arm motor command (Scarchilli and Vercher, 1999).

Methods

Twenty-six right-handed subjects ranging in age from 21 to 32 years, and a deafferented subject,

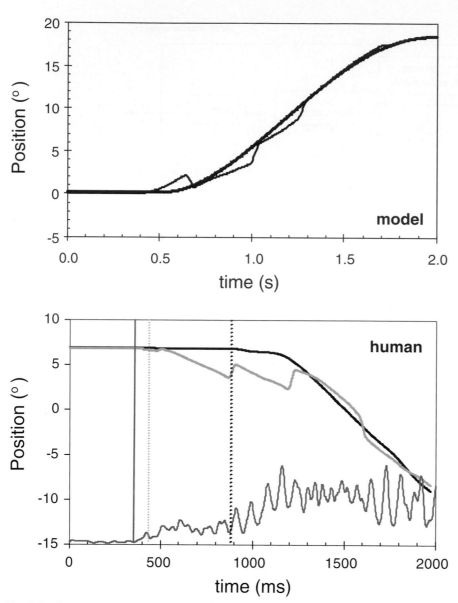

Fig. 5. Predicted (A) and recorded (B) kinematics of eye (gray trace) and arm (black trace) during eye tracking of a self-moved target, when a friction force was added to the manipulandum. On B is also represented the integrated and filtered EMG from the biceps muscle, showing that the eyes synchronize better with the arm–EMG than with the arm motion. Continuous lines, eye (gray) and arm positions (black). Gray line at bottom, rectified and integrated EMG of the biceps muscle. Vertical lines mark EMG (continuous dark), eye (dashed gray) and arm (dashed black) onsets, respectively. Vertical scales correspond to the position in degrees. There is no scale for the EMG signal amplitude, which values are in mV.

participated in the present study (10 subjects in experiment 1, 6 in experiment 2 and 10 in experiment 3). They were naive with regard to the aim of the study. They were also all exempt of known visual or oculomotor disorders.

Fig. 6 shows the experimental set-up used in these studies. A complete description can be found elsewhere (Vercher et al., 1996). Horizontal eye movements were recorded with an infrared corneal reflection device (Iris Skalar: bandwidth DC to 200

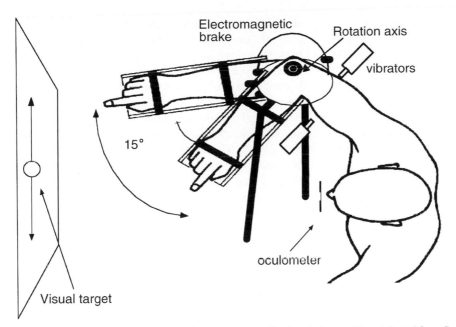

Fig. 6. Experimental set-up used to study eye–arm co-ordination during tracking. Adapted from Scarchilli and Vercher (1999).

Hz, resolution 1.5′ arc, linearity ±30°). Arm position was measured with a potentiometer at elbow level. The EMG activity of the moving arm biceps was recorded using surface electrodes (Meditrace, Graphic Controls) placed on the biceps brachialis. The EMG signal was pre-amplified ($\times 10{,}000$), and pre filtered (high pass 30 Hz, low pass 200 Hz). The shoulder was placed in abduction and flexion (about 30°), and the arm/forearm angle was near 100° to increase signal/noise ratio (Adamovich et al., 1994). The target, arm, eye and EMG signals were amplified, filtered (low pass 250 Hz) and digitized at 500 samples/s. An electromagnetic brake (Warner Electric, model TB 500, maximal torque 40 N m, tension range 0–20 V) was also positioned on the rotation axis. The brake torque was directly controlled by the computer through a digital-to-analogue converter, such that the generated friction was proportional to the voltage command. Thus, when the brake was off, the manipulandum needed a torque of 0.44 N m to be activated. On the other hand, the brake needed 2.66 N m when 3 V was applied (the relationship between the tension and the torque was near to linear in the range 1–17 V). Lacquaniti and Soechting (1986) showed that muscular activation is proportional to the perturbation force.

The subjects had to move their right arm back and forth and to track the hand-driven target with their eyes. At the beginning of each trial, the subject put the target on the right side of the screen and move the arm sinusoidally at about 0.3 Hz over 15° of amplitude. Subjects were required to maintain target fixation with their eyes. After receiving a 'ready' signal from the experimenter, the subject started to move the arm. The subject had 3 s to make the complete movement. The conditions were as follows.

- *Brake off (B-OFF).* The brake was attached to the manipulandum but not activated.
- *Brake on (B-ON).* Just before the arm movement, a passive friction was applied to the manipulandum. The subjects were instructed to try to maintain the velocity and the amplitude of arm movements in spite of the perturbation. There was no cue to indicate to the subject whether the brake was to be activated or not.

In experiment 1, the two conditions (B-OFF and B-ON) were randomly assigned to the subjects over a total of 120 trials. The brake was always attached to the manipulandum but activated during 1/3 of the trials only, on average.

In experiment 2, the perturbation was systematically applied. Subjects completed 100 consecutive trials in 3 blocks:

- PRE block (for pre exposure) — self-moved target tracking without perturbation (20 consecutive trials in the B-OFF condition);
- PER block (during exposure) — self-moved target tracking with perturbation (60 consecutive trials in the B-ON condition);
- POST block (for post-effect) — self-moved target tracking without perturbation (20 consecutive trials in the B-OFF condition).

In experiment 3, vibrations of the tendons of both the biceps and triceps muscles were applied during the exposure to the brake (PER block), in order to perturb the proprioceptive signal mediated by muscle spindle (Ia) fibers. Mechanical vibrations were applied by means of an electromagnetic vibrator (PA 25 E) to the triceps and biceps brachialis. The peak-to-peak amplitude was approximately 2 mm, whereas the frequency was 80 Hz (Ribot-Ciscar et al., 1998). The vibrators were fixed on an external bar, which allowed us to move and adapt the vibrators in such a manner that their heads were perpendicular, simultaneously to the distal tendon of the biceps and triceps muscles. The subjects were seated on a chair, their arm placed on a gutter. In order to insure optimal placement of the vibrator heads, each vibrator was turned on alternatively, and adjusted in position until the subject reported experiencing an illusion of movement of the forearm, in the direction opposite to the action of the vibrated muscle (flexion when the triceps was stimulated, and extension when the biceps was stimulated (Roll and Vedel, 1982). The simultaneous vibration of the agonist–antagonist muscles began 60 s before the first tracking trial of the PER session. When applied, the vibratory stimulation lasted 20 min. The applied frequency and amplitude were most effective in exciting muscle spindle primary endings (Roll and Vedel, 1982; Kasai et al., 1992), as well as to affect sensory afferents (Gilhodes et al., 1986). Each subject participated in two sessions, one during which no vibration was applied during the PER blocks, and another during which the vibration was applied to the two muscles.

In experiments 2 and 3, the subjects did not know when the change of condition was to occur; however, they did know that during the 100 trials, a constant perturbation (Brake-ON) would be applied. Analysis

started with digital low-pass filtering of all signals (cut-off frequency of 30 Hz, −3 dB). The latencies between target and smooth pursuit motion onsets, EMG burst and arm motion, EMG burst and smooth pursuit motion, arm and smooth pursuit motions were measured. For the determination of the smooth pursuit and arm movement onsets, we used a velocity acceleration criterion previously described (Vercher et al., 1996). For the determination of the EMG burst beginning, we used a similar technique, proposed by Hodges and Bui (1996), after rectifying and integrating the EMG signal. Maximal velocities of arm motion and smooth pursuit were also determined. In order to test the effect of condition, dependent variables (eye-to-arm latency, EMG-to-eye latency, EMG-to-arm latency, and smooth pursuit gain: ratio between eye velocity and arm–target velocity) were submitted to analysis of variance (ANOVA, S_{10} $\langle c_3 \rangle$) and a Student–Newman–Keuls post-hoc test was applied to the data. Since we were interested in smooth pursuit initiation, only the trials where eye motion began with smooth pursuit were analyzed. The others (e.g. starting with a saccade) were rejected. These latter trials represented less than 5% of the total.

Results

Parts of these data have been previously published (Scarchilli and Vercher, 1999; Scarchilli et al., 1999). Fig. 5B is an example from a control subject, during the Brake-ON condition in experiment 1. The figure shows a typical pattern of eyes and arm movement, similar to the simulation shown in Fig. 5A. Moreover, the integrated EMG from the biceps clearly shows that smooth pursuit is synchronized with the onset of arm EMG. The timing of the arm is delayed only due to an external factor, thus breaking the eye–arm synchrony. When the brake was OFF, the eye–hand synchrony was due to both the arm and the eyes lagging the arm muscle EMG onset by exactly the same amount of time: 90 to 100 ms. This lag is called in the literature the electromechanical delay. This time is much longer than the time needed to produce an eye movement from an oculomotor command. This means that the eyes are in some way 'waiting' for the arm, or take into account the properties of the arm.

When the brake was unexpectedly ON, the time between EMG and smooth pursuit is not affected, while the arm is delayed relative to the EMG onset. This results in an anticipation of the eyes relative to the arm. This anticipation can reach up to 300 ms.

If the perturbation was maintained over a long period of time, two types of adaptation were observed (Fig. 7): first, and rapidly, the arm motor command was more effective and the lag between the EMG and the arm motor command decreased (Fig. 7A). Over a longer period, the EMG-to-smooth pursuit latency increased slightly (Fig. 7B). The result was that after adaptation, when the brake was turned OFF, smooth pursuit and arm motion were again close to synchrony, smooth pursuit slightly lagging the arm motion, while before adaptation smooth pursuit was leading arm movement (a kind of overcompensation, or after-effect).

The observation is compatible with the model, the arm and the eyes have separate controls, which adapt differently: the arm onset is advanced, and the smooth pursuit onset is delayed. This results in a re-synchronization of the eyes and arm.

Fig. 8 (from Scarchilli et al., 1999) shows the gain of the smooth pursuit system (defined as the ratio between the eye velocity and the arm velocity) just before and during unpredictable activation of the brake, in control subjects and in a deafferented subject. We observed that when the arm is impeded, the smooth pursuit gain decreases in controls, but not in the deafferented subject. Our conclusion was that in control subjects, part of the gain of smooth pursuit is due to a non-visual process, which is affected by the change of arm dynamics, while in the deafferented subject, all the smooth pursuit gain is tributary to vision, thus it is not affected by the braking.

In the last experiment, in order to affect arm proprioception in control subjects, we used tendinous vibrations applied concomitantly to both the biceps and the triceps. We exposed the subject to continuous braking of the arm, and we measured the smooth pursuit latency and gain after the exposure session. Some subjects had some difficulty to perform the task during the PER block when vibrations were applied. However, all the subjects experienced the illusory arm movement, when vibration was applied to only one muscle.

Fig. 9A shows that the distribution of velocities of arm movement is not affected by exposure to the vibration during adaptation to the brake. This was an important point to check since our analysis was mostly based on gain (the ratio between eye velocity and arm velocity). The histogram of latencies between the arm and the eyes (Fig. 9B) shows a Gaussian distribution in PER and POST blocks, in both sessions. From a qualitative point of view the distributions look very similar, except for the POST block in the without-vibration condition, where the distribution is flatter and wider than in the others.

Quantitatively, mean eye-to-arm latency was affected by the exposure to the brake, only when no vibration was applied during the PER blocks (Fig. 10A). Mean latency is 14.38 ± 2.3 ms in the PRE block and 38.47 ± 4.34 ms in the POST block in the session without vibration, and 13.54 ± 3.05 ms in the PRE block and 15.05 ± 3.36 ms in the POST block in the session with vibration. There was no difference between the PRE blocks in the two sessions ($P > 0.05$) while there was a significant difference between the POST blocks ($P < 0.05$). PRE and POST blocks were significantly different in the session without vibrations ($F_{1,384} = 24.98$, $P < 0.0001$) but it was not significant in the session with vibration ($F_{1,384} = 0.11$, $P > 0.7403$).

The same observation applies to the gain. Mean gain was 0.78 ± 0.02 in the PRE block and 0.92 ± 0.04 in the POST block in the session without vibration, while it was 0.76 ± 0.02 in the PRE block and 0.72 ± 0.04 in the POST block in the session with vibration. There was a significant difference between PRE and POST conditions in the session without vibration ($F_{1,383} = 8.35$, $P < 0.0041$) while there was no difference in the session with vibration ($F_{1,377} = 126$, $P > 0.2623$).

Thus the results of the last experiment showed that when no vibration was applied during an adaptation session, the smooth pursuit latency and gain increased as an effect of adaptation to the brake, while when vibration was applied to both arm muscles, no change was observed.

Discussion and conclusion

Over the last two decades, we accumulated evidences that during eye tracking of a self-moved target, the

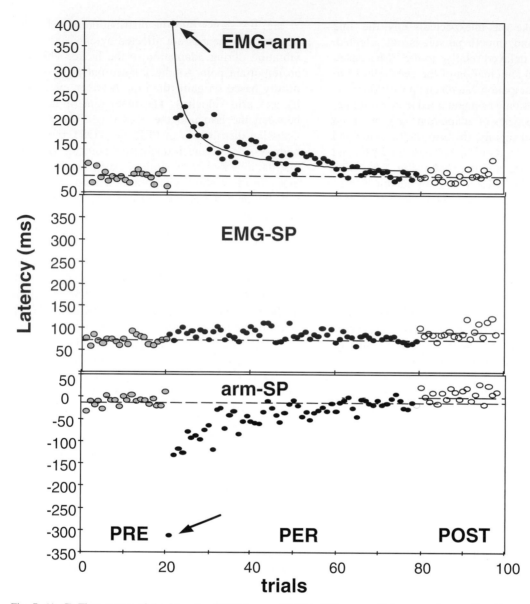

Fig. 7. (A–C) Time-course of the latencies (EMG-to-arm, EMG-to-SPi, arm-to-SPi) averaged over all subjects as a function of trial number. The vertical dashed lines show the transition from one block to the other. The horizontal dotted lines represent the average of the latencies in the PRE block. The horizontal dashed lines in the POST block represent the average latencies in the POST condition. The arrows indicate the first trial of the adaptation block. Adapted from Scarchilli and Vercher (1999).

smooth pursuit system and the arm motor system exchange information about their current states. It has been successively shown that (1) subjects can track their moving arm without vision (Gauthier and Hofferer, 1976), (2) smooth pursuit characteristics are changed in this condition as compared to eye-alone tracking (Gauthier et al., 1988; Vercher et al., 1993), (3) the lateral cerebellum is involved in this co-ordination (Vercher and Gauthier, 1988), (4) non-visual signals are involved in this co-ordination (Vercher et al., 1995), (5) arm motor command is responsible for the synchronization while arm proprioception is responsible for parametric adjustments (Vercher et al., 1996), and (6) adaptation of eye–arm

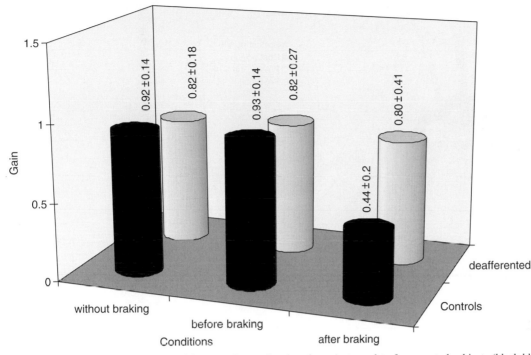

Fig. 8. Means and standard deviation of the smooth pursuit gain values. Average data from control subjects (black blocks) and from the deafferented subject (light blocks). The total number of trials for each subject is 90 for each of the controls (30 not perturbed and 60 perturbed) and 125 for the deafferented (42 and 83). A few trials were not included in the average. Adapted from Scarchilli et al. (1999).

co-ordination to external constraints (Vercher et al., 1997a,b; Guédon et al., 1998; Scarchilli and Vercher, 1999; Scarchilli et al., 1999). We designed a model, to simulate the above empirical data. It is also able to make some predictions, among which the need for the arm dynamics to be represented somewhere at the interface, or shared by both motor systems. This internal model should be able to adapt (to change its dynamics). It is clear to us that the simplest way to explain how the smooth pursuit can generate an eye trajectory similar to an arm motion when the arm movement is impeded (see Fig. 5) is that the smooth pursuit is using an internal model of the arm, and actually tracks a prediction of the arm path instead of the arm itself. Fig. 11, from Scarchilli et al. (1999) is a schematic representation showing the interaction between the arm and the eye through an internal model of the arm. This internal model receives a copy of the arm command, generates an estimate of arm movements, used by the smooth pursuit system to generate an eye movement. This internal model may also be used by the arm motor system in a sort

of internal feedback loop, as proposed by Wolpert et al. (1998). Both this forward internal model and the inverse model used to generate the command for the arm can be adapted when a mismatch between the intended and the actual motions is detected by the visual and/or the proprioceptive channel. The basic idea is that the co-ordination control system compares kinesthetic information from the arm to visual information. A dynamical matching between the two signals results in an increase of smooth pursuit dynamical properties. When they do not match, for instance when the arm impedance changes, if the perturbation is unexpected, this results in a degradation of the smooth pursuit performance. If the perturbation is sustained, then the system becomes adapted and recovers its performance. When proprioception is absent (temporary or definitely), this adaptive mechanism cannot play its role.

This latter point is supported by our previous studies with deafferented patients (Vercher et al., 1996, 1997a,b; Guédon et al., 1998; Scarchilli et al., 1999) and by the experiment reported here, where

218

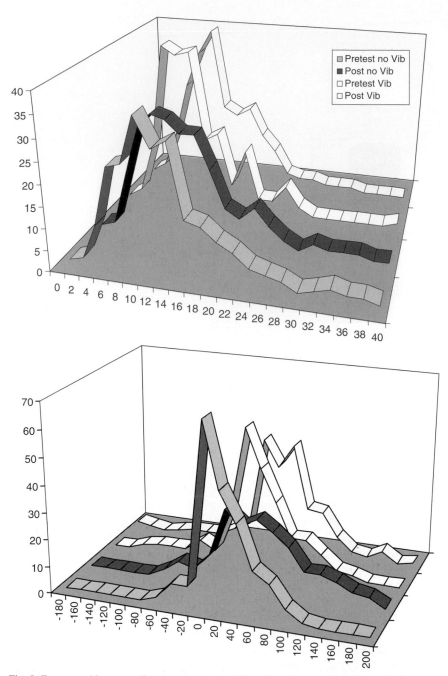

Fig. 9. Frequency histogram of arm mean velocity (A) and eye latency (B) before and after exposure and adaptation to the brake, with or without vibration.

we used vibrations to acutely alter the proprioceptive channel. Indeed, all the people who tested deafferented patients agree that these persons do not behave as controls, although they can in some experimental conditions reach a level of performance, not significantly and systematically different from controls. They have learned new strategies in order to use the information still available (mostly through vision)

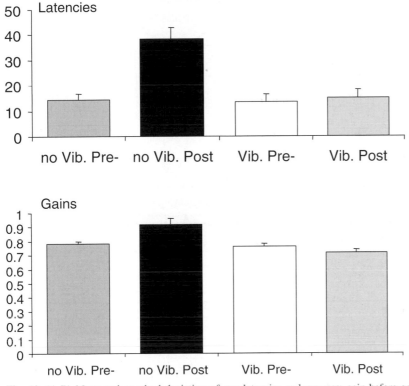

Fig. 10. (A,B) Mean and standard deviation of eye latencies and eye–arm gain before and after exposure and adaptation to the brake, with or without vibration

to compensate for their deficit. During the time of a session with vibrations, we may assume that our subjects did not have enough time to build up similar compensatory strategies.

The increase of latency observed in the session where no vibration was applied during exposure to the brake is compatible with the results of experiment 2 where we observed an increase of eye-to-arm latency as a result of adaptation. Before exposure to the brake the eyes and the arm movements were almost synchronized (the eyes were slightly ahead of the arm). During the first trials of exposure the eyes were largely leading the arm, this anticipation decreased along the exposure (see Fig. 7C); after exposure, the eyes were lagging the arm. The increase of gain is also compatible. During random exposure to the brake (Scarchilli et al., 1999), the gain decreased by 50% (see Fig. 8). Adaptation resulted in a

significant increase of gain, only when no vibration was applied to alter proprioceptive signals. The fact that when vibrations were applied, no change of gain occurred must be compared to the fact that during exposure to the brake, the deafferented subject did not show any change of smooth pursuit gain at all. Unfortunately, we were not able to perform the adaptation experiment in the deafferented subject: due to the particular experimental constraints (absence of direct vision of the arm) too much attentional demand made the experiment really exhausting for the subject as it was difficult to maintain his performance during the long time needed to reach adaptation in controls.

In conclusion, at this point, it is clear to us that the cybernetic approach used so far must be extended to other tools in order to take into account the adaptive capabilities shown. Indeed, the cybernetic approach

220

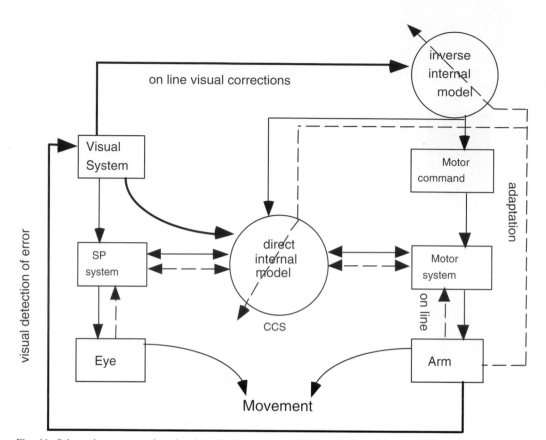

Fig. 11. Schematic representation showing the involvement of the internal model of arm dynamics as a way to predict arm motion. Continuous bold arrows represent the visual signal flow. Continuous thin arrows show the outflow and efferent copy signal flow. Dashed thin arrows indicate the proprioceptive signal flow. Diagonal arrows are used to indicate that the signal is used to update (adapt) the system. This is a simplified model: not all the features of the Coordination Control System are represented here. Adapted from Scarchilli et al. (1999).

is concerned with system input–output relationship. The neural network approach is commonly used now in neuro-computational studies dealing with motor adaptation and is a promising way to provide the model with auto-adaptive capabilities. Linking a cybernetic model to a neuro-mimetic model is not usual but does not present a major difficulty: most of the neuro-mimetic models proposed in the oculomotor research field are based on the same basic knowledge as more classical models.

Acknowledgements

We are grateful to the two deafferented subjects, GL and IW for their participation, to Profs. Yves Lamarre, Jacques Paillard and Jonathan Cole, for contributing to the studies involving the patients, and to a number of graduate students and colleagues, among which: Olivier Guédon, Stefano Lazzari, Denis Quaccia, Karine Scarchilli, and Michel Volle. This work has been supported by grants from the CNRS, the EU (BRAIN Program), the Human Frontier Science Program, the Fondation de France and the Fondation pour la Recherche Médicale.

References

Adamovich, S.V., Levin, M.F. and Feldman, A.G. (1994) Merging different motor patterns: coordination between rhythmical and discrete single joint movements. *Exp. Brain Res.*, 99: 325–337.

Duhamel, J.R., Colby, C.L. and Goldberg, M.E. (1992) The

updating of the representation of visual space in parietal cortex by intended eye movements. *Science*, 255: 90–92.

Engel, K.C. and Soechting, J.F. (2003) Interactions between ocular motor and manual responses during two-dimensional tracking. In: C. Prablanc, D. Pélisson and Y. Rossetti (Eds.), *Neural Control of Space Coding and Action Production. Progress in Brain Research*, Vol. 142. Elsevier, Amsterdam, pp. 141–153 (this volume).

Flanagan, J.R. and Wing, A.M. (1997) The role of internal models in motion planning and control: Evidence from grip force adjustments during movements of hand-held loads. *J. Neurosci.*, 17(4): 1519–1528.

Fuchs, A.F. (1967) Saccadic and smooth pursuit eye movements in the Monkey. *J. Physiol. (Lond.)*, 191: 609–631.

Gauthier, G.M. and Hofferer, J.M. (1976) Eye tracking of self-moved targets in absence of vision. *Exp. Brain Res.*, 26: 121–139.

Gauthier, G.M., Vercher, J.-L., Mussa Ivaldi, F. and Marchetti, E. (1988) Oculo-manual tracking of visual targets: control learning and co-ordination control model. *Exp. Brain Res.*, 73: 127–137.

Ghez, C., Gordon, J., Ghilardi, M.F., Christakos, C.N. and Cooper, S.E. (1990) Roles of proprioceptive input in the programming of arm trajectories. *Cold Spring Harbor Symp. Quant. Biol.*, 55: 837–847.

Gilhodes, J.C., Roll, J.P. and Tardy-Gervet, M.F. (1986) Perceptual and motor effects of agonist–antagonist muscle vibration in man. *Exp. Brain Res.*, 61: 395–402.

Guédon, O. (1998) Etude comportementale et modélisation de l'adaptation d'un opérateur humain soumis à une modification infographique de sa relation visuo-manuelle. Doctoral Thesis dissertation, Université d'Aix-Marseille III.

Guédon, O., Gauthier, G.M., Cole, J., Vercher, J.-L. and Blouin, J. (1998) The role of arm afferent information in the adaptation to altered visuo-manual relationships in a two dimensional tracking task. *J. Mot. Behav.*, 30: 234–248.

Hodges, P.W. and Bui, B.H. (1996) A comparison of computer-based methods for the determination of onset of muscle contraction using electromyography. Electromyography and motor control. *EEG Clin. Neurophysiol.*, 101: 511–519.

Ingram, H.A., Van Donkelaar, P., Cole, J., Vercher, J.L., Gauthier, G.M. and Miall, R.C. (2000) The role of proprioception and attention in a visuomotor adaptation task. *Exp. Brain Res.*, 132: 114–126.

Kasai, T., Kawanishi, M. and Yahagi, S. (1992) The effects of wrist muscle vibration on human voluntary elbow flexion–extension movements. *Exp. Brain Res.*, 90: 217–220.

Kawato, M. (1999) Internal models for motor control and trajectory planning. *Curr. Opin. Neurobiol.*, 9: 718–727.

Kawato, M., Kuroda, T., Imamizu, H., Nakano, E., Miyauchi, S., and Yoshioka, T. (2003). Internal forward models in the cerebellum: fMRI study on grip force and load force coupling. In: C. Prablanc, D. Pélisson and Y. Rossetti (Eds.), *Neural Control of Space Coding and Action Production. Progress in Brain Research*, Vol. 142. Elsevier, Amsterdam, pp. 171–188 (this volume).

Lacquaniti, F. and Soechting, J.F. (1986) EMG responses to load perturbations of the upper limb: effect of dynamic coupling between shoulder and elbow motion. *Exp. Brain Res.*, 61: 482–496.

Lazzari, S., Vercher, J.L. and Buizza, A. (1997) Manuo-ocular co-ordination in target tracking. I: a model simulating human performance. *Biol. Cybern.*, 77: 257–266.

Massion, J. (1997) *Cerveau et Motricité*. Presses Universitaires de France, Paris.

Miall, R.C., Weir, D.J., Wolpert, D.N. and Stein, J.F. (1993) Is the cerebellum a Smith predictor? *J. Mot. Behav.*, 25: 203–216.

Miall, R.C., Reckess, G.Z. and Imamizu, H. (2001) The cerebellum coordinates eye and hand tracking movements. *Nat. Neurosci.*, 4(6): 638–644.

Prablanc, C. and Martin, O. (1992) Automatic control during hand reaching at undetected two-dimensional target displacements. *J. Neurophysiol.*, 67: 455–469.

Prablanc, C., Desmurget, M. and Gréa, H. (2003). Neural control of on-line guidance of hand reaching movements. In: C. Prablanc, D. Pélisson and Y. Rossetti (Eds.), *Neural Control of Space Coding and Action Production. Progress in Brain Research*, Vol. 142. Elsevier, Amsterdam, pp. 155–170 (this volume).

Rashbass, C. (1961) The relationship between saccadic and smooth tracking eye movements. *J. Physiol.*, 159: 326–338.

Ribot-Ciscar, E., Rossi-Durand, C. and Roll, J.-P. (1998) Muscle spindle activity following muscle tendon vibration in man. *Neurosci. Lett.*, 258: 147–150.

Roll, J.P. and Vedel, J.P. (1982) Kinesthetic role of muscle afferents in man, studied by tendon vibration and microneurography. *Exp. Brain Res.*, 47: 177–190.

Scarchilli, K. and Vercher, J.-L. (1999) Oculo-manual co-ordination: taking into account the dynamical properties of the arm. *Exp. Brain Res.*, 124: 42–52.

Scarchilli, K., Vercher, J.-L., Gauthier, G.M. and Cole, J. (1999) Is the oculo-manual co-ordination control system using an internal representation of the arm dynamics? *Neurosci. Lett.*, 265: 139–142.

Schmidt, R.A. (1975) A schema theory of discrete motor skill learning. *Psychol. Rev.*, 82(4): 225–260.

Shadmehr, R. and Mussa-Ivaldi, F.A. (1994) Adaptive representation of dynamics during learning of a motor task. *J. Neurosci.*, 14(5): 3208–3224.

Van Donkelaar, P. and Lee, R.G. (1994) Interactions between the eye and hand motor systems: disruptions due to cerebellar dysfunction. *J. Neurophysiol.*, 72(4): 1674–1685.

Vercher, J.-L. and Gauthier, G.M. (1988) Cerebellar involvement in the co-ordination control of the oculo-manual tracking system: Effects of lesion of dentate nucleus. *Exp. Brain Res.*, 73: 155–166.

Vercher, J.-L., Volle, M. and Gauthier, G.M. (1993) Dynamics of human visuo-oculo-manual coordination control in target tracking tasks? *Aviat. Space Environ. Med.*, June: 500–506.

Vercher, J.-L., Quaccia, D. and Gauthier, G.M. (1995) Oculo-manual co-ordination control: Respective role of visual and non-visual information in ocular tracking of self-moved targets. *Exp. Brain Res.*, 103: 311–322.

222

Vercher, J.-L., Gauthier, G.M., Blouin, J., Guédon, O., Cole, J. and Lamarre, Y. (1996) Oculo-manual tracking in normal subjects and a deafferented patient: Respective role of arm motor efference and proprioception in initiation of smooth pursuit of self-moved targets. *J. Neurophysiol.*, 76: 1133–1144.

Vercher, J.-L., Gauthier, G.M., Cole, J. and Blouin, J. (1997a) Role of arm proprioception in calibrating the arm–eye temporal co-ordination. *Neurosci. Lett.*, 237: 109–112.

Vercher, J.-L., Lazzari, S. and Gauthier, G.M. (1997b) Manuo-ocular co-ordination in target tracking. II: comparing the model with the human behavior. *Biol. Cybern.*, 77: 267–275.

Westheimer, G. and Conover, D.W. (1954) Smooth eye movements in the absence of a moving visual stimulus. *J. Exp. Psychol.*, 47(4): 283–284.

Wolpert, D.M. and Kawato, M. (1998) Multiple paired forward and inverse models for motor control. *Neural Netw.*, 11: 1317–1329.

Wolpert, D.M., Ghahramani, Z. and Jordan, M.I. (1995) An internal model for sensorimotor integration. *Science*, 269: 1880–1882.

Wolpert, D.M., Miall, R.C. and Kawato, M. (1998) Internal models in the cerebellum. *Trends Cogn. Sci.*, 2(9): 338–347.

Normal and Pathological Spatial Representations

C. Prablanc, D. Pélisson and Y. Rossetti (Eds.)
Progress in Brain Research, Vol. 142
© 2003 Elsevier Science B.V. All rights reserved

CHAPTER 14

Delayed reaching and grasping in patients with optic ataxia

A.D. Milner [1,*], H.C. Dijkerman [2], R.D. McIntosh [1], Y. Rossetti [3] and L. Pisella [3]

[1] *Cognitive Neuroscience Research Unit, Wolfson Research Institute, University of Durham, Queen's Campus, University Boulevard, Stockton-on-Tees TS17 6BH, UK*
[2] *Psychological Laboratory, Helmholtz Research Institute, University of Utrecht, Heidelberglaan 2, 3584 CS Utrecht, The Netherlands*
[3] *Espace et Action, INSERM Unité 534, 16 avenue Lépine, 69676 Bron, France*

Abstract: A series of experiments documenting the reaching and grasping of two patients with optic ataxia is presented. We compare their immediate responses with their behavior when required to delay for a few seconds before responding. When the delayed response is 'pantomimed', i.e. made in the absence of the target object, their performance typically improves. This pattern was predicted from a two-visual-systems model in which the cortical dorsal stream mediates normal visually guided actions while the ventral stream deals with visual information that has to be held in memory. We further found that when a 'preview' task was used in which the patients could use memorized information to guide a response to a still-present target object, they did so in preference to using the visual information facing them.

Introduction

The great majority of studies of visually guided prehension have set out to characterize and explain the ways in which humans and animals make movements directly toward targets in their visual field. The ability to execute such skilled actions must have been one of the earliest and most critical adaptive changes in the evolution of the primate brain. There is evidence from a range of converging methodologies that these direct actions are guided through rather 'automatic' sensorimotor transformations mediated by circuits within the posterior parietal and premotor cortex, in close conjunction with brainstem and cerebellar nuclei (Jeannerod et al., 1995; Andersen et al., 1998; Milner and Dijkerman, 1998). The

* Correspondence to: A.D. Milner, Cognitive Neuroscience Research Unit, Wolfson Research Institute, University of Durham, Queen's Campus, University Boulevard, Stockton-on-Tees TS17 6BH, UK. Tel.: +44-1642-333850; Fax: +44-1642-385866;
E-mail: a.d.milner@durham.ac.uk

major visual input for these systems appears to filter through from V1 via the primate 'dorsal stream' of cortical processing (Milner and Goodale, 1995). This stream extends anteriorly to include the parietal areas that transform visual information into action coordinates. Dorsal-stream lesions in monkeys have long been known to result in a spectrum of visuomotor deficits, including deficits of reaching in space and of grasping small objects (Ferrier, 1890; Ettlinger, 1977; Faugier-Grimaud et al., 1978; Glickstein et al., 1998).

We have made a number of observations in recent years with two human subjects who have sustained fairly symmetrical bilateral parietal lesions. Both patients show 'optic ataxia' when using either hand to respond to either side of their peripheral visual field. The primary defining disorder in optic ataxia is a failure to point or reach accurately toward objects presented visually. Generally the pointing difficulty does not extend to non-visual targets, nor is it necessarily associated with a visuospatial perception deficit (Perenin and Vighetto, 1988). Indeed in his original description of optic ataxia in 1909, Bálint reported that his patient's inaccuracy of manual control was largely restricted to one hand. To enable successful reaching with the other hand, the relevant spatial information must have received adequate visual processing. Like the lesioned monkeys described by Ferrier and his 20th-century successors, patients with optic ataxia also have problems in orienting the wrist (Perenin and Vighetto, 1988), and scaling their grip appropriately during prehension (Jakobson et al., 1991; Jeannerod et al., 1994). These human parietal lesions appear to have disrupted visuomotor processing systems homologous to those identified in the dorsal stream of the monkey. Current lesion and functional neuroimaging evidence locates these systems superiorly in the human parietal lobe, in and around the intraparietal sulcus (Perenin and Vighetto, 1988; Binkofski et al., 1998; Culham and Kanwisher, 2001).

Not all investigators, however, have restricted themselves to examining *direct* prehension. In a pioneering set of experiments, Goodale and colleagues (1994) compared movements made by subjects in immediate and *delayed* grasping tasks. Their immediate task was straightforward: the subject had to reach out and pick up a rectangular block presented directly in front of him or her. To examine delayed grasping, Goodale et al. (1994) devised two tasks: 'delayed real grasping' and 'delayed pantomimed grasping'. In the former case, the subject examined the block for a short period, but had to refrain from responding until after a delay period, during which the block was kept out of sight. In pantomimed grasping, the block was no longer present after the delay (having been covertly removed), so that the subject had to reach out and *pretend* to grasp it. Grasping in the 'real' delayed task could thus be guided by external visual cues just like immediate grasping, since the object was visible at the time of responding. In contrast, pantomimed grasping could *only* be driven by information that was retained internally — presumably in working memory — since the object itself was no longer present.

A good indicator of efficient visual guidance during prehension is provided by the correlation between the maximum anticipatory finger–thumb opening during the reach and the actual width of the object (Jeannerod, 1981). Goodale et al. (1994) reported that when normal subjects performed the delayed pantomime task, their maximum grip size correlated highly with object width, even after delays as long as 30 s. However, systematic differences between the kinematics of the immediate and pantomimed actions led the authors to suggest that the latter were not driven by the normal visuomotor control systems that govern immediate actions. Adopting the theoretical framework presented by Goodale and Milner (1992; see also Milner and Goodale, 1993, 1995), they proposed that immediate grasping was implemented via dedicated visuomotor transformations within the dorsal stream. The pantomime task, in contrast, would have to rely on visual information outlasting that transiently available within the dorsal stream, specifically in the form of a stored perceptual representation of the target object. For this, they proposed that the services of the ventral visual stream would have to be enlisted.

In support of their interpretation, Goodale et al. (1994) presented data from the visual-form agnosic patient D.F. This patient presented with a profoundly impaired ability to perceive shape, size and orientation (Milner et al., 1991). Her perceptual disorder appears from functional MRI evidence to be due to bilateral damage of ventral stream visual areas, and/or a disconnection of these areas from contour processing systems in primary visual cortex (Murphy et al., 1998). D.F. nonetheless shows excellent scaling of her grip with respect to object width during immediate grasping (Goodale et al., 1991). Her intact visuomotor skills have been putatively attributed to a relatively intact dorsal stream (Milner and Goodale, 1995). Yet despite her preserved immediate grasping, D.F. showed no grip scaling in the pantomime task, even after a delay of only 2 s (Goodale et al., 1994). She dutifully opened her hand on each trial in her efforts to pretend to grasp the previewed block, but her grip size did not correlate with the width of the block she had been shown.

This selective failure in the delayed pantomime condition was attributed to D.F.'s inability to store, even for a few seconds, suitable information about the object to guide her grasping movements. Goodale et al. (1994) argued that only the perceptual system, in the ventral visual stream, could provide the necessary visual information for her working memory to use. Since in D.F. this perceptual system was unable to encode the target object's dimensions, no such visual information would be available to her working memory. In other words, the indirect route from vision to action via perceptual representations would be closed to D.F., because her brain could not form those intermediary perceptual representations.

Goodale et al.'s (1994) interpretation is attractive, but it relies on a single dissociation. Patient D.F. performed normally on the immediate grasping task and very poorly on the delayed task, but such a pattern could arise because delayed grasping is intrinsically more difficult than immediate grasping. On the other hand, if Goodale et al.'s hypothesis is correct, it should be possible to observe the converse pattern of performance in patients with damage to the immediate visuomotor system in the dorsal stream. Specifically, an optic ataxic patient, provided that her ventral stream remained relatively intact, might perform paradoxically *better* when tested on delayed pantomimed grasping than on immediate grasping. The reasoning behind this prediction is that some optic ataxic patients at least should be able to circumvent their damaged visuomotor system by bringing a relatively intact perceptual system into play to guide their actions, just as Goodale et al. (1994) postulated for healthy subjects. This secondary system, because of its slower operating constraints, would be unable, or much less able, to guide immediate grasping.

This line of argument need not be restricted to grasping behavior. By the same token, we might also predict improved *spatial* accuracy in optic ataxia, if the patient could be induced to delay a few seconds after target offset before initiating a pointing movement. In other words, the reaching disorder that is the defining essence of optic ataxia might be ameliorated when the action is delayed. In the present chapter we review relevant data from two patients with bilateral optic ataxia (A.T. and I.G.). Our aim was to look for changes in visually guided behavior when a delay was interposed between stimulus and response. We first describe two experiments in the domain of object size, and then our studies relating to spatial location.

The patients

Patient A.T. was aged between 44 and 46 at the times of testing, twelve years after an eclamptic attack which provoked a hemorrhagic softening in the territory of both parieto-occipital arteries (branches of the posterior cerebral arteries). Structural MR images early after the episode revealed bilateral parietal damage extending to the upper part of the occipital lobes and encroaching slightly into the medial part of the right premotor cortex. The calcarine area remained intact except for a part of the upper lip on the left side (see Fig. 1). Nevertheless, for the initial two weeks after the lesion, A.T. presented a severe visual deficit resembling cortical blindness. At the time of the current testing, A.T. continued to show the symptoms of Bálint's syndrome, including visual disorientation, simultanagnosia, and severe optic ataxia for targets in her peripheral visual field. On the other hand, she showed no clinical indications of occipito-temporal damage (e.g. alexia, object agnosia, achromatopsia, or prosopagnosia), and she was able to lead a surprisingly normal life despite her extensive lesions.

Patient I.G. had suffered bilateral parieto-occipital infarction 17 months before we began the present testing, during which she was aged 31 to 32. She initially presented with severe headache, dysarthria and bilateral blindness, which lasted for 3 days. Subsequently, bilateral optic ataxia and simultanagnosia became apparent (Pisella et al., 1999, 2000), but by the start of our testing her simultanagnosia had subsided, at least for presentations of two to three objects (Pisella et al., 2000). I.G. received a diagnosis of ischemic stroke, related to acute vasospastic angiopathy in the posterior cerebral arteries. MRI revealed a hyperintense signal on T2 sequences that was near-symmetrically located in the posterior parietal and upper and lateral occipital cortico-subcortical regions (see Fig. 2). Reconstruction of the lesion indicated that it involved mainly Brodmann's areas 7, 18, 19, the intraparietal sulcus, and part of area 39.

Studies of delayed grasping

We tested both patients on immediate grasping and pantomimed grasping, and in both cases found evidence for improved scaling of the grasp in the pantomime condition (Milner and Dijkerman, 2001). However, the results are clearer in I.G., and we will concentrate on those data here.

As in several previous studies (e.g. Goodale et al., 1991, 1994), we used rectangular blocks varying in

228

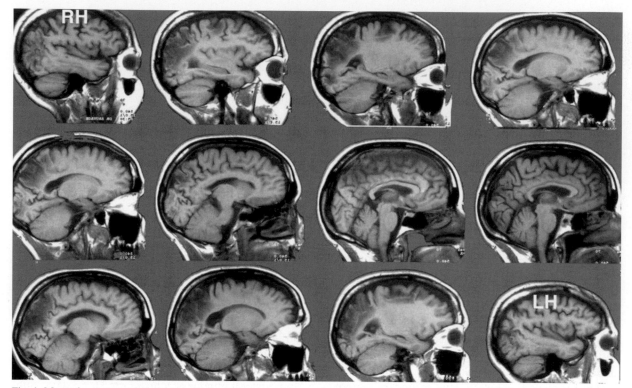

Fig. 1. Magnetic resonance images of A.T.'s brain. Twelve equi-spaced sagittal sections are shown, six from each side of the brain. There is symmetrical parietal lobe damage on the two sides of her brain, in the absence of damage to occipito-temporal lobe structures on either side.

width, but of constant surface area. Four different blocks were used, with the dimensions 5 cm × 5 cm, 4 cm × 6.25 cm, 3 cm × 8.3 cm, and 2 cm × 12.5 cm. They were made of dark gray plastic with a thickness of 1 cm, and were presented on a table against a white background. Due to the fact that I.G.'s optic ataxia chiefly affects non-foveal vision, we presented the objects eccentrically, using a central red fixation spot. The left edge of each object was positioned 6 cm (approximately 5°) to the right of this spot. Fixation was checked continually by an experimenter facing the patient. We recorded finger–thumb separation throughout all of the reaching and grasping movements, or for 1 s in the case of I.G.'s size judgments in the matching task (see below). The dependent variable of interest was the maximum grip aperture attained during reaching (MGA), or the mean finger–thumb aperture in the case of matching. Previous studies (Jeannerod, 1981; Jeannerod and Decety, 1990; Goodale et al., 1994) have shown that these measures are linearly related to object size in

healthy subjects in all of our tasks. For more details of this study, see Milner et al. (2001).

Experiment 1

In the first session, I.G. performed three tasks in the following order: (a) perceptual matching; (b) delayed real grasping; (c) delayed pantomimed grasping. The perceptual task required her to make a manual size estimate using her forefinger and thumb without reaching toward the object. In pantomimed grasping, I.G. was required to delay grasping the object for 5 s — during which the object was removed — and then to pretend to grasp it (see Fig. 3). In the delayed 'real' grasping task, the procedure was similar, except that the object remained present after the delay period and was available for grasping afterwards. This task was chosen for comparison with pantomimed grasping because it more closely mirrors the time-course of that task than does a straightforward immediate grasping task.

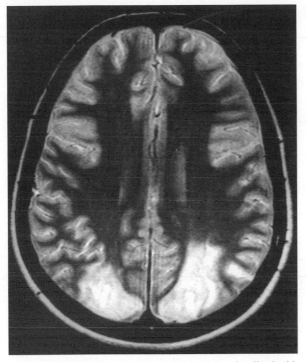

Fig. 2. A horizontal section through I.G.'s brain, visualized with structural MRI. Extensive damage is present bilaterally in the posterior parietal lobes.

The results are shown in Fig. 4. I.G. reliably varied her finger–thumb grip in proportion to the object size in the perceptual task (Fig. 4a), as has been reported before in optic ataxic patients (Jakobson et al., 1991; Jeannerod et al., 1994). As predicted, she also showed reliable grip scaling in the delayed pantomime task (Fig. 4c). Thus I.G. could tailor her grip to the size of an object both in an explicitly perceptual task (matching), and in one that relied on visual memory (pantomimed grasping). Yet much as expected, there was only weak evidence of grip scaling in the delayed *real*-grasping task (Fig. 4b).

These data demonstrate the predicted improvement of grip scaling when the stimulus was no longer present, as compared with when it was. Nevertheless, there was still a mild trend for grip scaling in the delayed real-grasping task, a trend that had not been predicted. We therefore tested I.G. in a second session in which we compared delayed real grasping with immediate real grasping.

In this second session, I.G. performed the following tasks, presented in an 'abccba' design: (a) immediate grasping, (b) delayed real grasping, and (c) delayed pantomimed grasping. We found no significant grip scaling during immediate grasping. In delayed real grasping, however, grip scaling was now evident, with I.G. opening her hand significantly less wide for the narrowest object than for the other three objects (Fig. 5b). Finally, clear grip scaling was again found in the delayed pantomimed-grasping task (Fig. 5c). There was also a general reduction in I.G.'s initially exaggerated grip apertures from the first to the second testing blocks.

Thus I.G. was unable to scale her grip size when an immediate grasp was required for a new object: yet when she could preview the object 5 s *before* grasping, she could adjust her grip quite well. Of course, in contrast to the immediate or pantomimed tasks, for which only one source of visual information could be used, both present *and* past visual information were potentially available in the delayed real grasping task. We had assumed that the prior information would be entirely superseded by the new sensory information available to guide action on-line, as has been shown in healthy subjects in a different context for proprioceptive targets (Rossetti and Pisella, 2002). I.G.'s relative success in pantomimed grasping, however, suggests that prior information might actually provide her with better visual guidance than current information. Therefore she might have used such stored information in the delayed real-grasping task, rather than relying on the currently visible object. We set out to test directly which of these two sources of visual information she used during delayed real grasping. To do this, we created a new series of delayed real-grasping trials in which occasional 'incongruent' test trials were embedded.

Experiment 2

In this experiment, only delayed real grasping was tested. However, although the usual four objects were used throughout, half of the trials with the widest and narrowest objects were made into incongruent test trials. On these occasions, the narrowest (2 cm) object was covertly replaced during the delay interval by the widest (5 cm), or the widest replaced

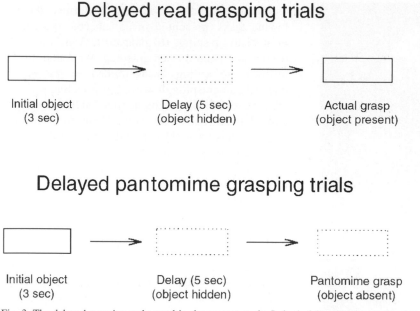

Delayed real grasping trials

Initial object
(3 sec)

Delay (5 sec)
(object hidden)

Actual grasp
(object present)

Delayed pantomime grasping trials

Initial object
(3 sec)

Delay (5 sec)
(object hidden)

Pantomime grasp
(object absent)

Fig. 3. The delayed grasping tasks used in the present study. In both delayed tasks (real and pantomimed), the object was first viewed for 3 s, and then shielded from view for 5 s. In delayed real grasping, the subject then had to reach out and grasp the object. In pantomimed grasping, however, the subject had to *pretend* to reach out and grasp the object after this delay, as it had been covertly removed during the delay period.

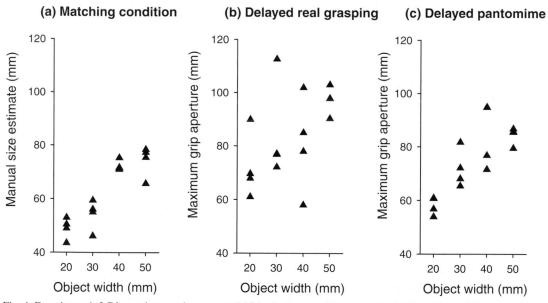

(a) Matching condition   **(b) Delayed real grasping**   **(c) Delayed pantomime**

Fig. 4. Experiment 1: I.G.'s maximum grip aperture (MGA) during a perceptual matching task and two delayed prehension tasks.

by the narrowest (see Fig. 6). In addition to I.G., six age-matched right-handed healthy control subjects were also tested.

We confirmed that our control subjects scaled their grip in accordance with the size of the object facing them (Fig. 7). It made no difference whether they had

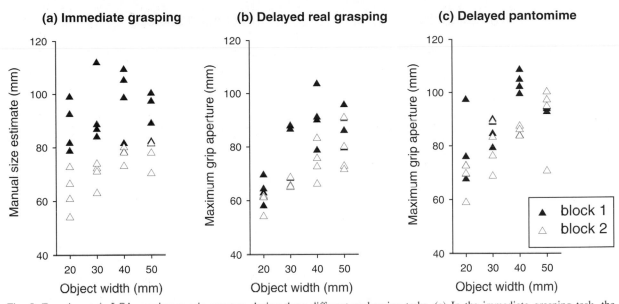

Fig. 5. Experiment 1: I.G.'s maximum grip aperture during three different prehension tasks. (a) In the immediate grasping task, the subject simply had to reach out to pick up the target object, front to back, using forefinger and thumb, as soon as it became visible. (b) During delayed real grasping, however, clearly significant grip scaling was observed. (c) As expected, highly significant grip scaling was also found in the delayed pantomimed grasping task.

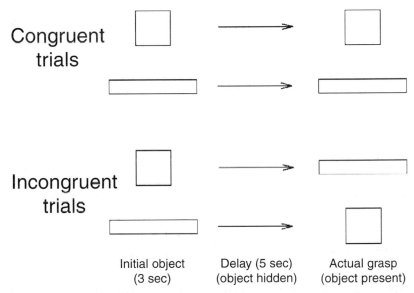

Fig. 6. Schematic of Experiment 2. In a quarter of all trials, the widest object (50 mm) was covertly replaced by the narrowest (20 mm), or vice versa, during the delay period (incongruent trials, bottom). In another quarter of the trials the narrowest and widest objects remained unchanged (congruent trials, top). In the remaining half of the trials, objects of intermediate widths were used (30 and 40 mm, not depicted here), and remained unchanged throughout each trial (congruent filler trials).

been shown the same or a different block 5 s earlier. In contrast, I.G. opened her hand widely whenever the wide object had been previewed, even when reaching out to grasp the narrow one (Fig. 7, left). Evidently I.G. used a memory-based route to by-pass her visuo-motor deficit, while the controls never did this.

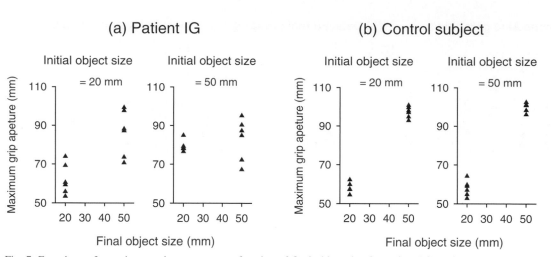

Fig. 7. Experiment 2: maximum grip aperture as a function of final object size for patient I.G. and one representative control subject. When the initial object was 5 cm wide and covertly replaced by the 2 cm wide object, I.G. programmed her grip size on the basis of the initial large object width. All of the six control subjects always used the final object size for programming their MGA, irrespective of whether it had changed during the trial.

On the incongruent trials where the narrow object was replaced by the wide one, however, I.G.'s grip did reach an appropriately wide aperture (Fig. 7, left). Presumably, the initially programmed small grip aperture had to be corrected during the course of the reach in order for her to eventually grasp the wide object, and this would be reflected in the measured maximum grip aperture. In support of this interpretation, we found that the velocity profile of handgrip opening differed reliably on these narrow-to-wide incongruent trials from that seen on congruent 'wide' trials. During the incongruent reaches, the rate of grip opening was significantly slower, and it reached its peak significantly later in the movement, presumably reflecting late perceptually based adjustments made to the initially programmed small aperture. These findings counter the objection that I.G. might simply have reacted to the uncertainty introduced by the incongruent trials by adopting a conservative strategy of opening her hand wide on all trials. In any case, this argument could not account for her appropriately small grip apertures on congruent trials with the small object.

Two visual routes to grasping

We established in Experiment 1 that I.G.'s visuomotor difficulties included the misgrasping of objects of different widths presented in peripheral vision. At the same time we showed that, like patient A.T. (Jeannerod et al., 1994), I.G. *perceived* the object widths quite accurately, and could signal these percepts manually. Most crucially, we confirmed our prediction that she should show an improvement in her grasping movements when performing a pantomime task. Taken together with the data from D.F. (Goodale et al., 1994), these findings complete a double dissociation. They are consistent with the idea that posterior parietal visuomotor systems are part of the neural circuitry for mediating normal immediate grasping, while not being essential for *delayed* responses of an ostensibly similar kind (Rossetti, 1998; Rossetti and Pisella, 2002).

Independent support for the idea that a delay interposed in a grasping task causes a change from direct visuomotor control to a perception-based control of grip formation, has been provided in a recent study by Hu and Goodale (2000). These authors used a virtual-reality technique in which an irrelevant larger or smaller object was present in the visual array along with the target object. As expected, there was a substantial size-contrast illusion in a perceptual report task: a given target was judged to be smaller when paired with a larger object, than when paired with a smaller one. Yet immediate grasping was immune to this illusion. Most importantly, after a delay of 5 s, grip size when reaching for the target object now did become subject to the illusion. In other words, in this test situation healthy subjects showed a qualitative difference in the nature of their visual grip scaling during delayed as compared with immediate responding.

In our study, we successfully predicted good *pantomimed* grasping by I.G.; but we did not expect that her *real* grasping behavior would improve when she had seen the object a few seconds earlier. We had assumed that I.G. would use the information present in her visual field whenever she attempted to grasp a real object. Instead, she improved when a preview was given. Experiment 2, however, showed that her manner of achieving good delayed real grasping was quite different from that of normal observers. Interspersing incongruent trials within a delayed real-grasping test session confirmed that healthy control subjects completely disregarded the previewed information. In sharp contrast, I.G. pre-programmed her grasp on the basis of this prior information, without regard to the current visual scene. Consequently when a wide object was covertly replaced by a narrow one, she opened her hand too widely for the object in front of her.

The present data are consistent with Goodale et al.'s (1994) proposal that vision can guide grasping actions through the perceptual processing networks in the ventral stream as well as through the visuo-motor systems of the parietal lobe. These networks evidently allowed I.G.'s grasping difficulties to be circumvented, albeit by taking a slower and more circuitous route from vision to action. While less unequivocal, the data we obtained from testing the older and more severely brain-damaged patient A.T. in a similar fashion supports the same conclusion (Milner and Dijkerman, 2001).

Studies of delayed pointing in optic ataxia

A parallel set of predictions can be made for delayed pointing. A number of studies have indicated that healthy subjects use a different form of spatial coding when they use remembered information about target location to guide the action. It has been proposed that for immediate motor guidance the brain uses a spatial code that is tied to an ego-centric frame of reference, but for delayed actions a quite different, context-based form of spatial coding is employed. In this latter type of coding, the location of a stimulus is computed with respect to other visual stimuli in the environment, which the brain assumes to be stable (Paillard, 1987; Milner and Goodale, 1995; Bridgeman et al., 1997; Rossetti, 1998). Since this system is sensitive to visual context, it can be deceived easily: for example, a stationary stimulus enclosed by a frame that is rapidly displaced appears to shift in the converse direction. Quick reaching movements to the target location do not fall prey to this or related illusions (Bridgeman et al., 1981, 1997, 2000). However, studies of both normal and brain-damaged subjects suggest that our movements become dominated by such context-relative spatial coding when a delay of 2 s or more is interposed between stimulus and response (Rossetti, 1998; Bridgeman et al., 2000). This time-based switchover between spatial coding systems bears an unmistakable family resemblance to that inferred for shape processing by Goodale et al. (1994) and Hu and Goodale (2000).

Relevant evidence is again available from patient D.F. When we assessed her on immediate and delayed pointing, we found that her performance was as accurate as for normal subjects when responding immediately to the target. However, when the target was turned off and a delay of 10 s was interposed, D.F. became highly inaccurate, making pointing errors twice as large as those of the controls (Milner et al., 1999b). This result is consistent with D.F.'s poor performance on certain non-delay tasks that demand the visual perception of spatial relationships (Dijkerman et al., 1998; Murphy et al., 1998). The suggestion therefore is not that D.F. has a specific impairment of spatial memory, but rather that her perceptual disorder deprives her working memory of crucial visual information. Again, this hypothesis predicts that a complementary dissociation should be possible in optic ataxia, such that the pointing responses of optic ataxic patients might *improve* under conditions of delayed responding. Our reasoning was that they might be able to base their delayed reaching on the context-based spatial system, assuming that this 'perceptual' route was relatively unscathed by their parietal-lobe damage. We tested both A.T. and I.G. to assess this prediction.

234

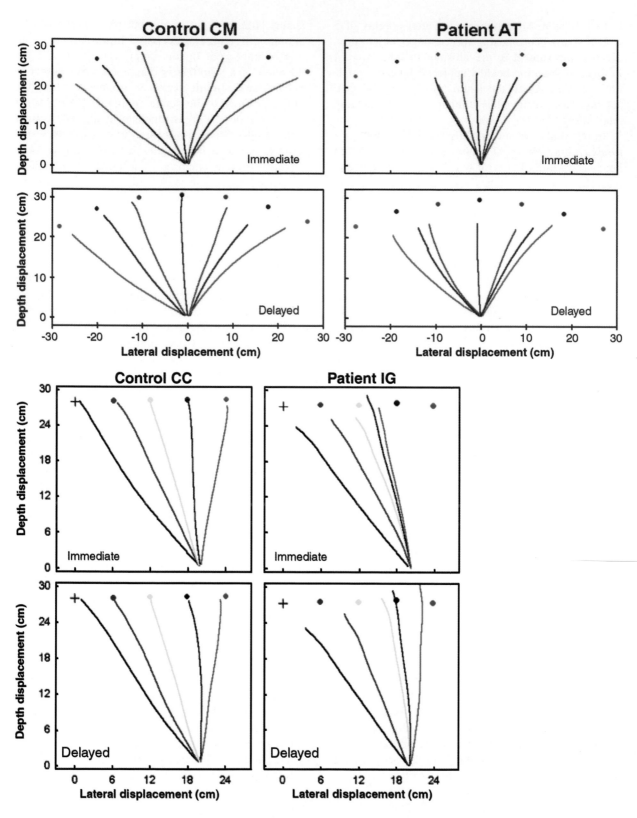

Experiment 3: immediate and delayed pointing

Our initial study of pointing was carried out with patient A.T. We presented a red target LED at one of 7 different locations, while she fixated a green LED placed 2.5 cm in front of the central target location. The LEDs were embedded in black Plexiglas, and were visible only when illuminated. They were arranged in an arc of 55 cm radius around the center of A.T.'s body at eccentricities of $-30°$, $-20°$, $-10°$, 0, $+10°$, $+20°$ and $+30°$ with respect to her body center.

In the immediate pointing condition, a viewing period of 2 s was followed by a tone cueing A.T. to point to the target, while maintaining central fixation. The target remained visible throughout the reach. In the delayed condition, we presented the LED for 2 s only, and asked A.T. to wait until she heard a tone 5 s later before pointing to the target location, again maintaining fixation. Since the target was no longer present, this delayed task was effectively one of 'pantomimed pointing'. For more details, see Milner et al. (1999a).

In immediate pointing, A.T. responded very inaccurately, except for targets close to the center of her visual field (cf. Jeannerod et al., 1994). However, when A.T. was required to delay before pointing, her errors reduced dramatically, particularly at the most peripheral locations (see Milner et al., 1999a). In sharp contrast, all three healthy controls were *less* accurate in the delayed than in the immediate condition. A.T.'s pointing responses were predominantly medial to and short of the targets. Interestingly, her improvement in the delayed condition was specific to the directional component of her responses (errors of movement amplitude were not significantly altered).

These directional effects are clearly evident in Fig. 8, which shows spatially averaged trajectories (with lateral displacement normalized against depth displacement) for A.T. and a control subject, C.M.

It is important to note that each average trajectory in Fig. 8 is plotted only for depth displacements common to all responses in that condition, so that each plot goes no further than its shortest component trajectory. Thus the endpoint of each average trajectory does not represent the mean endpoint of the responses comprising it. Fig. 8 illustrates that A.T.'s reaches have an abnormally strong directional bias toward the midline right from the outset. In other words, a severe disorder in calibrating the initial heading direction of her reaches constitutes a major component of A.T.'s misreaching behavior. A.T.'s reduced directional bias in the delayed condition is also present from the outset of the reach.

In a subsequent study, we compared immediate and delayed pointing in patient I.G., but here we used only four peripheral target locations, all within the right visual field. Throughout each trial, fixation was maintained on a 5-mm diameter red spot, 20 cm to the left of the hand start position and at a depth of 28 cm with respect to the start position. Peripheral targets were located at the same depth as the fixation spot and 6, 12, 18 or 24 cm to the right of fixation.

I.G.'s immediate pointing responses were directed accurately when made to the fixation point, but became progressively less accurate with increasing eccentricity. Her responses to targets close to fixation tended to be less accurate following a delay, but for the most peripheral locations, where her optic ataxia was most severe, I.G. pointed significantly *more* accurately following a delay. When I.G.'s absolute errors were analyzed in terms of directional and amplitude components, the beneficial effects of delay were found to be specific to the directional component, exactly as noted earlier in patient A.T. These directional effects are evident in Fig. 9, which shows spatially averaged trajectories for I.G., created in the same way as for A.T. (see above).

Just as previously observed for A.T., I.G.'s pointing responses are misdirected from their outset and

---

Fig. 8. (Top) Immediate and delayed pointing trajectories in patient A.T. and the control subject C.M., averaged only over the depth points common to all reaches. A.T.'s medial errors are present throughout her reach, and the improvements conferred by the delay condition are also evident throughout the trajectories.

Fig. 9. (Bottom) Immediate and delayed pointing trajectories in patient I.G. and the control subject C.C., averaged only over the depth points common to all reaches. I.G.'s medial (i.e. leftward) errors are clearly present throughout her reach, as are the changes induced by the delay condition.

veer markedly toward fixation for targets at the most peripheral locations. Similarly, the differences between I.G.'s immediate and delayed reaches are most pronounced at peripheral locations and are present throughout the entire trajectories. These results indicate that I.G.'s optic ataxic errors cannot be due solely to her known inability to apply rapid on-line corrections to an ongoing movement (Pisella et al., 2000; Gréa et al., 2002). As with A.T., her errors seem to result in large part from a faulty calibration of the initial reach parameters. This miscalibration remains, but becomes smaller, under conditions of delayed responding.

These delayed pointing data show very similar patterns in our two optic ataxic patients. Both patients responded with greater directional accuracy when making delayed rather than immediate pointing responses to locations in the peripheral visual field. This improvement under conditions of delayed responding is particularly striking given that healthy controls show the opposite pattern (Milner et al., 1999a).

Experiment 4

The observed pattern of superior performance for delayed over immediate pointing prompted us once more to test whether our patients might use memorized information (in this case about target location) in preference to that available on-line. To do this, we used a delayed *real* pointing task, in which both immediate and previewed location information were available and were occasionally brought into conflict. We used the same layout as for patient I.G. in Experiment 3 (see Fig. 9), though only the four rightmost target locations were used, with fixation maintained at the leftmost location throughout all trials. As before, a warning tone sounded on each trial, and a target was exposed (at location 1) for 2 s. The display was then occluded for a 5-s delay, whereupon the target was re-exposed (at location 2). The subject was required to point immediately to the target at this second location. 75% of the trials were congruent, with the target retaining its location during the delay period, i.e. locations 1 and 2 were the same. The remaining trials were incongruent, with the target location being changed covertly during the delay period. Incongruent trials involved

the near and far target positions only. On half of the incongruent trials the target was presented initially at the near position and re-appeared at the far position following the delay (near → far), and on the others the reverse sequence was used (far → near). While all reaches were recorded, only those trials (congruent and incongruent) involving the near and/or the far target positions were analyzed. We tested both A.T. and I.G. on this task.

Fig. 10 shows spatially averaged trajectories for three control subjects and for the two patients, with lateral displacement normalized against depth displacement. Control subjects were uninfluenced by the location of the target seen prior to the delay (location 1), and responded exclusively to the target shown at the time of response (location 2). However, this was not the case for the optic ataxic patients, both of whom were influenced strongly by location 1. Fig. 10 shows that the influence of location 1 was dominant in the early part of the reach and that location 2 gained progressively in influence as the reach unfolded. Additionally, there is a strong suggestion of an interaction between the effects of the two targets, such that target 2 had more influence in the far → near condition than in the near → far condition. To assess the development of these patterns over the spatial course of the reaches, multiple ANOVAs were performed for each subject. The heading angle of the right index finger with respect to its starting position was used as the dependent variable, and separate ANOVAs by target 1 (near vs. far) and target 2 (near vs. far) were performed at several different depth displacements. These were focused particularly on the early part of the reach (i.e. depth displacements of 5 cm and less).

The analyses showed that during the initial portion of the reach (the first 1–2 cm), both patients' responses were determined predominantly by the target location prior to the delay and presumably memorized (location 1). Only as the trajectory unfolded did the influence of the physically present target (location 2) develop in strength. Moreover, the influence of the physically present target was stronger when it lay close to fixation than when it lay far from fixation. This latter interaction was highly significant for patient A.T., although it only approached significance for patient I.G. ($p < 0.1$ from a depth displacement of 4 cm onward). It seems that our

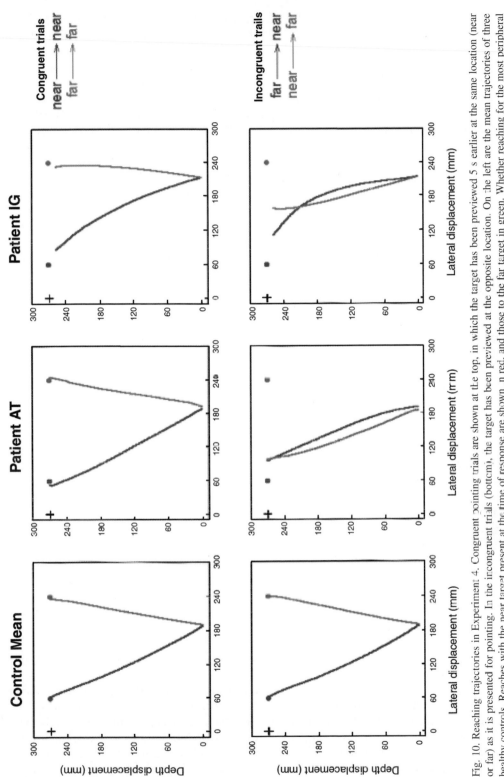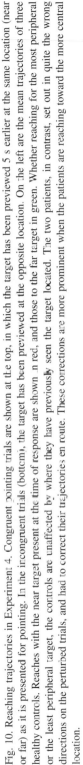

Fig. 10. Reaching trajectories in Experiment 4. Congruent pointing trials are shown at the top, in which the target has been previewed 5 s earlier at the same location (near or far) as it is presented for pointing. In the incongruent trials (bottom), the target has been previewed at the opposite location. On the left are the mean trajectories of three healthy controls. Reaches with the near target present at the time of response are shown in red, and those to the far target in green. Whether reaching for the most peripheral or the least peripheral target, the controls are unaffected by where they have previously seen the target located. The two patients, in contrast, set out in quite the wrong directions on the perturbed trials, and had to correct their trajectories en route. These corrections are more prominent when the patients are reaching toward the more central location.

optic ataxic patients were both better able to make use of on-line sensory information to guide their actions if this information was from a visual location closer to fixation. Thus, the severity of the immediate pointing deficit was greatest at the most peripheral locations, the benefits of delayed responding were most apparent at those locations, and the influence of current visual location information was weakest there.

Two visual routes to pointing

The main results of these pointing experiments are clear. Both of our optic ataxic patients responded more accurately when making delayed rather than immediate pointing responses to peripheral targets. This general pattern of improvement under conditions of delayed responding is opposite to that seen in patient D.F. (Milner et al., 1999b), and to the prevailing pattern in controls (Milner et al., 1999a). These results are difficult to explain on the assumption of a unique representation of visual space in the parietal lobe, damage to which might be thought to cause the localization difficulties characteristic of optic ataxia. If that were so, then no improvement should be possible with delay. In addition, the benefits of pointing on the basis of stored location information were clearly exploited by both A.T. and I.G. in a real delayed pointing task, i.e. *even though the target was still present to guide action after the delay*. The evidence for this is provided by Experiment 4, in which we covertly shifted the location of the target between preview and pointing. Both patients programmed their reaches initially on the basis of the previewed target location, and so had to modify their initial heading direction on-line, presumably using an intact but slow 'intentional' correction system (Pisella et al., 2000).

This dissociating pattern of visuospatial impairments in optic ataxia and visual-form agnosia supports the conclusions arrived at from a number of studies of normal individuals (Rossetti, 1998; Bridgeman et al., 2000). It seems that there are at least two separate systems for spatial representation in the brain, each specialized for broadly different purposes. One system is dedicated for the immediate guidance of action, and hence uses spatial information coded in egocentric coordinates. It is almost certainly embodied in the superior parts of the parietal lobe. The other system is designed for the longer-term coding of spatial relationships for perceptual and cognitive purposes, and seems to lie in a more inferior (probably temporo-parietal) location in the human brain, predominantly in the right hemisphere (Milner and Goodale, 1995). This system could operate on a contextual basis in the present delay task by computing the target location relative to the fixation point. The present evidence that this second system can function relatively well in patients with extensive bilateral parietal damage is consistent with its receiving information about spatial relationships through the ventral (occipito-temporal) visual stream. In support of this idea, relative coding of stimulus location within a visual array has recently been physiologically demonstrated in neurones in the monkey's temporal neocortex (Missal et al., 1999; Baker et al., 2000).

When reaching rapidly toward targets within the visual array, A.T. and I.G. cannot, like healthy subjects, use the dorsal-stream visuomotor system effectively, yet there is insufficient time to engage the ventral system fully. The result is that they make large errors. The ventral system's normal role in spatial orientation would only be to signal the general 'ball-park' location of a target in relation to other stimuli, in contrast to the high absolute accuracy of the dorsal system. This lesser accuracy is apparent in the delayed pointing of controls, in this as in previous studies (e.g. Elliott and Madalena, 1987; Berkinblit et al., 1995; Milner et al., 1999b). Due to their brain damage, A.T. and I.G. no longer have ready access to the dedicated visuomotor system, and so have lost the advantage that immediate responding would normally offer. As a result, they show a paradoxical improvement when a time delay allows their more general-purpose perceptual system to come into full operation.

The nature of the pointing bias in optic ataxia

Experiment 3 allowed us to determine the extent to which the misreaches that were made to targets outside the central part of the visual field by AT. and I.G. were due to failures to correct their movements, as opposed to failures to initially direct the movements accurately (see also Prablanc et al., 2003, this volume). Despite the different set-ups used, Figs. 8 and 9 show very similar patterns for the two patients. It is clear that the pattern of medially biased errors is present right from the very start of the reaches. This bias remains present during delayed pointing, though it becomes less severe in both patients. Our data thus indicate that as well as having a problem with making rapid on-line corrections (Pisella et al., 2000; Gréa et al., 2002), patients with optic ataxia also make large initial directional errors when reaching for targets in peripheral vision. Their failure to apply on-line corrections is likely to compound this deficit, and indeed the immediate pointing trajectories plotted in Figs. 8 and 9 give no hint of on-line corrections.

What is the nature of these directional errors in optic ataxia? Their most obvious characteristic is their medial bias, in both A.T. and I.G.: A.T. was fixating centrally and veered inwards on both sides, while I.G. was fixating to the left and so tended to err leftwards. This medial misreaching is not a new observation: it was noted some years ago both in monkeys with posterior parietal lesions (Bates and Ettlinger, 1960; Lamotte and Acuña, 1978) and in unilateral optic ataxic patients (Perenin and Vighetto, 1983). It is as if the arm movements are drawn inwards toward the line of sight from either side, somewhat reminiscent of the 'magnetic misreaching' behavior described by Carey et al. (1997). Their patient was so severely affected that she was unable to reach to targets located away from the fixated object at all, her hand always being drawn to the fixation point instead of to the target object. A similar patient has been described by Buxbaum and Coslett (1997). Both patients had superior damage to the parietal lobes bilaterally, but there was additional cortical damage elsewhere in both cases. These reports may give a clue to the nature of the residual visual guidance retained by more typical optic ataxic patients like A.T. and I.G.

Magnetic misreaching can perhaps be regarded as a 'primitive' form of reaching, in which the hand automatically follows the eye. Even healthy subjects, while reaching toward a fixated object, cannot re-orient gaze to a new target during the movement: instead their saccades are delayed until after the end of the reach (Neggers and Bekkering, 2000, 2001). This tendency for fixation and reaching to be coupled to the same stimulus may be embodied in hard-wired subcortical circuitry. For example, there are visuomotor neurons in the superior colliculus and adjacent midbrain tegmentum that fire when a monkey reaches toward a fixated target (Werner et al., 1997a,b). It might well be that without any cortical modulation, this subcortical system would produce magnetic misreaching as a kind of default behavior. An important role of the superior parietal cortex may therefore be to exercise inhibitory control over this midbrain mechanism, allowing the normal person to make hand movements elsewhere than to the object currently fixated. In effect, this downstream modulation would free the brain to transform visual location information directly into limb coordinates when programming a reach, instead of having to rely on the saccadic system as an intermediary. Damage to the parietal visuomotor system would diminish this downstream inhibition, causing reaching to be more influenced by the subcortical system. Reaches would therefore tend to stray toward the center of gaze, accounting for the medial biases shown by A.T. and I.G.

However, despite these biases, both patients still make reaching movements that correlate highly with target location. There are two alternative ways of understanding this preserved visual guidance. First, it is possible that in both patients there is some spared function in the visuomotor systems of the posterior parietal cortex. On this hypothesis, their immediate reaching behavior would still receive partial visual guidance through the normal dorsal-stream route, but this would be supplemented by a significant contribution from the subcortical system. By this way of thinking, magnetic misreaching might be seen in cases where the parietal damage is more complete than that present in A.T. or I.G., so that reaching becomes entirely 'subcortical'. This account, however, would incorporate no role for the ventral stream in guiding action. Therefore it would have difficulty explaining why there is a qualitatively similar pattern of reaching errors in our patients when response is delayed, since in this case we have argued that the ventral stream is guiding reaching.

The second possibility is that the preserved visual guidance seen in our patients, even in immediate reaching, is provided entirely by the ventral processing stream (in association with the right inferior parietal cortex), without any reference to the damaged (superior parietal) dorsal system. This temporo-parietal spatial representation system, in tandem with frontal structures, may itself be able to partially suppress the subcortical reach system, though less completely than an intact dorsal stream. This possibility is supported by the known presence of heavy projections to the superior colliculus from frontal areas in the monkey. Again this account could explain the medial biases observed in A.T. and I.G. when pointing to peripheral targets. One could further argue that *optic ataxia with magnetic misreaching* would result if this temporo-parietal route was itself disrupted along with damage to the dorsal stream, leaving only the subcortical system in control.

Our initial predictions were based on the assumption that imposing a delay before making a reaching response would allow our optic ataxic patients to improve their accuracy by use of the ventral visual stream, thus circumventing the disrupted dorsal stream. This assumption is supported by the results we have reported. However, the delay turned out only to have the effect of reducing the medial bias, which still remained present throughout the trajectories. This was true in both of our patients. This persistence of the medial bias is more consistent with the second hypothesis set out above. Although the ventral stream would come fully to the fore during delayed reaching, it would be parsimonious to assume that it was also providing (partial) visual information to guide action in the immediate reaching task as well.

Our proposal then is that in both immediate and delayed reaching, the ventral stream provides the visual information to program reaching movements in optic ataxic patients. The difference is that the ventral route is better able to resist the influence of the subcortical reach system in the delayed case. In the immediate reaching task, the rather slow ventral route would not have time to become fully functional, and thus not be able to inhibit the subcortical system so effectively. Of course in the normal individual, the ventral stream would have little or no influence on the visuomotor control of immediate reaching, due to the pre-emptive action of the faster dorsal stream (see Rossetti, 1998; Rossetti and Pisella, 2002).

Our suggestion of a subcortical system supporting reaching to fixated objects would explain the central sparing in A.T. and I.G., because targets near to fixation would not need to rely so much on the dorsal stream. It would also explain why delayed responding benefited reaching most clearly at peripheral locations. Finally it would explain why in our last experiment, in which target location was perturbed on some trials, the influence of current target location information was weakest in the periphery.

A related idea that has been developed in a different context concerns the 'covert orienting' of visual attention (Posner, 1980), a crucial element of which is the disengagement of attention away from fixation. There is strong evidence that the posterior parietal cortex plays a crucial role in this process (Posner et al., 1984; Robinson et al., 1995; Corbetta et al., 2000; Goldberg et al., 2002). Indeed a severe difficulty in switching attention away from fixation was described by Bálint (1909) as part of the biparietal syndrome exhibited by his original patient. According to the 'premotor theory' of visual attention (Rizzolatti et al., 1994), covert orienting is embodied in the same visuomotor systems that guide overt orienting movements. These similar notions of disengagement would merit fuller comparative discussion in another context.

We have tentatively suggested that it is the ventral stream, rather than the damaged dorsal stream, which provides the residual visual guidance for immediate reaching in optic ataxia. One way to test this idea would be to see whether such reaching is influenced by context-based visual illusions such as the Roelofs effect (Bridgeman et al., 1997, 2000). Rapid reaching is resistant to this illusion in intact individuals, presumably because it is controlled by the dorsal stream; but if reaching in optic ataxia is controlled by the ventral stream instead, it should now become vulnerable to the illusion. The present account also makes a prediction about the behavior of magnetic misreaching patients, whose use of either cortical stream for guiding reaching is assumed to be disrupted. If that is so, then their misreaching should remain unchanged after a delay — that is, their pointing errors should fail to improve, since we have argued that a delay serves only to maximize the ventral stream's role in guiding reaching.

Acknowledgements

The authors thank A.T. and I.G. for their patience, co-operation, and good humor. They also thank several colleagues whose willing help has been crucial for the work described here, including Marc Jeannerod, François Michel, Yves Paulignan, Caroline Tilikete, and Alain Vighetto. The authors are also grateful to the Wellcome Trust (grant No. 052443), the Leverhulme Trust (grant No. F00128C), and INSERM Progrès (grant No. 4P012E) for their support.

References

Andersen, R.A., Snyder, L.H., Batista, A.P., Buneo, C.A. and Cohen, Y.E. (1998) Posterior parietal areas specialized for eye movements (LIP) and reach (PRR) using a common coordinate frame. In: G.R. Bock and J. Goode (Eds.), *Sensory Guidance of Movement*. Wiley, Chichester, pp. 122–128.

Baker, C.I., Keysers, C., Jellema, T., Wicker, B. and Perrett, D.I. (2000) Coding of spatial position in the superior temporal sulcus of the macaque. *Curr. Psychol. Lett.*, 1: 71–87.

Bálint, R. (1909) Seelenlähmung des 'Schauens', optische Ataxie, räumliche Störung der Aufmerksamkeit. *Monatsschr. Psychiatrie Neurol.*, 25: 51–81.

Bates, J.A.V. and Ettlinger, G. (1960) Posterior parietal ablations in the monkey. *Arch. Neurol.*, 3: 177–192.

Berkinblit, M.B., Fookson, O.I., Smetanin, B., Adamovich, S.V. and Poizner, H. (1995) The interaction of visual and proprioceptive inputs in pointing to actual and remembered targets. *Exp. Brain Res.*, 107: 326–330.

Binkofski, F., Dohle, C., Posse, S., Stephan, K.M., Hefter, H., Seitz, R.J. and Freund, H.-J. (1998) Human anterior intraparietal area subserves prehension. A combined lesion and functional MRI activation study. *Neurology*, 50: 1253–1259.

Bridgeman, B., Kirch, M. and Sperling, A. (1981) Segregation of cognitive and motor aspects of visual function using induced motion. *Percept. Psychophys.*, 29: 336–342.

Bridgeman, B., Peery, S. and Anand, S. (1997) Interaction of cognitive and sensorimotor maps of visual space. *Percept. Psychophys.*, 59: 456–469.

Bridgeman, B., Gemmer, A., Forsman, T. and Huemer, V. (2000) Processing spatial information in the sensorimotor branch of the visual system. *Vis. Res.*, 40: 3539–3552.

Buxbaum, L.J. and Coslett, H.B. (1997) Subtypes of optic ataxia: reframing the disconnection account. *Neurocase*, 3: 159–166.

Carey, D.P., Coleman, R.J. and Della Sala, S. (1997) Magnetic misreaching. *Cortex*, 33: 639–652.

Corbetta, M., Kincade, J.M., Ollinger, J.M., McAvoy, M.P. and Shulman, G.L. (2000) Voluntary orienting is dissociated from target detection in human posterior parietal cortex. *Nat. Neurosci.*, 3: 292–297.

Culham, J.C. and Kanwisher, N.G. (2001) Neuroimaging of cognitive functions in human parietal cortex. *Curr. Opin. Neurobiol.*, 11: 157–163.

Dijkerman, H.C., Milner, A.D. and Carey, D.P. (1998) Grasping spatial relationships: failure to demonstrate allocentric visual coding in a patient with visual form agnosia. *Conscious. Cogn.*, 7: 424–437.

Elliott, D. and Madalena, J. (1987) The influence of premovement visual information on manual aiming. *Q.J. Exp. Psychol.*, 39A: 541–559.

Ettlinger, G. (1977) Parietal cortex in visual orientation. In: F.C. Rose (Ed.), *Physiological Aspects of Clinical Neurology*. Blackwell, Oxford, pp. 93–100.

Faugier-Grimaud, S., Frenois, C. and Stein, D.G. (1978) Effects of posterior parietal lesions on visually guided behavior in monkeys. *Neuropsychologia*, 16: 151–168.

Ferrier, D. (1890) *Cerebral Localisation. The Croonian Lectures*. Smith, Elder, London.

Glickstein, M., Buchbinder, S. and May, J.L. (1998) Visual control of the arm, the wrist and the fingers: pathways through the brain. *Neuropsychologia*, 36: 981–1001.

Goldberg, M.E., Bisley, J., Powell, K.D., Gottlieb, J. and Kusunoki, M. (2002) The role of the lateral intraparietal area of the monkey in the generation of saccades and visuospatial attention. *Ann. N. Y. Acad. Sci.*, 956: 205–215.

Goodale, M.A. and Milner, A.D. (1992) Separate visual pathways for perception and action. *Trends Neurosci.*, 15: 20–25.

Goodale, M.A., Milner, A.D., Jakobson, L.S. and Carey, D.P. (1991) A neurological dissociation between perceiving objects and grasping them. *Nature*, 349: 154–156.

Goodale, M.A., Jakobson, L.S. and Keillor, J.M. (1994) Differences in the visual control of pantomimed and natural grasping movements. *Neuropsychologia*, 32: 1159–1178.

Gréa, H., Pisella, L., Rossetti, Y., Desmurget, M., Tilikete, C., Grafton, S., Prablanc, C. and Vighetto, A. (2002) A lesion of the posterior parietal cortex disrupts on-line adjustments during aiming movements. *Neuropsychologia*, 40: 2471–2480.

Hu, Y. and Goodale, M.A. (2000) Grasping after a delay shifts size-scaling from absolute to relative metrics. *J. Cogn. Neurosci.*, 12: 856–868.

Jakobson, L.S., Archibald, Y.M., Carey, D.P. and Goodale, M.A. (1991) A kinematic analysis of reaching and grasping movements in a patient recovering from optic ataxia. *Neuropsychologia*, 29: 803–809.

Jeannerod, M. (1981) Intersegmental coordination during reaching at natural visual objects. In: J. Long and A. Baddeley (Eds.), *Attention and Performance XI*. Erlbaum, Hillsdale, NJ, pp. 153–168.

Jeannerod, M. and Decety, J. (1990) The accuracy of visuomotor transformation: an investigation into the mechanisms of visual recognition of objects. In: M.A. Goodale (Ed.), *Vision and Action: The Control of Grasping*. Ablex, Norwood, pp. 33–48.

Jeannerod, M., Decety, J. and Michel, F. (1994) Impairment of grasping movements following bilateral posterior parietal lesion. *Neuropsychologia*, 32: 369–380.

Jeannerod, M., Arbib, M.A., Rizzolatti, G. and Sakata, H. (1995) Grasping objects: the cortical mechanisms of visuomotor transformation. *Trends Neurosci.*, 18: 314–320.

242

Lamotte, R.H. and Acuña, C. (1978) Deficits in accuracy of reaching after removal of posterior parietal cortex in monkeys. *Brain Res.*, 139: 309–326.

Milner, A.D. and Dijkerman, H.C. (1998) Visual processing in the primate parietal lobe. In: A.D. Milner (Ed.), *Comparative Neuropsychology*. Oxford University Press, Oxford, pp. 70–94.

Milner, A.D. and Dijkerman, H.C. (2001) Direct and indirect visual routes to action. In: B. De Gelder, E. De Haan and C.A. Heywood (Eds.), *Out of Mind: Varieties of Unconscious Processes*. Oxford University Press, Oxford, pp. 241–264.

Milner, A.D. and Goodale, M.A. (1993) Visual pathways to perception and action. *Prog. Brain Res.*, 95: 317–337.

Milner, A.D. and Goodale, M.A. (1995) *The Visual Brain in Action*. Oxford University Press, Oxford.

Milner, A.D., Perrett, D.I., Johnston, R.S., Benson, P.J., Jordan, T.R., Heeley, D.W., Bettucci, D., Mortara, F., Mutani, R., Terazzi, E. and Davidson, D.L.W. (1991) Perception and action in 'visual form agnosia'. *Brain*, 114: 405–428.

Milner, A.D., Paulignan, Y., Dijkerman, H.C., Michel, F. and Jeannerod, M. (1999a) A paradoxical improvement of optic ataxia with delay: new evidence for two separate neural systems for visual localization. *Proc. R. Soc. Lond. B*, 266: 2225–2230.

Milner, A.D., Dijkerman, H.C. and Carey, D.P. (1999b) Visuospatial processing in a pure case of visual-form agnosia. In: N. Burgess, K.J. Jeffery and J. O'Keefe (Eds.), *The Hippocampal and Parietal Foundations of Spatial Cognition*. Oxford University Press, Oxford, pp. 443–466.

Milner, A.D., Dijkerman, H.C., Pisella, L., McIntosh, R.D., Tilikete, C., Vighetto, A. and Rossetti, Y. (2001) Grasping the past: delay can improve visuomotor performance. *Curr. Biol.*, 11: 1896–1901.

Missal, M., Vogels, R., Li, C.-Y. and Orban, G.A. (1999) Shape interactions in macaque inferior temporal neurons. *J. Neurophysiol.*, 82: 131–142.

Murphy, K.J., Carey, D.P. and Goodale, M.A. (1998) The perception of spatial relations in a patient with visual form agnosia. *Cogn. Neuropsychol.*, 15: 705–722.

Neggers, S.F.W. and Bekkering, H. (2000) Ocular gaze is anchored to the target of an ongoing pointing movement. *J. Neurophysiol.*, 83: 639–651.

Neggers, S.F.W. and Bekkering, H. (2001) Gaze anchoring to a pointing target is present during the entire pointing movement and is driven by a non-visual signal. *J. Neurophysiol.*, 86: 961–970.

Paillard, J. (1987) Cognitive versus sensorimotor encoding of spatial information. In: P. Ellen and C. Thinus-Blanc (Eds.), *Cognitive Processes and Spatial Orientation in Animal and Man, Volume II. Neurophysiology and Developmental Aspects*. Nijhoff, Dordrecht, pp. 43–77.

Perenin, M.-T. and Vighetto, A. (1983) Optic ataxia: a specific disorder in visuomotor coordination. In: A. Hein and M. Jeannerod (Eds.), *Spatially Oriented Behavior*. Springer-Verlag, New York, NY, pp. 305–326.

Perenin, M.-T. and Vighetto, A. (1988) Optic ataxia: a specific disruption in visuomotor mechanisms, I. Different aspects of the deficit in reaching for objects. *Brain*, 111: 643–674.

Pisella, L., Tiliket, C., Rode, G., Boisson, D., Vighetto, A. and Rossetti, Y. (1999) Automatic corrections prevail in spite of an instructed stopping response. In: M. Grealy and J.A. Thomson (Eds.), *Studies in Perception and Action*. Erlbaum, Hillsdale, NJ, pp. 275–279.

Pisella, L., Gréa, H., Tilikete, C., Vighetto, A., Desmurget, M., Rode, G., Boisson, D. and Rossetti, Y. (2000) An 'automatic pilot' for the hand in human posterior parietal cortex: toward reinterpreting optic ataxia. *Nat. Neurosci.*, 3: 729–736.

Posner, M.I. (1980) Orienting of attention. *Q.J. Exp. Psychol.*, 32: 3–25.

Posner, M.I., Walker, J.A., Friedrich, F.J. and Rafal, R.D. (1984) Effects of parietal lobe injury on covert orienting of attention. *J. Neurosci.*, 4: 1863–1874.

Prablanc, C., Desmurget, M. and Gréa, H. (2003) Neural control of on-line guidance of hand reaching movements. In: C. Prablanc, D. Pélisson and Y. Rossetti (Eds.), *Neural Control of Space Coding and Action Production. Progress in Brain Research*, Vol. 142. Elsevier, Amsterdam, pp. 155–170 (this volume).

Rizzolatti, G., Riggio, L. and Sheliga, B.M. (1994) Space and selective attention. In: C. Umiltà and M. Moscovitch (Eds.), *Attention and Performance, XV. Conscious and Nonconscious Information Processing*. MIT Press, Cambridge, MA, pp. 231–265.

Robinson, D.L., Bowman, E.M. and Kertzman, C. (1995) Covert orienting of attention in macaques, II. Contributions of parietal cortex. *J. Neurophysiol.*, 74: 698–712.

Rossetti, Y. (1998) Implicit short-lived motor representations of space in brain damaged and healthy subjects. *Conscious. Cogn.*, 7: 520–558.

Rossetti, Y. and Pisella, L. (2002) Several 'vision for action' systems: a guide to dissociating and integrating dorsal and ventral functions. In: W. Prinz and B. Hommel (Eds.), *Attention and Performance, XIX. Common Mechanisms in Perception and Action*. Oxford University Press, Oxford, pp. 62–119.

Werner, W., Dannenberg, S. and Hoffmann, K.-P. (1997a) Arm-movement-related neurons in the primate superior colliculus and underlying reticular formation: comparison of neuronal activity with EMGs of muscles of the shoulder, arm and trunk during reaching. *Exp. Brain Res.*, 115: 191–205.

Werner, W., Hoffmann, K.-P. and Dannenberg, S. (1997b) Anatomical distribution of arm-movement-related neurons in the primate superior colliculus and underlying reticular formation in comparison with visual and saccadic cells. *Exp. Brain Res.*, 115: 206–216.

C. Prablanc, D. Pélisson and Y. Rossetti (Eds.)
Progress in Brain Research, Vol. 142
© 2003 Elsevier Science B.V. All rights reserved

CHAPTER 15

Conscious visual representations built from multiple binding processes: evidence from neuropsychology

Glyn W. Humphreys *

Behavioural Brain Sciences Centre, School of Psychology, University of Birmingham, Birmingham, B15 2TT, UK

Abstract: I review neuropsychological evidence, from patients with selective brain lesions, indicating that there can be several kinds of binding in vision. Damage to early processes within the ventral visual stream impairs the binding of contours into shapes. This impairment can leave unaffected a more elementary operation of binding form elements into contours. Thus the process of binding elements into a contour is distinct from the process of binding contours into more wholistic shapes. In other patients with damage to the parietal lobe, there can be poor binding of shape to surface information in objects. This problem in turn can co-exist with a relatively intact process of binding of contours into shapes. These findings suggest that there are multiple stages of binding in vision, including binding to derive shape descriptions (in the ventral visual stream) and binding shape and surface detail together (involving interactions between the ventral and dorsal streams). I also discuss evidence for transient binding based on common onsets of stimuli. I conclude that the unity of consciousness is derived from several separable neural processes of binding.

Introduction

Our conscious perception of the visual world is unitary in nature. We perceive figures segmented against the perceptual ground, with visual elements being given their appropriate assignment within this organized percept. The figures and ground are usually given their correct surface properties, and feature elements are not 'free floating' or ambiguously assigned to more than one object. However, this unitary perception is dependent on neural processes that decompose the image in various ways, with the elements making up shapes and surfaces being processed independently, in different neural areas. How then do we come to perceive a coherent world? One view of this is that perceptual coherence is dependent on a single process of 'binding', which 'glues'

features together; a form of reversed 'big bang', in which independent elements are put together again. Contrary to this, I argue that there are multiple stages involved in binding together visual features, several of which can be isolated by the selective effects of brain damage on human perception. I consider first the evidence for visual features being coded independently in the brain. Subsequently I discuss neuropsychological disorders that seem specifically to affect the binding of features. Finally I discuss the implications of this idea of multiple forms of visual binding for understanding the nature of conscious visual perception.

The need for binding in vision

Damage to areas of the brain concerned with visual processing can lead to selective disorders of visual perception affecting the perception of some but not other aspects of the visual world. An example of this is the disorder cerebral achromatopsia, in which patients can have selective loss of colour vision

* Correspondence to: G.W. Humphreys, Behavioural Brain Sciences Centre, School of Psychology, University of Birmingham, Birmingham, B15 2TT, UK.
E-mail: g.w.humphreys@bham.ac.uk

without necessarily having an impairment of form perception or motion vision (Heywood and Cowey, 1999). In contrast to this, other patients can have a gross impairment in motion vision without consequent deficits in colour perception (Heywood and Zihl, 1999). The neural processes underlying colour perception seem distinct from those mediating motion vision. Likewise there can be marked damage to form perception along with a preserved ability to reach and grasp objects, or, in the opposite case, impaired reaching and grasping from vision along with spared object perception (e.g., for reviews, see Milner and Goodale, 1995; Jeannerod, 1997; see also Milner et al., 2003, this volume). This neuropsychological evidence suggests that visual processing is fractionated at a neural level, with different regions specialized for coding colour, motion, form and location information. Convergent evidence comes from neurophysiology, where cells in different cortical areas show selective response preferences for the different visual attributes (e.g., colour in area V4, motion in area MT, and so forth; see Desimone and Ungerleider, 1989; Zeki, 1993), and from functional imaging data in humans, based on selective activation of different cortical sites according to the visual property involved (e.g., see Watson et al., 1993; Ungerleider and Haxby, 1994; Tootell et al., 1995). Indeed, even within the domain of form perception, there is evidence that multiple cells at early stages of vision code the image independently and in parallel. To code coherent representations of whole objects, activity must be integrated across these cells, so that local image features group into the shapes that we recognize and act upon. I will use the term 'visual binding' to describe this process of integrating image features, both between and within visual dimensions. In this chapter I will argue that binding in vision does not happen in a single step but instead decomposes into multiple stages, each of which may take place in separate neural areas.

'One shot' accounts of binding

At least two major solutions have been put forward to explain binding in vision. One is that features are linked on the basis of time. The best known account of this kind is that binding is contingent on temporal synchrony in the firing of neurons (e.g., see

Singer and Gray, 1995; Eckhorn, 1999). A temporal code may be used to solve the binding problem if neurons responsive to the features of a single object fire together, whilst those responsive to the features in different objects fire at another time. This account is supported most strongly by physiological evidence showing time-locked firing of cells when stimulus elements group (for a review see Singer and Gray, 1995), though there is also behavioural evidence that temporal synchronization in the input being important for feature binding in humans (e.g., Fahle, 1993; Elliott and Muller, 1998). I will discuss neuropsychological evidence for temporal binding at the end of the chapter.

A second account is that binding is determined by visual processing 'going spatially serial'. For instance, attention applied serially to the location of each object in the field may enhance activation for all the features there, whilst decreasing the activation for features falling at unattended locations. Since only the features of attended objects will be active together, these features can be used to activate stored knowledge without fear that features from other objects in the field will join in this process. There is certainly evidence that attention to a location can increase the activation of features that fall there (Hillyard et al., 1998; Brefczynski and de Yoe, 1999), and it can also reduce activation associated with stimuli at unattended regions (e.g., Moran and Desimone, 1985). Hence the visual system is armed with mechanisms for binding by spatial attention. This idea, of spatial binding by attention, is expressed most elegantly in the well-known Feature Integration Theory of visual attention (Treisman and Gelade, 1980; Treisman, 1998). To explain why the features of a whole object become bound, though, a more elaborated account may be needed. For example, if attention falls on just a part of a stimulus, feedback from processes concerned with object coding may be needed so that features are integrated across the complete form (e.g., see Humphreys and Riddoch, 1993 and Vecera and Farah, 1994, for this proposal).

These accounts of binding are not mutually inconsistent of course. For example, attention may generate a competitive advantage on processing by improving the synchrony of firing for features at an attended location. Nevertheless proponents of both the attentional and temporal synchrony accounts have tended to discuss binding as a unitary process that happens in a single 'shot', by attention to the location of a stimulus or by synchronous firing of cells. The neuropsychological data I now proceed to discuss will counter this view, suggesting instead that different binding processes can be separated, both functionally and neurally (in terms of their localization in the brain).

Fractionating the binding process in form perception

The term 'integrative agnosia' has been used to describe patients who seem to have difficulty in binding form elements into coherent shapes (Riddoch and Humphreys, 1987; Humphreys, 1999). For example, the integrative agnosic patient HJA, when given a black and white photograph of a paintbrush remarked that "it appears to be two things close together; a longish wooden stick and a shorter, darker object, though this can't be right or you would have told me" (that there were two objects rather than one present) (see Humphreys and Riddoch, 1987). Butter and Trobe (1994) reported a similar patient who thought that line drawings of single objects depicted multiple items. Indeed, such patients may identify silhouettes (lacking such details) more accurately than drawings, because the internal edges in line drawings are used to segment objects apart (Riddoch and Humphreys, 1987; Butter and Trobe, 1994; Lawson and Humphreys, 1999). This fits with there being a problem in the inter play between grouping and segmentation. If the grouping of parts into wholes is relatively weak, when compared with segmentation processes, then recognition of the whole can be impaired. Further evidence for this comes from studies showing abnormal reductions when overlapping forms are presented (Riddoch and Humphreys, 1987; DeRenzi and Lucchelli, 1993; Butter and Trobe, 1994) and when forms are fragmented (Boucart and Humphreys, 1992).

These deficits in integrative agnosia demonstrate that object recognition depends on processes that bind edge contours into their correct spatial relations, and that facilitate segmentation of elements into 'figure' and 'ground'. These patients typically have lesions to their ventral visual systems (e.g., bilateral damage to the lingual and fusiform gyri, in the case of patient HJA; Riddoch et al., 1999). This is consistent with these brain regions mediating the grouping and segmentation of visual form.

Recently, Giersch et al. (2000) provided evidence that the processes leading to form binding can be fractionated. They presented targets formed by local collinear edges (appearing then like a fragmented line), presented amongst distractor edges set at random orientations. The difficulty of discriminating the target was graded by gradually adding distractors to the displays so that, eventually, even control subjects had difficulty in discriminating targets (see Kovacs, 2000). Interestingly, Giersch et al. found that the threshold for detecting the collinear targets was intact in patient HJA. Apparently the process of binding local elements into collinear contours was preserved.

This last result contrasts with HJA's performance on other tasks in which contours had to be integrated into more wholistic shapes. HJA was presented with the stimulus configuration shown at the top of each shape triplet in Fig. 1 (presented here within a single box) followed by the two other stimuli presented below (these were shown on the screen below where the original shape triplet had appeared). HJA had to match the original configuration to one of the two subsequent ones. The stimuli appeared as either overlapping line drawings (SUP), occluded shapes (OCC), silhouettes (SIL) or spatially separated shapes (SEP). HJA was impaired at this matching task, but particularly with occluded shapes, even relative to the more complex stimuli in which all contours were depicted (condition SUP). This impairment was most evidence when just a small area was occluded. This suggests that HJA computed the occluded edges of the background shapes, but these edges somehow disrupted performance. An indication of why this disruption occurred is provided by HJA's performance on simple copying tasks. Fig. 2 shows some examples of HJA's copies of both non-occluded (Fig. 2a) and occluded shapes (Fig. 2b). With non-occluded shapes HJA performed well, making no errors. However with occluded shapes HJA sometimes mistakenly drew in the occluded line as if it were visible in the front shape (see Fig. 2b (i) and 2c (ii)). This demonstrates that HJA computed the occluded edge in the background shape, but this 'virtual' line was some-

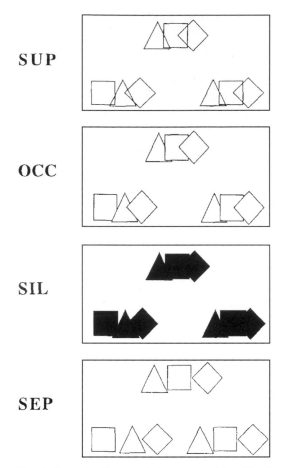

SUP

OCC

SIL

SEP

Fig. 1. Example displays of the type used by Giersch et al. (2000). On each trial the top shapes in each box were presented first, followed by the lower shapes on the left and right of the screen. The task was to choose which of the bottom shapes matched the top one.

times used as if it were really present. Other errors in copying occluded shapes included segmenting a background shape when T junctions were formed between the foreground and background shapes, and inappropriate linking of foreground contours to join background contours (Fig. 2b (ii), (iii)). Also, with some complex background shapes (as in Fig. 2c (i)), there were some apparent failures to group collinear edges, so the edges were depicted incorrectly as non-collinear. These data indicate a range of problems for this patient when dealing with occlusion. Apparently, occluded edges are completed but then are 'labelled' incorrectly by HJA's visual system, in terms

of whether they are physically present or not and whether they are in the front or background shape. Consequently, occluded lines are sometimes represented as visible in the foreground, and sometimes they are used to segment parts. It is interesting here that HJA has no general problem in depth perception, despite the deficit in depicting depth relations from line drawings. HJA can perceive stereoscopic depth (Humphreys and Riddoch, 1987) and he uses the depth cues of stereopsis and motion parallax, from head movements, to help him identify real objects (Chainay and Humphreys, 2001).

These data suggest two things. First, there is a distinction between the binding of local oriented elements into edges and the binding edge elements into wholistic shapes. In HJA the initial process is intact and the second impaired. Second, the process of contour completion (with occluded stimuli) must operate before figure–ground relations are coded; were this not so, it would be difficult to understand how occluded contours could be represented as part of a foreground shape, as we see in HJA's drawings. HJA's deficits also suggest one additional conclusion, that the binding of contours into wholistic shapes takes place in conjunction with figure–ground coding. As a consequence, HJA's lesion impairs both figure–ground assignment and the contour assignment process. However, this conclusion should remain cautious, since it rests on an associated pair of deficits in a patient (for a discussion, see Humphreys and Price, 2001).

Binding form and binding surface detail

A contrasting set of deficits to those found in patients with ventral lesions can be observed in cases with parietal damage. Unlike patients with ventral lesions, parietal patients typically have relatively intact object recognition but they have difficulties in binding together shape and surface detail. For example, Friedman-Hill et al. (1995) reported that patient RM, with Balint's syndrome [1] following bilateral parietal

---

[1] The term Balint's syndrome is applied to patients showing two primary behavioural symptoms: poor identification of multiple visual stimuli ('simultanagnosia') and poor visual localization, following the first description of such a case by Balint (1909).

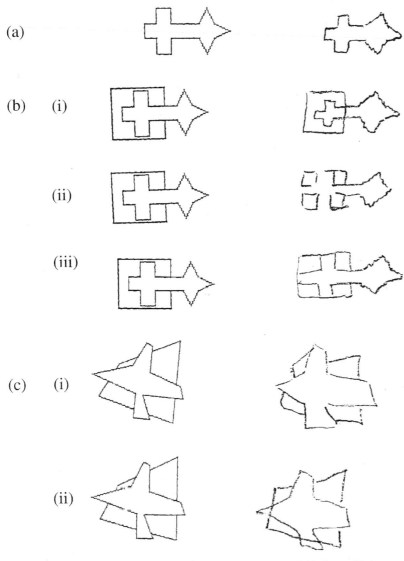

Fig. 2. Examples of the stimuli given to HJA for copying (on the left) along with some example copies (on the right).

damage, made abnormally large numbers of 'illusory conjunction' (IC) errors when asked to identify multiple coloured letters. Given a red X and a blue O, RM might report that there was a red O and a blue X, even when the stimuli appeared for long durations. Cohen and Rafal (1991) reported similar results when stimuli were presented to the contralesional field of patients with unilateral parietal damage. Normal subjects can also generate ICs when stimuli appear briefly (e.g., Treisman and Schmidt, 1982; though see Donk, 1999), but not under the pro-

longed viewing durations used with parietal patients. These results suggest that the parietal lobe plays a role in integrating shape and surface detail. The binding of parts of shapes, though, seems relatively preserved.

An example of form binding continuing to operate after parietal damage comes from studies of visual extinction, where grouping can dictate whether patients consciously perceive stimuli. Visual extinction occurs when patients can report single stimuli presented in their contralesional field but cannot report (or sometimes even detect) the same stimulus when it is presented simultaneously with an ipsilesional stimulus (e.g., Karnath, 1988). Extinction to stimuli on one side of space may occur because parietal damage induces a spatial bias in attention, so that an ipsilesional item is given greater 'weight' than a contralesional one when stimuli are selected for report. Despite this, spatial extinction can be reduced by grouping between the ipsi- and contralesional stimuli. A wide variety of grouping effects have now been reported, involving bottom-up cues such as collinearity, connectedness and common shape (see Humphreys, 1998). There is also evidence for extinction being reduced if stimuli activate a common stored representation (e.g., when two letters activate a common representation for a word, compared with when the letters make a non-word, when bottom-up cues to grouping should be equated; Kumada and Humphreys, 2001). All these results suggest that form binding can be relatively preserved even when the integration of form and surface detail is impaired (evidenced by the abnormally high numbers of ICs in patients of this type).

Humphreys et al. (2000) directly examined the relations between binding in the form dimension and binding of surface detail to form. The patient they studied, GK, showed left-side extinction under conditions of double simultaneous stimulation. This was modulated by grouping between the form elements, so that extinction was weaker when the items grouped than when they did not (Gilchrist et al., 1996; Humphreys, 1998; Boutsen and Humphreys, 2000). The effects of grouping on both spatial and non-spatial extinction indicate that some forms of binding continued to operate. In contrast to this GK showed poor binding when asked to report the surface and shape properties of multiple items in the field. When asked to report the colour and identity of a letter at fixation surrounded by two flanking letters, GK made about 32% illusory conjunction responses, miscombining either the shape or colour of the central letter with one of the other stimuli. There were few errors with single items.

To compare the binding of form and of form and surface detail, Humphreys et al. (2000) presented GK with shapes such as those depicted in Fig. 3. Stimuli fell to the left or right of fixation, and when two shapes were present they could group by common

shape [two squares (same shape and aligned collinear edges) or two circles (same shape only)], common contrast polarity (both white, both black vs. one white and one black, against a grey background), and connectedness (connected vs. unconnected). GK was asked to report the shapes and letters present. The results were clear (see Fig. 3). Single shapes were reported at a relatively high level (87% and 90% correct for shapes in the left and right fields). On trials with two stimuli, there was better identification when the shapes were the same, when they had the same rather than opposite contrast polarities and when they were connected relative to when they were unconnected. For stimuli with different shapes and contrast polarities, there was extinction on 67% of the trials with unconnected shapes. When the same stimuli were connected, however, there was extinction on just 33% of the trials.

In addition to making extinction errors, GK sometimes reported both items but made errors on their features (e.g., black square, white circle → white square, black circle). We termed these 'feature exchange' errors. Feature exchange errors were compared with the number of feature misidentifications made in other conditions where 'feature exchange' errors could not occur because the two stimuli shared one of the critical attributes (e.g., the stimuli had the same colour or the same shape). On these trials, unambiguous feature misidentifications could be made by reporting an attribute not present in the display (e.g., white square, black square → white square, black circle; here the response 'circle' can be classed as a feature misidentification, since this shape was not present). The chance likelihood of feature exchange errors can be estimated from the probability that two feature misidentifications errors would occur together on the same trial (based on the rate of unambiguous feature misidentifications). We found that feature exchange errors were much more likely than chance feature misidentifications, consistent with feature exchanges being true illusory conjunctions of shape and surface properties from different stimuli.

These data suggest that GK has problems in binding shape and surface detail together, but this problem occurs after shapes have been bound into perceptual groups (so that grouping influences the basic rate of extinction). Since shape-grouping has

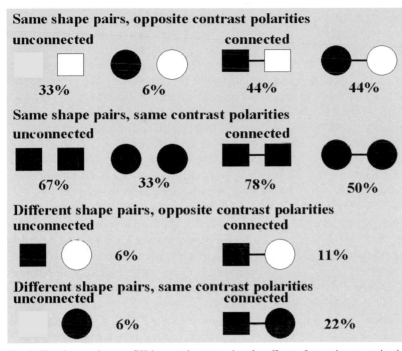

Fig. 3. The shapes given to GK in a study comparing the effects of grouping on extinction and illusory conjunctions. On each trial, only one pair of shapes was presented, against the background of a complete grey screen. One shape fell to the left and one to the right of fixation.

already taken place, surface properties migrate between whole shapes. The illusory conjunction errors could arise for several reasons. One possibility is that there is impaired attention to the location of shapes, a process which, normally, ensures that surface and form information are bound together correctly and not confused between stimuli (e.g., Treisman, 1998). GK's parietal lesions may disrupt his attention to the common location occupied by shape and surface detail, with the result that shapes and surface details from different objects are available for combination. Another possibility is that the parietal lesions disrupt location coding itself, with the result that surface detail and shape were misaligned during the integration process. Whichever account holds, the binding of local elements into shape seems to be unimpeded by deficits in attention and explicit location coding.

Parallel binding in normal vision?

The neuropsychological data suggest that there are several forms of binding in vision: binding local elements into contour, binding edges into more wholistic shapes, and binding shapes to surface detail. The finding that grouping influences extinction in turn indicates that some binding processes operate unconsciously; indeed patients can be unaware of stimuli unless they group with other items that are consciously represented in the field.

There is supportive evidence for these conclusions from work on normal vision. Kellman and Shipley (1991) and Shipley and Kellman (1992), for example, have argued that both visible and occluded contours are computed from local, oriented operators, and the outputs of these operators are then used to compute more global shape representations. In a patient such as HJA, the local operators may still compute occluded contours, but there is then an impairment in integrating the contours with more wholistic shape representations (Giersch et al., 2000). HJA's case can also be used to argue for the locus of these processes in the brain. HJA has bilateral damage affecting the lingual and fusiform gyri and the inferior posterior temporal gyrus, so that these regions appear to support the integration of contours into shapes. Indeed by competitively weighting one emerging perceptual group against others these regions may be fundamental to both object segmentation and figure–ground coding (see also Riddoch and Humphreys, 1987). In contrast, the intact grouping of oriented fragments into edges, in HJA, may rely on preserved regions of early visual cortex (V1/V2). This fits also with physiological studies on non-human primates and fMRI studies with humans, which converge in showing that these early regions of visual cortex are activated by illusory contours (Redies et al., 1986; Von der Heydt and Peterhans, 1989; Grosof et al., 1993; Sheth et al., 1996; Mendola et al., 1999), and that global perceptual structures can emerge from long-range interactions between the neurons in these regions (Gilbert and Wiesel, 1989; Gilbert et al., 2000).

The evidence from patient GK also fits with the argument that binding in the form system takes place within the ventral cortex, since this is relatively spared in his case. Nevertheless GK is grossly impaired at selecting multiple shapes and at localizing stimuli, once selected (see Humphreys et al., 1994). Explicit localization of visual elements is not necessary for form binding to operate.

The evidence on grouping in extinction is contrary to the idea that binding is dependent on serial attention being applied to a spatial region, to favour those features over others in the field, as suggested by Feature Integration Theory (Treisman, 1998). Nevertheless the effects of binding on extinction have typically been shown using relatively simple visual displays where, when the elements group, only a single object is present. Serial, spatial attention may be useful (and perhaps even necessary) when multiple shapes are present, when there is increased competition for selection of the features between the different objects. Against this, there is evidence for parallel binding of form elements in normal observers even with multiple stimuli present. For example, search for targets defined by a combination of form elements can be efficient when the distractors are homogeneous and form an independent group from the conjunction target (Duncan and Humphreys, 1989; Humphreys et al., 1989). Search is also efficient if the elements group into a single two- or three-dimensional object (Donnelly et al.,

1991; Humphreys and Donnelly, 2000), or if, once grouped, the target and distractors have different three-dimensional orientations (Enns and Rensink, 1991). These effects seem to arise from parallel grouping between the multiple items present. This can yield representations of the whole display as a 'single object', which is useful when the different object representations discriminate targets from distractors (Duncan and Humphreys, 1989). However the opposite may also apply, if grouping binds together targets and distractors (see Rensink and Enns, 1995); then attention may help to segment the stimuli (e.g., by activating features within some spatial regions over others). On this view, pre-attentive binding, within the ventral visual system, must normally operate together with attentional segmentation, to enable individual objects to be identified in complex (multi-object) scenes. This last process may be damaged in patients such as GK, with the result that sometimes separate shapes 'run into one another', so that their surface properties also become confused.

Computational models of vision

The argument that there are separate processes for the binding of form information, and the binding of surfaces to forms, fits with the assumption made in computational models of vision, such as the FAÇADE model of Grossberg and colleagues (e.g., Grossberg and Mingolla, 1985; Grossberg and Pessoa, 1998). FAÇADE distinguishes two stages of visual coding. A first process of boundary formation operates within a 'boundary contour system' (BCS), where grouping processes such as collinearity and good continuation are used to form bounded contours of shapes. Subsequently a 'feature contour system' (FCS) fills in the spatial regions within the closed boundaries of shapes to generate the surface properties of objects. In terms of this model, a patient such as GK may have a relatively intact BCS but an impaired FCS; there is feature binding to form shapes but poor integration of shape and surface detail. In contrast, patients such as HJA would have damage to the BCS, disrupting the correct representation of complex visual shapes.

We can also ask whether the binding of shape and surface detail is contingent on attention (as in Feature Integration Theory), or whether it is based simply on co-registration of the locations of features within some explicit representation of space, presumably within the parietal lobe? As we have noted, the data on illusory conjunctions in patients with can be explained by either account. Nevertheless, there is evidence that surface detail and shape can be combined even without attention to their common location. For instance, in normal subjects reaction times to find one of multiple targets can be faster than the fastest times to detect a single target (when present), even when targets are defined by a combination of colour and form (Mordkoff et al., 1990; Linnell and Humphreys, 2001). This is consistent with conjunctions of form and colour being coded in a spatially parallel manner. Similarly there is also 'super-additivity' in segmentation tasks when form and colour boundaries coincide (Kubovy et al., 1999). These results would follow if binding were based on co-registration of features rather than serial attention. In either case though the parietal lobe may be crucial, either for directing visual attention or for holding a 'master map' (cf. Treisman, 1998) for co-registering features.

Temporal binding

Although I have argued that there are distinct binding processes in vision, it remains possible that they are all under-scored by a single mechanism, such as synchronous firing between neurons (cf. Singer and Gray, 1995). Recent work in our laboratory provides some neuropsychological evidence that temporal binding can be important for visual selection. Again this work has been conducted with patient GK. Earlier we noted evidence for extinction in this patient. Extinction effects have typically been found when the stimuli are exposed for relatively long durations (500 ms or longer). In contrast to this, Humphreys et al. (2002) reported very different results when the stimuli were exposed for shorter durations. Example data are shown in Fig. 4. There are two important things to point out: (1) GK was better at reporting a single letter in his right field relative to when it fell in his left field, but there was some improvement in report over time for both left and right letters; (2) in contrast, GK's report of two letters was initially *better* than his ability to report a single letter on the left, but then it decreased as the

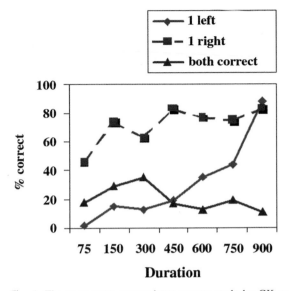

Fig. 4. The percentage correct letter reports made by GK as a function of the stimulus exposure duration.

stimulus exposure increased. At the longer stimulus durations (above 450 ms), there was an extinction effect: the report of a single left letter was better than the report of the left letter on two-letter trials. But, at briefer durations (300 ms or less), the opposite result occurred. There was better report of the left letter in a two-letter pair than a single letter on the left.

This last pattern of performance (two items > one item) has been reported once previously in a patient with parietal damage, by Goodrich and Ward (1997). They term it 'anti-extinction', to contrast it with the more usual extinction effect (two items < one item). Goodrich and Ward suggested that anti-extinction was produced by a form of response-based grouping, when the same task was applied to bilaterally presented stimuli. This account is insufficient to explain our data, however, since the same task was always applied but performance changed from anti-extinction to extinction as a function of stimulus duration. In addition, we have failed to find effects of having different or the same task applied to the stimuli used on bilateral trials (Humphreys et al., 2002). An alternative account is that there is temporary binding between the bilateral stimuli, generated by the forms onsetting at the same time. However, binding by common onset is transient. When stimuli are presented for longer durations, more sustained processes of binding need to come into play. This more sustained process is affected by factors such as shape similarity and connectedness, which influence recovery from extinction under long durations with GK (Humphreys et al., 2000). Consistent with the view that common onsets are necessary for the effect, we failed to find evidence for anti-extinction in studies that had the stimuli defined by offsets of contours from pre-masks.

One other proposal is that the anti-extinction effect is due to the common onsets cueing attention to an area or field containing both left and right field items. Due to this, both items can sometimes be available for report. However, when the stimuli remain for longer durations another form of attentional bias may influence performance, for instance, GK may make an eye movement to the rightmost letter, and this disrupts report of the left-side item. We assessed this last proposal by measuring GK's eye movements when he performed the letter report tasks. Surprisingly, eye movements had little impact on the anti-extinction effect: the effect occurred even on trials where GK made an eye movement to the rightmost letter (i.e., he remained able to report the left-side letter, provided the stimuli were presented briefly). Subsequently, we presented GK with three letters on a trial, two flankers created by new onsets and a third central letter created by offsets from a central pre-mask (see Fig. 5). The task was again to name all the letters present. Our idea was that, if the letter onsets cue GK's attention, then he should be able to report all the stimuli. Indeed since he typically reports from right to left, then he should

name the central (offset) letter before the left (onset letter). On the other hand, if stimuli bind by common onset, then GK might report the onset letters first and sometimes extinguish the central (offset) letter, as it is not part of the same group. This was what we found. The data are consistent with a temporal binding account, rather than an account in terms of cueing attention. In a further study we examined GK's report of briefly presented letters that were presented simultaneously or successively, at different time intervals. There was relatively good report of two letters presented simultaneously, but not when the letters were staggered over time. We conclude that there is a temporary binding based on common onset. However, this binding is not stable unless supported by a more sustained binding process, which may itself be contingent on attention (see below). For a patient such as GK, there is a spatial bias in the more sustained binding process, either due to a spatial bias in attention or to poor co-registration of features (see above).

Visual binding, consciousness and probabilistic interpretations

There are implications from these arguments for understanding the nature of our conscious representation of the visual world. One implication is that our conscious representation of a world of objects with attached surfaces is only derived after the several binding processes have taken place; earlier forms of binding take place unconsciously. Recent studies of the phenomenon of 'change blindness', however, suggest that any bindings that are formed unconsciously can be dissolved and are unavailable to direct perceptual report unless 'fixed' by attention (e.g., Rensink, 2000; Simons, 2000). Consequently, we are able to detect change taking place in only a very limited number of attended object representations, even if multiple representations are formed unconsciously. To reconcile the evidence for unconscious binding, along with poor detection of changes in multiple bindings (in change blindness), we can think of bindings operating probabilistically rather than being fully formed in a single shot. For example, co-incident activity states in neurons may represent the likelihood that two visual elements are part of the same object. The application of attention

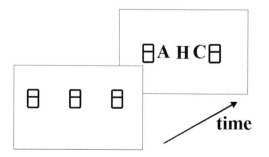

Fig. 5. The 3-letter displays used in the study of temporal grouping and anti-extinction. The two flanker letters were created by luminance onsets (black on a white screen). The central letter was created by offsetting contours from a pre-mask presented at fixation.

to these elements may lead to a further commitment of the visual system to a particular representation, reinforcing the binding of attended elements at the expense of binding between other elements in the field. Attention may be directed in either a bottom-up or a top-down manner, based on grouping between elements or on intention (one example being the effects of endogenous attentional cueing in visual neglect; e.g., Riddoch and Humphreys, 1983). On this view, attention stands as a kind of doorway to conscious representation, mediating between the formation of probabilistic representations and the commitment to particular descriptions, out of the many present, in consciousness. Of course, this side-steps the issue of what comprises attention in the first place. In my view this is a false question, since attention is not 'one' thing. Rather attention may be conceived of as an emergent property formed from top-down mechanisms that regulate competition between visual elements; these top-down mechanisms would include goal-directed activation from the frontal lobes, the programming of a motor response to a stimulus and so forth. In each case, the net result would be a commitment of the system to a particular object representation that may finally be maintained in visual short-term memory (VSTM). This then becomes an interactive account. A first stage of processing leads to the formation of probabilistic bindings, these interact with goal- and action-directed biases leading eventually to object representations being committed to VSTM. This then defines the context of visual consciousness.

Acknowledgements

This work was supported by grants from the European Union and from the Medical Research Council, UK. I am extremely grateful to HJA and GK for all their time and for their ability to make research fun as well as interesting. My thanks go also to all of my colleagues who contributed to the different parts of the work reported here: Muriel Boucart, Caterina Cinel, Anne Giersch, Dietmar Hienke, Nikki Klempen, Taksune Kumada, Illona Kovacs, Gudrun Nys, Andrew Olson, Jane Riddoch, and Jeremy Wolfe.

References

Balint, R. (1909) Seelenahmung des 'Schauens': Optische ataxie, raumliche Storung der Aufmerkamsamkeit. *Monatsschr. Psychiatrie Neurol.*, 25: 51–81.

Boucart, M. and Humphreys, G.W. (1992) The computation of perceptual structure from collinearity and closure: Normality and pathology. *Neuropsychologia*, 30: 527–546.

Boutsen, L. and Humphreys, G.W. (2000) Axis-based grouping reduces visual extinction. *Neuropsychologia*, 38: 896–905.

Brefczynski, J.A. and de Yoe, E.A. (1999) A physiological correlate of the 'spotlight' of visual attention. *Nat. Neurosci.*, 2: 370–374.

Butter, C.M. and Trobe, J.D. (1994) Integrative agnosia following progressive multifocal leukoencephalopathy. *Cortex*, 30: 145–158.

Chainay, H. and Humphreys, G.W. (2001) The real object advantage in agnosia: Evidence of a role for shading and depth in object recognition. *Cogn. Neuropsychol.*, 18: 175–191.

Cohen, A. and Rafal, R.D. (1991) Attention and feature integration: Illusory conjunctions in a patient with a parietal lobe lesion. *Psychol. Sci.*, 2: 106–110.

DeRenzi, E. and Lucchelli, F. (1993) The fuzzy boundaries of apperceptive agnosia. *Cortex*, 29: 187–215.

Desimone, R. and Ungerleider, L.G. (1989) Neural mechanisms of visual processing in monkeys. In: E. Boller and J. Grafman (Eds.), *Handbook of Neuropsychology, II*. Elsevier, Amsterdam, pp. 267–299.

Donk, M. (1999) Illusory conjunctions are an illusion: The effects of target–nontarget similarity on conjunction and feature errors. *J. Exp. Psychol. Hum. Percept. Perform.*, 25: 1207–1233.

Donnelly, N., Humphreys, G.W. and Riddoch, M.J. (1991) Parallel computation of primitive shape descriptions. *J. Exp. Psychol. Hum. Percept. Perform.*, 17: 561–570.

Duncan, J. and Humphreys, G.W. (1989) Visual search and stimulus similarity. *Psychol. Rev.*, 96: 433–458.

Eckhorn, R. (1999) Neural mechanisms of visual feature binding investigated with microelectrodes and models. *Vis. Cogn.*, 6: 231–266.

Elliott, M.A. and Muller, H.M. (1998) Synchronous information presented in 40 Hz flicker enhances visual feature binding. *Psychol. Sci.*, 9: 277–283.

Enns, J. and Rensink, R.A. (1991) Preattentive recovery of three-dimensional orientation from line drawings. *Psychol. Rev.*, 98: 335–351.

Fahle, M. (1993) Figure–ground discrimination from temporal information. *Proc. R. Soc. Lond. B Biol. Sci.*, 254: 199–203.

Friedman-Hill, S., Robertson, L.C. and Treisman, A. (1995) Parietal contributions to visual feature binding: Evidence from a patient with bilateral lesions. *Science*, 269: 853–855.

Giersch, A., Humphreys, G.W., Boucat, M. and Kovacs, I. (2000) The computation of occluded contours in visual agnosia: evidence for early computation prior to shape binding and figure-ground coding. *Cog. Neuropsychol.*, 17: 731–759.

Gilbert, C. and Wiesel, T.N. (1989) Columnar specificity of intrinsic horizontal and corticocortical connections in cat visual cortex. *J. Neurosci.*, 9: 2432–2442.

Gilbert, C., Ito, M., Kapadia, M. and Westheimer, G. (2000) Interactions between attention, context and learning in primary visual cortex. *Vis. Res.*, 40: 1217–1226.

Gilchrist, I., Humphreys, G.W. and Riddoch, M.J. (1996) Grouping and extinction: Evidence for low-level modulation of selection. *Cogn. Neuropsychol.*, 13: 1223–1256.

Goodrich, S.J. and Ward, R. (1997) Anti-extinction following unilateral parietal damage. *Cogn. Neuropsychol.*, 14: 595–612.

Grosof, D.H., Shapley, R.M. and Hawken, M.J. (1993) Macaque V1 neurons can signal 'illusory' contours. *Nature*, 257: 219–220.

Grossberg, S. and Mingolla, E. (1985) Neural dynamics of form perception: Boundary completion, illusory figures, and neon colour spreading. *Psychol. Rev.*, 92: 173–221.

Grossberg, S. and Pessoa, L. (1998) Texture segregation, surface representation and figure–ground separation. *Vis. Res.*, 38: 2657–2684.

Heywood, C.A. and Cowey, A. (1999) Cerebral achromatopsia. In: G.W. Humphreys (Ed.), *Case Studies in the Neuropsychology of Vision*. Psychology Press, London, pp. 17–40.

Heywood, C.A. and Zihl, J. (1999) Motion blindness. In: G.W. Humphreys (Ed.), *Case Studies in the Neuropsychology of Vision*. Psychology Press, London, pp. 1–16.

Hillyard, S.A., Vogel, E.K. and Luck, S.J. (1998) Sensory gain control (amplification) as a mechanism of selective attention: Electrophysiological and neuroimaging evidence. *Philos. Trans. R. Soc. Lond. B Biol. Sci.*, 353: 1257–1270.

Humphreys, G.W. (1998) Neural representation of objects in space: A dual coding account. *Philos. Trans. R. Soc. Lond. B Biol. Sci.*, 353: 1341–1352.

Humphreys, G.W. (1999) Integrative agnosia. In: G.W. Humphreys (Ed.), *Case Studies in the Neuropsychology of Vision*. Psychology Press, London, pp. 41–58.

Humphreys, G.W. and Donnelly, N. (2000) 3D constraints on spatially parallel shape processing. *Percept. Psychophys.*, 62: 1060–1085.

Humphreys, G.W. and Price, C.J. (2001) Cognitive neuropsychology and functional brain imaging: Implications for functional and anatomical models of cognition. *Acta Psychol.*, 107: 119–153.

Humphreys, G.W. and Riddoch, M.J. (1987) *To See or Not to See: A Case Study of Visual Agnosia*. Lawrence Erlbaum Associates, London.

Humphreys, G.W. and Riddoch, M.J. (1993) Interactions between object and space vision revealed through neuropsychology. In: D.E. Meyer and S. Kornblum (Eds.), *Attention and Performance, XIV*. MIT Press, Cambridge, MA, pp. 143–162.

Humphreys, G.W., Quinlan, P.T. and Riddoch, M.J. (1989) Grouping processes in visual search: Effects with single- and combined-feature targets. *J. Exp. Psychol. Gen.*, 118: 258–279.

Humphreys, G.W., Romani, C., Olson, A., Riddoch, M.J. and Duncan, J. (1994) Non-spatial extinction following lesions of the parietal lobe in humans. *Nature*, 372: 357–359.

Humphreys, G.W., Cinel, C., Wolfe, J., Olson, A. and Klempen, N. (2000) Fractionating the binding process: Neuropsychological evidence distinguishing binding of form from binding of surface features. *Vis. Res.*, 40: 1569–1596.

Jeannerod, M. (1997) *The Cognitive Neuroscience of Action*. Oxford University Press, Oxford.

Karnath, H.-O. (1988) Deficits of attention in acute and recovered visual hemi-neglect. *Neuropsychologia*, 26: 27–43.

Kellman, P.J. and Shipley, T.F. (1991) A theory of visual interpolation in object perception. *Cogn. Psychol.*, 23: 141–221.

Kovacs, I. (2000) Human development of perceptual organization. *Vis. Res.*, 40: 1301–1310.

Kubovy, M., Cohen, D.J. and Hollier, J. (1999) Featured integration that routinely occurs without focal attention. *Psychon. Bull. Rev.*, 6: 183–203.

Kumada, T. and Humphreys, G.W. (2001) Lexical recovery from extinction: Interactions between visual form and stored knowledge modulate visual selection. *Cogn. Neuropsychol.*, 18: 465–478.

Lawson, R. and Humphreys, G.W. (1999) The effects of view in depth on the identification of line drawings and silhouettes of familiar objects. *Vis. Cogn.*, 6: 165–196.

Linnell, K.J. and Humphreys, G.W. (2001) Spatially parallel processing of within-dimension conjunctions. *Perception*, 30: 49–60.

Mendola, J.D., Dale, A.M., Fischl, B., Liu, A.K. and Tootell, R.B.H. (1999) The representation of illusory and real contours in human cortical visual areas revealed by functional magnetic resonance imaging. *J. Neurosci.*, 19: 8560–8572.

Milner, A.D. and Goodale, M.A. (1995) *The Visual Brain in Action*. Oxford University Press, Oxford.

Milner, A.D., Dijkerman, H.C., McIntosh, R.D., Rossetti, Y. and Pisella, L. (2003) Delayed reaching and grasping in patients with optic ataxia. In: C. Prablanc, D. Pélisson and Y. Rossetti (Eds.), *Neural Control of Space Coding and Action Production. Progress in Brain Research*, Vol. 142. Elsevier, Amsterdam, pp. 225–242 (this volume).

Moran, J. and Desimone, R. (1985) Selective attention gates visual processing in the extra-striate cortex. *Science*, 229: 782–784.

Mordkoff, J.T., Yantis, S. and Egeth, H.E. (1990) Detecting conjunctions of colour and form in parallel. *Percept. Psychophys.*, 48: 157–168.

Redies, C., Crook, J.M. and Creutzfeldt, O.D. (1986) Neural response to borders with and without luminance gradients in cat visual cortex and dorsal lateral geniculate nucleus. *Exp. Brain Res.*, 61: 49–81.

Rensink, R.A. (2000) Visual search for change: A probe into the nature of attentional processing. *Vis. Cogn.*, 7: 345–376.

Rensink, R.A. and Enns, J. (1995) Pre-emption effects in visual search: Evidence for low-level grouping. *Psychol. Rev.*, 102: 101–130.

Riddoch, M.J. and Humphreys, G.W. (1983) The effect of cueing on unilateral neglect. *Neuropsychologia*, 21: 589–599.

Riddoch, M.J. and Humphreys, G.W. (1987) A case of integrative visual agnosia. *Brain*, 110: 1431–1462.

Riddoch, M.J., Humphreys, G.W., Gannon, T., Blott, W. and Jones, V. (1999) Memories are made of this: The effects of time on stored knowledge in a case of visual agnosia. *Brain*, 122: 537–559.

Sheth, B.R., Sharma, J., Rao, S.C. and Sur, M. (1996) Orientation maps of subjective contours in visual cortex. *Science*, 274: 2110–2115.

Shipley, T.F. and Kellman, P.J. (1992) Perception of partly occluded objects and illusory figures: Evidence for an identity hypothesis. *J. Exp. Psychol. Hum. Percept. Perform.*, 18: 106–120.

Simons, D.J. (2000) Current approaches to change blindness. *Vis. Cogn.*, 7: 1–16.

Singer, W. and Gray, C.M. (1995) Visual feature integration and the temporal correlation hypothesis. *Annu. Rev. Neurosci.*, 18: 555–586.

Tootell, R.B.H., Reppas, J.B., Kwong, K., Malach, R., Born, R.T., Brady, T.J., Rosen, B.R. and Belliveau, J.W. (1995) Functional analysis of human MT and related visual cortical areas using magnetic resonance imaging. *J. Neurosci.*, 15: 3215–3230.

Treisman, A. (1998) Feature binding, attention and object perception. *Philos. Trans. R. Soc. Lond. B Biol. Sci.*, 353: 1295–1306.

Treisman, A. and Gelade, G. (1980) A feature-integration theory of attention. *Cogn. Psychol.*, 12: 97–136.

Treisman, A. and Schmidt, H. (1982) Illusory conjunctions in the perception of objects. *Cogn. Psychol.*, 14: 107–141.

Ungerleider, L.G. and Haxby, J.V. (1994) 'What' and 'where' in the human brain. *Curr. Opin. Neurobiol.*, 4: 157–165.

Vecera, S.P. and Farah, M.J. (1994) Does visual attention select objects or locations? *J. Exp. Psychol. Gen.*, 123: 146–160.

Von der Heydt, R. and Peterhans, E. (1989) Mechanisms of contour perception in monkey visual cortex, I. Lines of pattern discontinuity. *J. Neurosci.*, 9: 1731–1748.

Watson, J.D.D., Myers, G.R., Frackowiak, R.S.J., Hajnal, V.J., Woods, R.P., Mazziota, J.C., Ship, S. and Zeki, S. (1993) Area V5 of the human brain: Evidence from a combined study using positron emission tomography and magnetic resonance imaging. *Cereb. Cortex*, 3: 79–84.

Zeki, S. (1993) *A Vision of the Brain*. Blackwell, Oxford.

C. Prablanc, D. Pélisson and Y. Rossetti (Eds.)
Progress in Brain Research, Vol. 142
© 2003 Elsevier Science B.V. All rights reserved

CHAPTER 16

Modulation and rehabilitation of spatial neglect by sensory stimulation

Georg Kerkhoff [*]

*EKN – Clinical Neuropsychology Research Group, Department Neuropsychology, Hospital Bogenhausen, Dachauerstrasse 164,
D-80992 Munich, Germany*

Abstract: After unilateral cortical or subcortical, often parieto-temporal lesions, patients exhibit a marked neglect of their contralateral space and/or body side. These patients are severely disabled in all daily activities, have a poor rehabilitation outcome and therefore require professional treatment. Unfortunately, effective treatments for neglect are just in the process of development. The present chapter reviews three aspects related to the rehabilitation of neglect. The first part summarizes findings about spontaneous recovery in patients and experimental animals with neglect. The second part deals with techniques and studies evaluating *short-term* sensory modulation effects in neglect. In contrast to many other neurological syndromes spatial neglect may be modulated transiently but dramatically in its severity by sensory (optokinetic, neck proprioceptive, vestibular, attentional, somatosensory–magnetic) stimulation. In part three, current treatment approaches are summarized, with a focus on three novel techniques: repetitive optokinetic stimulation, neck vibration training and peripheral somatosensory–magnetic stimulation. Recent studies of repetitive optokinetic as well as neck vibratory treatment both indicate significantly greater as well as multimodal improvements in neglect symptomatology as compared to the standard treatment of neglect. This clear superiority might result from the partial (re)activation of a distributed, multisensory vestibular network in the lesioned hemisphere. Somatosensory–magnetic stimulation of the neglected or extinguishing hand provides another feasible, non-invasive stimulation technique. It may be particularly suited for the rehabilitation of somatosensory extinction and unawareness of the contralesional body side. Finally, pharmacological approaches for the treatment of neglect are shortly addressed. Isolated drug treatment of neglect is currently no successful rehabilitation strategy due to inconsistent results as well as possible side effects. However, combined behavioural and drug treatments might yield better results. This has to be tested empirically in patient studies. In conclusion, the findings obtained in short-term sensory stimulation studies led to the development of effective techniques for the long-term rehabilitation of neglect. Future rehabilitation studies should evaluate effective treatment *combinations* considering all possible techniques and devices (behavioural, pharmacological, prosthetic or physiological).

Introduction

Neglect (synonymous with *hemispatial neglect, hemi-inattention, hemisensory neglect, hemineglect*) denotes the impaired or lost ability to react to or

* Correspondence to: G. Kerkhoff, EKN – Clinical Neuropsychology Research Group, Department Neuropsychology, Hospital Bogenhausen, Dachauerstrasse 164, D-80992 Munich, Germany. Tel.: +49-89-154-057; Fax: +49-89-156-781;
E-mail: georg.kerkhoff@extern.lrz-muenchen.de

process sensory stimuli (visual, auditory, tactile, olfactory) presented in the hemispace contralateral to a lesion of the human right or left cerebral hemisphere. Besides the aforementioned aspects of *sensory* neglect, *motor* neglect may occur and manifest itself as the reduced use or nonuse of a contralateral extremity (arm, leg) during walking or bimanual activities. Finally, neglect may occur in the imagination of spatial scenes (*representational* neglect). By definition neglect is not merely the result of elementary sensory (i.e. hemianopia, hemisensory loss), motor (i.e. hemiparesis) or cognitive/emotional disorders (i.e. reduced intelligence, depression). After a short description of the clinical and anatomical aspects of neglect the chapter will deal consecutively with the following three topics of neglect: spontaneous recovery, short-term modulation using sensory stimulation, and long-term stimulation for the permanent rehabilitation of patients with spatial neglect. A final synopsis and outlook finishes the chapter.

Anatomy

The most frequent etiological cause of neglect in humans are (often large) infarctions in the territory of the right, less often the left middle cerebral artery (MCA; Vallar, 1993; Karnath et al., 2001), causing lesions which centre on the inferior parietal cortex (*Brodmann areas*, BA 40, 7) and the superior temporal cortex. Accompanying damage to adjacent structures such as the optic radiations, the insula, dorsolateral frontal cortex (BA 4, 6, 44, 45, 46) and superior temporal cortex (BA 22, 37) is frequently apparent (Smania et al., 1998). Furthermore, neglect occurs after posterior thalamic (nc. pulvinaris) or basal ganglia lesions (nc. caudatus; Karnath et al., 2002) as a result of intracerebral bleedings, but has never been described following pure occipital lesions. Occasionally, neglect after lateral frontal lesions has been reported where similar lesions in animals regularly lead to contralesional neglect (Deuel and Collins, 1984). Neglect may also result from tumours or traumatic injuries of the aforementioned areas. In general, severe and multimodal neglect is caused by very large right-sided lesions which encroach on parietal, temporal, and regions of occipital or frontal cortex as well as subcortical structures (Vallar, 1993).

Frequency

Contralesional neglect occurs in some 33% of left--hemisphere and more than 50% of right-hemisphere lesioned patients [1] (Stone et al., 1991) when tested

---

[1] Since left-sided neglect after right cerebral lesions is the most frequent type of neglect the term 'neglect' in this review refers always to left-sided neglect in humans if not indicated otherwise. Of course, this does not exclude the fact that right-sided neglect after uni- or bilateral lesions may occur (more rarely) as well.

immediately (within 7 days) after lesion onset. The absolute percentage of neglect depends critically on the criterion or test used but the asymmetry in the occurrence of contralesional neglect has been found across different samples and methods. Recovery is considerably quicker and more complete in neglect after left-hemisphere lesions as opposed to right-hemisphere lesions (Stone et al., 1991). Thus, there is a clear hemispheric asymmetry showing that neglect is more frequent, more severe and more permanent following right-hemispheric lesions. However, *transient* right-sided neglect occurs infrequently after unilateral left-sided lesions or bilateral cerebral lesions.

Recovery

Recovery from the most obvious signs of neglect (i.e. the tendency to orient to the ipsilesional side and the lack of visual exploration in the contralesional hemispace) has been noted in the majority of patients within the first 6 months (Hier et al., 1983). In the remaining 25% neglect may persist up to years and performance in tasks which are sensitive to neglect may decline again after cessation of apparently successful rehabilitation treatment in the clinic (Paolucci et al., 1998). As mentioned above recovery from neglect is more likely after left- compared with right-sided cerebral lesions (Stone et al., 1991). Furthermore, recovery from 'frontal' neglect is more rapid and more complete in humans than from the classical 'parietal' neglect syndrome. Substantial recovery is less likely after large lesions and in those patients with diffuse brain atrophy in addition to the focal right-hemispheric lesion (Levine et al., 1986).

Little is known about the mechanisms guiding spontaneous recovery and/or those enabling treatment-guided improvements during rehabilitation. Pantano et al. (1992) reported a concomitant increase in regional cerebral blood flow (rCBF) in the posterior areas of the damaged right hemisphere and the anterior areas of the intact, left hemisphere probably including the frontal eye fields after a specific neglect treatment in their patients. Only the left frontal activation, in the region of the frontal eye fields, covaried with improved visual scanning behaviour after treatment. The authors concluded that the left (intact) frontal eye fields are crucial for recovery of visual scanning in neglect. In a later PET study with three neglect patients this finding was not uniformly replicated (Pizzamiglio et al., 1998). In this study behavioural recovery seemed to covary with improved blood flow in surviving areas of the *lesioned* hemisphere.

Similar results have been obtained in primate studies where neglect was induced by lesioning the frontal polysensory association cortex. Metabolic mapping for local glucose utilization (2-DG) showed a widespread reduction of glucose in ipsilesional striatal and partially thalamic nuclei connected with the frontal lobe whereas no reductions were found in cortical areas connected to the frontal lobe (Deuel and Collins, 1984). Behavioural recovery of visual, somatosensory and motor neglect was paralleled by a normalization of glucose metabolism in these subcortical circuits of the lesioned hemisphere (Deuel and Collins, 1984). To summarize, as in the few human imaging studies neglect after focal right-sided lesions of the frontal or parietal cortex is associated with widespread depressions of metabolic activity in the same hemisphere. Behavioural recovery is paralleled (or enabled) by a normalization of activity in this neural network for spatial attention that includes cortical and subcortical areas. This widespread depression of activity helps to explain why neglect occurs after cortical and subcortical lesions of many different anatomical structures.

Short-term modulation of neglect, extinction and unawareness by sensory stimulation

A variety of different techniques (see Kerkhoff, 2001, for a detailed review) has been used to influence neglect behaviour (Fig. 1, Table 1). The basic idea underlying all sensory stimulation manoeuvres in neglect patients is that neglect results from a disrupted representation and/or transformation of spatial coordinates into a common frame of reference necessary for accurate orientation of the subject in space. Since many sensory and proprioceptive data are fed into such a hypothetical reference frame, many of these input channels have been used to manipulate the neglect symptomatology by varying sensory or proprioceptive input.

Caloric stimulation

Cold water (caloric) stimulation of the contralesional ear (usually the left) or warm water stimulation of the ipsilesional ear (the right in patients with left neglect) stimulates the horizontal ear canal of the vestibular system and leads to a tonic deviation of the eyes towards the contralesional hemispace thereby reducing sensory neglect for some 10–15 min (see Fig. 1A). This procedure also improves neglect-related disturbances of the body scheme and postural disturbances as well (Rode et al., 1998) and in some cases transiently relieves the patient from his/her anosognosia for the left hemiplegia (time course 10–15 min; Rode et al., 1992). Caloric stimulation also improves the deviation of the subjective visual straight ahead (Karnath, 1994) and improves somatosensory neglect phenomena for a similar time period (Vallar et al., 1997; see also Vallar et al., 2003, this volume). Hence, this type of sensory stimulation exerts multimodal positive effects on many aspects of the neglect syndrome. Caloric stimulation in healthy subjects leads to a strong activation of a large cortico-subcortical network including parietal, temporal, insular and subcortical regions of the hemisphere contralateral to the stimulated ear (Bottini et al., 1994, 2001). Despite its short-term effectiveness, caloric stimulation has not been evaluated as a tool for long-term or repetitive stimulation. This is largely due to the vestibular habituation phenomenon associated with repeated caloric stimulation. The typical side effects of this stimulation like vertigo and vomiting encountered in normal subjects are not experienced by neglect patients (Rode et al., 1998).

Optokinetic/large-field visual motion stimulation

A more tolerable stimulation procedure is optokinetic or visual motion stimulation with large-field visual displays containing stimuli all moving coherently to the left or right. Leftward motion (in case of left neglect) temporarily reduces the ipsilesional line bisection error (Pizzamiglio et al., 1990; Mattingley et al., 1994). Similarly, slow motion stimulation towards the neglected hemispace reduces the 'size' and 'space' distortions transiently (cf. Fig. 1B, adapted from Kerkhoff, 2000) and reduces tactile extinction of the contralesional hand temporarily. Occasionally, negative effects have also been observed with this procedure in a line extension task with leftward optokinetic stimulation (Bisiach et al., 1996). This negative effect might be explained by the fact that *fast* optokinetic stimulation (OKS) leads to constant changes in eye position which may render a percep-

tual task more difficult for a patient, thus aggravating the deficit. We have found in a series of experiments that *slow* motion stimulation (velocity 7.5°/s) is fully sufficient to observe full normalization in a variety of visual neglect tasks (cf. Fig. 1B, adapted from Kerkhoff, 2000). Obviously, the motor component of the optokinetic nystagmus obtained with high-speed

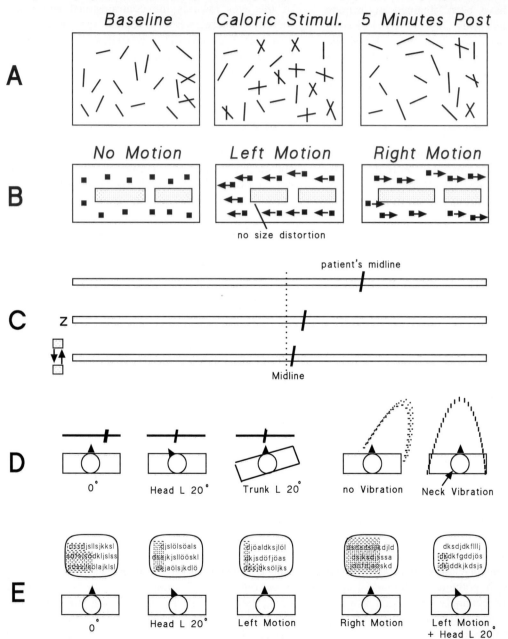

stimulation is not crucial for the modulatory effect on neglect (Mattingley et al., 1994). Hence, optokinetic stimulation seems to affect nearly all aspects of the neglect syndrome transiently. Surprisingly, the effects of long-term OKS have rarely been studied systematically.

Imaging studies in normal subjects using OKS show activation of a large cortico-subcortical network including vestibular cortex, oculomotor areas and visual motion sensitive areas in temporo-parietal-occipital cortex as well as in the basal ganglia of both hemispheres (Dieterich et al., 1998).

Cueing

Another simple stimulation is 'cueing' the patient to attend to stimuli in the contralesional hemispace (Fig. 1C). Cueing may simply be the verbal command to look further to the left or to require the patient to read a letter located on the left side of a line before he is allowed to attempt bisection or to display flickering stimuli in the contralesional hemispace (Riddoch and Humphreys, 1983; Butter et al., 1990). Lin et al. (1996) have recently elaborated this cueing paradigm. They showed that circling of a digit at the left end of a line and the tracing of the complete line with the right index finger was the most effective cueing procedure. This led to a complete normalization of the line bisection error in left ne-

glect. Obviously, the use of a visuomotor component (manual tracing) was most effective, probably by involving fronto-parietal neuronal networks crucial for visuomotor control.

Neck vibration/head rotation

Vibration of the contralesional neck muscles leads to a temporary shift of the visual subjective straight ahead (SSA) towards the contralesional hemispace (Karnath et al., 1993) and reduces neglect-related omissions of visual stimuli in this hemispace. Neck vibration activates mainly contralateral insular and secondary somatosensory cortices (Bottini et al., 2001) as well as some other regions. Both regions are often damaged in patients with neglect. A similar, transient effect as with neck vibration can be achieved through selective rotation of the head or leftward trunk rotation while visual fixation remains straight ahead (Fig. 1D,E; see Kerkhoff, 2001 for further details and references). Similar effects have been reported with different body positions (upright vs. supine). The activity of the otoliths of the vestibular system is reduced in a supine body position. Positioning neglect patients in a supine position reduces neglect (see Vallar et al., 1997). As with optokinetic stimulation, we will return to the effects of repetitive neck vibration as a possible treatment strategy for neglect in the next section.

Fig. 1. Effects of short-term sensory stimulation on different neglect phenomena. (A) Line cancellation performance before (baseline), immediately after caloric (cold water) stimulation of the contralesional horizontal ear canal, and 5 min after stimulation. Note the significant reduction of omissions (uncrossed lines) in the left part of the display during stimulation. (B) Effect of linear visual background motion during a horizontal, visual size judgment test in neglect. When the background stimuli are stationary (no motion) the left bar is reproduced too large as compared to the right bar on the screen. Left motion alleviates this size distortion while right-sided background motion (velocity 7.5°/s) produces similar effects as no motion. (C) Cueing of attention to the left, contralesional side. Having the patient identify the letter on the left of the bisection line (z) prior to bisection reduces the ipsilesional deviation in line bisection. Display of apparent movement of a light at the contralesional end of the line (squares with arrows) has a similar beneficial effect on line bisection, even if this phi-movement is not consciously perceived due to an additional left-sided field defect. (D) Effect of head orientation (circle, black triangle indicating nose, and thus head direction) and trunk rotation to the left (L, 20° rotation) on line bisection judgments. Leftward head orientation (with the trunk straight ahead) and leftward trunk orientation (with the head straight ahead) both lead to a normalization of the line bisection error. Effect of vibrating the left posterior neck muscles in left-sided visual neglect leads to an ocular exploration pattern in total darkness that is organized more symmetrically around the body midline (rightmost plot). Note, in contrast, the ipsilesionally (to the right) deviated exploration pattern in the condition without vibration. (E) Effects of head-on-trunk-rotation (circles, black arrows indicating head orientation) and visual background motion are displayed on a computer screen while neglect patients read a text displayed on the same screen. The shaded area indicates approximately the omitted words (= neglect dyslexia). Note that left-sided head rotation (20°, without visual background motion) as well as left visual background motion (with the head and trunk remaining straight) both reduce neglect dyslexia; the strongest reduction of omissions is seen when both conditions are combined, indicating a summation of both effects. For further details and references see text. (Reproduced by permission from Pergamon/Elsevier from Kerkhoff (2001), fig. 10, page 18.)

TABLE 1

Summary of short-term sensory stimulation procedures for the modulation of neglect and extinction (see text for more details and references)

Sensory stimulation	Basic modulating principle	Results
Caloric stimulation	improvement of neglect by caloric (cold water) stimulation of the horizontal ear canal (contralesional ear) or warm-water stimulation of the ipsilesional ear	marked improvements in perceptual neglect and unawareness; transient effects (15 min); uncomfortable
Optokinetic stimulation	activation of a large parieto-temporo-occipital and subcortical multisensory network involved in spatial processing; activation leads to multimodal improvements	positive modulatory effects on nearly every neglect deficit, effects disappear shortly after cessation of stimulation (ca. 5 min following stimulation)
Cueing	reduction of neglect by verbal, visual or auditory stimulation; this facilitates attentional shifts towards the contralesional hemispace	easily applicable procedure with small but short-lived effects; cueing in combination with arm movements most effective
Neck muscle vibration	vibration of left dorsal neck muscles leads to a shift of subjective space towards the contralesional hemispace and to a normalization of the eye movement pattern in neglect patients	strong effects on visual neglect and eye movements which does not require conscious awareness of the patient
Limb activation	improvement of visual neglect by acting with the contralesional arm (usually the left) in the contralesional hemispace; such activities are believed to activate attentional circuits in the lesioned hemisphere	easy to use in clinic and at home; demonstrated transfer to daily activities; often not applicable due to severe contralesional sensorimotor deficits (arm/hand)
Peripheral magnetic stimulation	application of high-speed peripheral magnetic stimulation of the contralesional dorsal hand; stimulation gives somatosensory afferent inflow and leads to activation of the primary and secondary somatosensory cortices in the lesioned hemisphere	non-painful stimulation that requires special technical facilities; positive and enduring effects on tactile extinction; effects persist up to 24 h after a single stimulation session
TENS	transcutaneous electroneural stimulation of the left neck muscles by low-voltage current	easy to realize, portable, low-cost; small effects in cancellation tasks; small effects compared to other stimulation methods
Prisms	exploiting the sensorimotor recalibration effect during readaptation after a previous prism exposure	significant, multimodal effects (up to 72 h); repeated prism exposure might yield enduring effects

Limb activation

Apart from passive arm or body positioning active movements of the contralesional, left arm or shoulder (which is often easier to perform for neglect patients with residual hemiparesis) in left hemispace leads to a temporary reduction of sensory neglect phenomena (summarized in Robertson, 1999). Another influential factor is cueing with alerting stimuli, i.e. a sudden beep. This leads to an immediate alertness reaction and temporarily improves visual neglect (Robertson, 1999).

Transcutaneous electroneural stimulation (TENS)

This technique is widely used in physiotherapy, i.e. to treat stays or to stimulate muscles. TENS of the left hand has a small but significant effect on perceptual neglect (Vallar et al., 1997) but this effect is weaker than vibration of the left neck. In contrast, Guariglia et al. (1998) reported small, but significant improvements in representational neglect and drawing after left-sided TENS and deteriorations after right-sided TENS of the neck, thus suggesting a more lateralized effect.

All these different methods show that neglect is considerably influenced by sensory, attentional or gravitational factors. This elucidates mechanisms crucial to the genesis of neglect and extinction. However, not all manoeuvres described herein to obtain transient modulatory effects are as well suitable for long-term rehabilitation.

Long-term rehabilitation approaches

Despite recovery of the most obvious signs of hemineglect a considerable portion of neglect patients — especially those with *large* right-hemispheric lesions — remain severely impaired in functional activities of daily living (ADL), i.e. dressing, eating, transfers from bed to the wheelchair, wheelchair navigation or reading. Neglect patients have a delayed recovery from hemiplegia, postural problems, and require further ambulant treatment after discharge from the hospital (Paolucci et al., 1998). Few neglect patients recover in a way that allows them to live independently or even return to their previous job. Neglect is therefore a major negative predictor of recovery from brain lesions (Katz et al., 1999), and consequently effective, novel treatment methods are urgently required.

Scanning/visual exploration treatment

Early treatment approaches for neglect began in the seventies (Diller and Weinberg, 1977). They were mainly based on clinical experience and were less theory-driven than more recent approaches to the syndrome. Since disturbed visual exploration of space is one of the most obvious deficits in neglect patients this was one that received most attention in treatment studies (Diller and Weinberg, 1977). Later studies have implemented a similar approach and compared the training of visual scanning strategies in neglect patients with nonspecific cognitive training (Antonucci et al., 1995) or combined it with specific visuospatial training. While specific visual exploration training ameliorates reading and visual search, cognitive training has only minor effects on neglect. Table 2 summarizes current long-term treatment approaches in spatial neglect.

Pharmacological treatment

As in other areas of neurorehabilitation pharmacological treatments have been suggested for treatment. Improvement of neglect with dopamine agonists was prompted by the observation that experimental reduction of dopamine unilaterally in monkeys and rats (Carli et al., 1985; Apicella et al., 1991) causes neglect-like deficits in these animals. Heilman et al. (1978) first described hypoarousal and emotional indifference in patients with left neglect following large right-hemispheric lesions. Consequently, pharmacological reduction of hypoarousal and emotional indifference might reduce the neglect symptomatology. Fleet et al. (1987) reported improved scanning in two neglect patients following application of a dopamine agonist. However, the opposite effect (aggravation of neglect) was reported in a recent study with the same drug (Grujic et al., 1998). In another recent study (Lehmann et al., 2001) positive effects on visual scanning were obtained after treatment with a well-known noradrenergic antidepressant (Imipramin). Evidently, the neuropharmacological basis of spatial neglect is not fully understood at present. Hence, firm conclusions concerning pharmacological treatment in neglect are premature since few systematic studies have been conducted in these patients. One obvious problem with drug treatments specifically in neglect patients resides in the fact that neglect cannot be considered solely as a 'single-receptor-type disease', as for instance Parkinson's disease. As the lesions of neglect patients are typically involving a large cortico-subcortical network, and consequently many different types of neurons responsive to a wide variety of pharmacological substances, any medication will inevitably affect numerous sensory and cognitive abilities, and not always positively. Side effects like fatigue, increased seizure frequency or raised irritability are more likely in pharmacological therapy as compared to behavioural treatments of neglect and compromise the desired benefits of the drug. Furthermore, some drugs are not to be prescribed for prolonged periods (i.e. amphetamine) which may create a problem after cessation of the application. Hence, it seems at present unlikely that isolated pharmacological stimulation is a successful therapy for neglect. A more promising approach might be to evaluate short-term

TABLE 2

Summary of long-term treatment techniques designed for the *permanent* rehabilitation of patients with spatial neglect (see text for more details and references)

Treatment	Basic therapeutic principle	Efficiency, practicability, transfer
Visual exploration	improvement of search strategy and speed using paper–pencil and wide-field projection devices; reduction of critical omissions by systematic strategy	easy to realize in a rehabilitation setting; limited transfer to daily activities; needs numerous training sessions (i.e. 40)
Pharmacology	application of dopaminergic or noradrenergic substances to activate attentional (putative right-hemispheric) networks	effects of dopaminergic stimulation are contradictory; positive effects of noradrenergic treatment on visual scanning and visual attention
Repetitive optokinetic stimulation	activation of a large parieto-temporo-occipital and subcortical multisensory network involved in spatial processing; activation leads to multimodal improvements	easy to realize in a rehabilitation setting; no side effects; requires some technical facilities; strong effects after only five treatment sessions
Neck muscle vibration	vibration of left dorsal neck muscles leads to a shift of subjective space towards the contralesional hemispace	easy to use in different daily situations (i.e. self-care); transfer to non-trained activities and to the tactile modality; some patients do not experience the vibration illusion
Limb activation	improvement of visual neglect by acting with the contralesional arm (usually the left) in the contralesional hemispace; such activities are believed to activate attentional circuits in the lesioned hemisphere	easy to use in clinic and at home; demonstrated transfer to daily activities; often not applicable due to severe contralesional sensorimotor deficits (arm/hand)
Attention training	amelioration of neglect phenomena by activating sustained, non-lateralized attentional capacities using stimuli which have an alerting quality (i.e. brisk tone)	easy to use in clinic and at home; transfer to non-trained activities; stability of improvements questionable
TENS	transcutaneous electroneural stimulation of the left neck muscles by low-voltage current	easy to realize, portable, low-cost; very small or nonsignificant effects in treatment as compared to other treatments

modulatory effects of certain drugs on multimodal neglect to establish which components are activated by which medication. Coull et al. (2000) described noradrenergically mediated activation of a large attentional neuronal network during an attention task in normal subjects. Delivery of the drug led to an increase in the modulatory effect of frontal cortex on projections from subcortical (locus coeruleus) to cortical (parietal cortex) brain regions. If similar effects could be obtained in neglect patients it is very likely that attentional aspects of the neglect syndrome would be improved by noradrenergic medication.

Another idea is to evaluate the efficacy of *combined* pharmacological and behavioural treatments. In such a combined therapy a drug may be chosen to increase the general arousal level so that the patient might be more susceptible to the effects of a certain behavioural treatment like optokinetic or neck vibration treatment. One crucial question here is whether the obtained improvements remain stable after cessation of the medication.

Repetitive optokinetic stimulation (R-OKS)

Based on the manifold positive, but transient effects of OKS summarized above we conducted a pilot study with three neglect patients to evaluate the long-term effects of repetitive optokinetic stimulation (R-OKS) as a treatment for neglect (Kerkhoff et al., 2001). Three patients with multimodal left-sided neglect (two severe, one moderate, all with right parietal lesions, chronicity 3–6 months postlesion) were subjected to a single-subject baseline design. All subjects received standard visual exploration training (three sessions per week) throughout the complete course of the pilot study. During a 2-week baseline period all subjects were tested four times in a variety of neglect tests to exclude effects of spontaneous recovery and/or test repetition. During this period, no significant improvements in any test were seen (despite the visual exploration training being performed). After the fourth baseline test, repetitive optokinetic stimulation was given for five sessions (45 min each, delivered in a period of 10–14 days). After OKS training, auditory neglect and neglect dyslexia were substantially improved (see Fig. 2). These improvements remained stable after a 2-week follow-up in all cases. Interestingly, these improvements were obtained in two modalities of neglect (vision and audition) which underlines the multimodal efficiency of OKS as already documented with short-term optokinetic stimulation. These encouraging results suggest that R-OKS may be an effective treatment for *multimodal* neglect symptoms (Fig. 2). It must be conceded that five treatment sessions were not sufficient to improve all aspects of neglect up to a level that enabled the patients to regain complete functional independence. However, the multimodal effects on visual and especially auditory neglect are worth extending this treatment in larger patient groups and with more treatment sessions.

Regarding the crucial mechanisms for the improvements we can only speculate. It is likely that some parts of the neuronal network activated by OKS (see above) survived the lesion and could be reactivated by repetitive OKS. Imaging studies support the idea that surviving islands in a right-hemispheric cortical network mediate behavioural recovery from spatial neglect (Pizzamiglio et al., 1998). Apart from the physiological basis of the recovery enabled by R-OKS some other aspects of the treatment itself deserve further evaluation. Hence, it is well-known that performing smooth pursuit eye movements activates the right parieto-temporal cortex. Since the patients in our treatment study performed smooth pursuit eye movements while being stimulated by the visual motion pattern on the screen it is possible that the observed improvements resulted either from the stimulation with multiple moving stimuli, from the performance of pursuit eye movements, or from both components. The separate contributions of both mechanisms to the treatment have to be tested experimentally in subsequent studies. Another *clinically* relevant question is whether the effect of R-OKS can be enhanced by using very large visual motion displays, i.e. 80° horizontal and 60° vertical stimulation field instead of 40° horizontal and 30° vertical as used in our pilot study.

Neck vibration treatment

Based on the positive effects of short-term neck vibration on visual neglect phenomena summarized above we evaluated in a controlled crossover rehabilitation study whether repetitive application of contralesional neck vibration in combination with standard visual exploration training is superior to visual exploration training given *without* neck vibration (Schindler et al., 2002). Twenty neglect patients were randomly allocated to two groups ($n = 10$ each). Each group received 15 sessions of the respective training for 3 weeks (5 per week), after which the two treatments were reversed and another 15 treatment sessions with the other treatment were given (crossover design). The results show uniformly larger treatment gains during the neck vibration + exploration training (regardless of the time when it was received) as compared to exploration training without concomitant neck vibration. Significant improvements in the visual straight ahead, cancellation and reading were obtained after the combined treatment. Furthermore, the improvements transferred to a tactile search task in peripersonal space thus showing multimodal efficacy. Moreover, the improvements were also evident in several activities of daily living as rated before and after the treatment blocks by the nurses who were involved in the care of the patients but who were 'blind' to the neuropsychological treatment. According to these ratings, combined neck vibration and optokinetic treatment led to greater improvements in reaching, grasping, transfers from/to bed and wheelchair, and dressing as compared to pure visual exploration treatment.

One possible limitation of neck vibration in some neglect patients may reside in the fact that not all subjects respond as vigorously to the illusion created by the vibration of the posterior neck muscles (see Karnath et al., 1993, for more details of the technique). Nevertheless, the clear superiority of this treatment in contrast to the relatively smaller effects of standard visual exploration training argue for a wider use of this treatment technique.

Visuomotor prism adaptation

Without going into the details of this approach (Rode et al., 2003) it can be said that the manifold improvements seen after a single 30-min visuomotor prism adaptation in patients with left visual neglect (Rossetti et al., 1998) as well as similar improvements found in patients with 'postural neglect' using the same technique (Tiliket et al., 2001) and the improvements obtained in auditory extinction are impressive evidence for the efficacy of this technique. As with all novel treatment approaches long-term treatment studies are urgently required to compare the effects of prism adaptation over a longer treatment period, and in comparison to other neglect treatments.

Sensory training in extinction

In contrast to the variety of stimulation and rehabilitation procedures that have been proposed for neglect very little is known about how extinction can be treated. Since it persists even when the most overt neglect signs have recovered treatments of extinction clearly would be of practical importance. Goldmann (1966) desribed impressive and stable improvements in 20 brain-damaged patients with tactile extinction after a teaching strategy. The aim of this cueing strategy was to direct the patient's attention to the extinguished stimulus and to the 'twoness' of the stimuli. Surprisingly, this treatment study has been completely neglected in the extinction literature. In summary, the allocationof attention (cueing) is also helpful in extinction and might be combined with other treatment techniques.

Repetitive peripheral magnetic stimulation (RPMS) in extinction

Another, more physiologically oriented treatment approach is somatosensory magnetic stimulation of the contralesional hand. The basic idea behind this procedure is based on the observation that some 90% of neglect patients are hemiparetic/-plegic on their left body side, and therefore are deprived of somatosensory input (i.e. touch, object surfaces, warm vs. cold stimuli) for months or years after their brain lesion. Consequently, it is not surprising that patients with tactile extinction show decreased activity (as measured with PET) in the ipsilesional secondary somatosensory cortex related to the extinguishing hand (Remy et al., 1999). How can this activity be increased, and would that reduce tactile extinction of the contralesional hand? Peripheral repetitive magnetic stimulation (RPMS) provides a powerful and non-painful somatosensory stimulation of the dorsal hand surface. It leads to strong activations of the primary and secondary somatosensory cortices. In a first study, we tested in 14 right-brain-damaged patients, all showing left-sided tactile extinction, whether one single session of RPMS (for 20 min, including 4000 single-pulse magnetic stimulations) leads to a significant improvement in tactile extinction. Subjects were randomly allocated to a RPMS stimulation group ($n = 7$) and a control group ($n = 7$). The control group did not receive magnetic

Fig. 2. Effects of repetitive optokinetic stimulation (5 sessions of 40 min each applied over a time period of 10 days) on neglect dyslexia (top figure) and the auditory straight ahead in azimuth in front space (lower figure). Single graphs of three patients in a pilot study and the arithmetic mean are displayed for both figures (see legend). Note the stability of neglect in reading and the marked deviation of the auditory straight ahead to the ipsilesional, right side during the baseline period in all patients. R-OKS treatment required the patients to look at a computer-generated random display of 30–70 dots on a dark background, all moving coherently towards the left, contralesional hemispace with a speed of 7.5–50°/s, varying from trial to trial to keep attention engaged. Subjects were encouraged to make smooth pursuit movements towards the direction of the motion. Marked improvements in reading and the auditory straight ahead were obtained during the R-OKS treatment, but not during the baseline period. All improvements remained stable in the follow-up period which was as long as the baseline and treatment period. (Adapted with permission from Hippocampus Verlag (Germany) from Kerkhoff et al., 2001, figs. 3 and 4, page 183.)

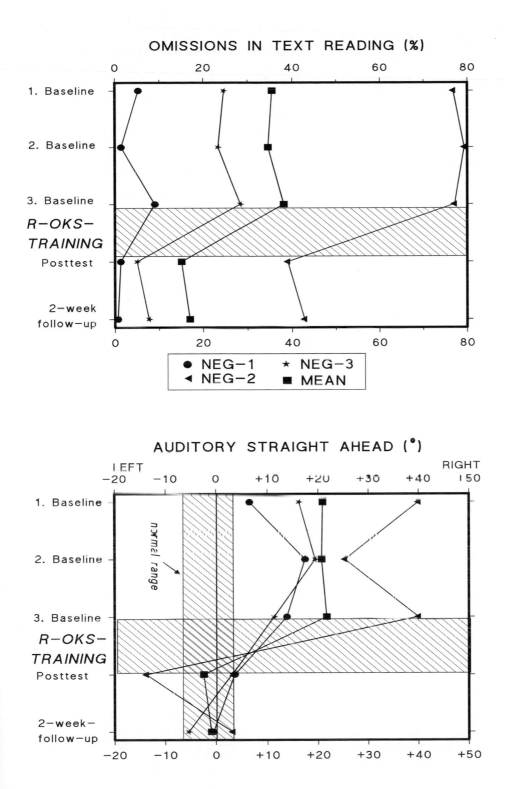

OMISSIONS IN TEXT READING (%)

1. Baseline
2. Baseline
3. Baseline

R-OKS-TRAINING

Posttest

2-week follow-up

● NEG−1   ★ NEG−3
◄ NEG−2   ■ MEAN

AUDITORY STRAIGHT AHEAD (°)

LEFT   RIGHT

1. Baseline
2. Baseline
3. Baseline

R-OKS-TRAINING

Posttest

2-week follow-up

normal range

stimulation but simply performed the tests in the same temporal sequence. After a single RPMS session an increase in the identification rate in bilateral tactile stimulation by 28% on average was achieved in the experimental group whereas no effects were observed in the nonstimulated group (Heldmann et al., 2000; cf. Fig. 3). As the testing took place some 30 min after the end of the magnetic stimulation this indicates that the effect is not merely a short-lived 'on/off' stimulation effect but obviously has enduring effects overlasting the stimulation period. Another beneficial side effect of the stimulation was the informal observation that four out of seven stimulated patients reported days after the RPMS that "they felt more in their left hand/arm". This feeling included being more aware of tactile stimuli on that side, of their different temperatures as well as being more aware of the spatial position of their contralesional arm in space (i.e. arm position sense). None of the control patients reported any of such subjective feelings. Although these are only subjective and informal observations, RPMS might contribute to an increased awareness of the contralesional limbs in patients with extinction and/or neglect. Furthermore, multiple sessions of RPMS might yield larger and more permanent effects.

Critical summary and future perspectives

Despite the improvements that have been made in the last decade in the development of theory-based treatment techniques for neglect and extinction the patients often remain moderately impaired at the end

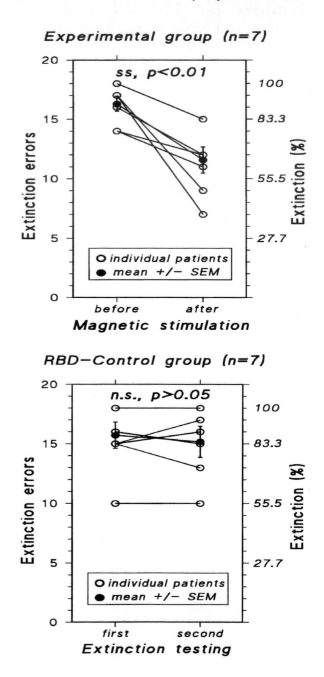

Fig. 3. Effects of a single magnetic stimulation session (20 min, 4000 magnetic impulses) of the contralesional, left ('extinguishing') hand on tactile extinction scores in an experimental ($n = 7$) and a control patient group ($n = 7$), all with chronic right-hemispheric lesions (mean chronicity 10.5 and 8.5 months postlesion). Subjects had to discriminate five different tactile surfaces while being stimulated bilaterally on their dorsal hand either with the same or two different materials. Both patient groups were matched appropriately for age, gender, severity of extinction, months since lesion, as well as associated deficits. Note the significant reduction of left-hand tactile extinction scores in the RPMS group and the stable extinction scores in the nonstimulated group. Right-hand extinction scores (not shown here) remained on an identical level in both subject groups, thus excluding a simple shift of attention towards the neglected left hand with a cost-effect on the right, ipsilesional hand. Figure based on results reported by Heldmann et al. (2000).

of clinical rehabilitation. This shows that the efforts so far are only partially effective. Therefore, the scientific development of effective treatment techniques in this field is urgently required. Obviously, spatial neglect is a multicomponent and multimodal syndrome resulting from damage to a large number of cortical and subcortical structures, and hence neural circuits relevant for sensory, motor and cognitive functioning in the brain. Consequently, the search for *multimodally* effective treatments is probably the most important task for the near future. Furthermore, as in other areas of medicine, effective combinations of treatments are to be sought, since the time available for stationary or ambulant treatment is critically limited (often less than 6 or even 4 weeks). Since 6 weeks of treatment with a single therapy technique often are not sufficient to fully rehabilitate patients with severe neglect, treatment combinations with different physiological and/or behavioural activity profiles might yield a better outcome. Such combinations could include all types of behavioural treatments, drugs, prostheses or medical interventions like TMS (transcortical magnetic stimulation). The increasing physiological, anatomical, neuropsychological and cognitive knowledge concerning sensory, motor and representational aspects of space coding in health and pathology will undoubtedly assist in developing such treatments for these severely disabled patients. The promising results of repetitive neck vibration, optokinetic stimulation, prism adaptation and magnetic stimulation show that the basic idea of sensory modulation and stimulation emerges into the scientific development of novel treatments for neglect. In exchange, the results obtained with such new methods will gain additional insights into normal and pathological space coding in the human brain.

Abbreviations

MCA	middle cerebral artery
BA	Brodmann area
SSA	subjective straight ahead
CT	computerized cranial tomography
(f)MRI	(functional) magnetic resonance imaging of the brain
2-DG	2-desoxyglycose
rCBF	regional cerebral blood flow
PET	positron emission tomography of the brain
OKS	optokinetic stimulation
R-OKS	repetitive optokinetic stimulation
TENS	transelectroneural stimulation

Acknowledgements

I am grateful to the following colleagues who were involved in several of the studies described in this chapter (listed alphabetically): Georg Goldenberg, Peter Havel, Barbara Heldmann, Thomas Jahn, Melanie Jonas, Ingo Keller, Christian Marquardt, Vera Ritter, Igor Schindler, Alfons Struppler and Wolfram Ziegler. Furthermore, I am grateful for helpful comments by an anonymous reviewer.

References

Antonucci, G., Guariglia, C., Judica, A., Magnotti, L., Paolucci, S., Pizzamiglio, L. and Zoccolotti, P. (1995) Effectiveness of neglect rehabilitation in a randomized group study. *J. Clin. Exp. Neuropsychol.*, 17: 383–389.

Apicella, P., Legallet, E., Nieoullon, A. and Trouche, E. (1991) Neglect of contralateral visual stimuli in monkeys with unilateral striatal dopamine depletion. *Behav. Brain Res.*, 46: 187–195.

Bisiach, E., Pizzamiglio, L., Nico, D. and Antonucci, G. (1996) Beyond unilateral neglect. *Brain*, 119: 851–857.

Bottini, G., Sterzi, R., Paulesu, E., Vallar, G., Cappa, S.F., Erminio, F., Passingham, R.E., Frith, C.D. and Frackowiak, R.S.J. (1994) Identification of the central vestibular projections in man: a positron emission tomography activation study. *Exp. Brain Res.*, 99: 164–169.

Bottini, G., Karnath, H.O., Vallar, G., Sterzi, R., Frith, C.D., Frackowiak, R.S.J. and Paulesu, E. (2001) Cerebral representations for egocentric space. *Brain*, 124: 1182–1196.

Butter, C.M., Kirsch, N.L., and Reeves, G. (1990) The effect of lateralized dynamic stimuli on unilateral spatial neglect following right hemisphere lesions. *Restorative Neurol. Neurosci.*, 2: 39–46.

Carli, M., Evenden, J.L. and Robbins, T.W. (1985) Depletion of unilateral striatal dopamine impairs initiation of contralateral actions and not sensory attention. *Nature*, 313: 679–682.

Coull, J.T., Büchel, C., Friston, K.J. and Frith, C.D. (2000) Noradrenergically mediated plasticity in a human attentional neuronal network. *NeuroImage*, 10: 705–715.

Deuel, R.K. and Collins, R.C. (1984) The functional anatomy of frontal lobe neglect in the monkey: behavioral and quantitative 2-deoxyglucose studies. *Ann. Neurol.*, 15: 521–529.

Dieterich, M., Bucher, S.F., Seelos, K. and Brandt, T. (1998)

Horizontal or vertical optokinetic stimulation activates visual motion-sensitive, ocular motor and vestibular cortex areas with right hemispheric dominance. An fMRI study. *Brain*, 121: 1479–1495.

Diller, L. and Weinberg, J. (1977) Hemi-inattention in rehabilitation: The evolution of a rational remediation program. *Adv. Neurol.*, 18: 63–82.

Fleet, W.S., Valenstein, E., Watson, R.T. and Heilman, K.M. (1987) Dopamine agonist therapy for neglect in humans. *Neurology*, 37: 1765–1770.

Goldman, H. (1966) Improvement of double simultaneous stimulation perception in hemiplegic patients. *Arch. Phys. Med. Rehabil.*, 63: 681–687.

Grujic, Z., Mapstone, M. and Gitelman, D.R. (1998) Dopamine agonists reorient visual exploration away from neglected hemispace. *Neurology*, 51: 1395–1398.

Guariglia, C., Lippolis, G. and Pizzamiglio, L. (1998) Somatosensory stimulation improves imagery disorders in neglect. *Cortex*, 34: 233–241.

Heilman, K.M., Schwarz, H.D. and Watson, R.T. (1978) Hypoarousal in patients with the neglect syndrome and emotional indifference. *Neurology*, 28: 229–232.

Heldmann, B., Kerkhoff, G., Struppler, A. and Jahn, Th. (2000) Repetitive peripheral magnetic stimulation alleviates tactile extinction. *NeuroReport*, 11: 3193–3198.

Hier, D.B., Mondlock, J. and Caplan, L.R. (1983) Recovery of behavioral abnormalities after right hemisphere stroke. *Neurology*, 33: 345–350.

Lehmann, V., Hildebrandt, H., Olthaus, O. and Sachsenheimer, W. (2001) Medikamentöse Beeinflussung visuo-räumlicher Aufmerksamkeitsstörungen bei rechtshirnigen Mediainfarkten. *Aktuelle Neurol.*, 28: 176–181.

Karnath, H.-O. (1994) Subjective body orientation in neglect and the interactive contribution of necke muscle proprioceptive and vestibular stimulation. *Brain*, 117: 1001–1012.

Karnath, H.-O., Christ, W. and Hartje, W. (1993) Decrease of contralateral neglect by neck muscle vibration and spatial orientation of trunk midline. *Brain*, 116: 383–396.

Karnath, H.-O., Ferber, S. and Himmelbach, M. (2001) Spatial awareness is a function of the temporal not the posterior parietal lobe. *Nature*, 411: 950–953.

Karnath, H.O., Himmelbach, M. and Rorden, C. (2002) The subcortical anatomy of human spatial neglect: putamen, caudate nucleus and pulvinar. *Brain*, 125: 350–360.

Katz, N., Hartman-Maeir, A., Ring, H. and Soroker, N. (1999) Functional disability and rehabilitation outcome in right hemisphere damaged patients with and without unilateral spatial neglect. *Arch. Phys. Med. Rehabil.*, 80: 379–384.

Kerkhoff, G. (2000) Multiple perceptual distortions and their modulation in patients with left visual neglect. *Neuropsychologia*, 38: 1073–1086.

Kerkhoff, G. (2001) Hemispatial neglect in man. *Prog. Neurobiol.*, 63: 1–27.

Kerkhoff, G., Kriz, G., Keller, I. and Marquardt, C. (1999) Head direction and optokinetic stimulation modulate space-based but not word-based neglect dyslexia. *Neural Plast., Suppl.*, 1: 155–156.

Kerkhoff, G., Marquardt, C., Jonas, M. and Ziegler, W. (2001) Repetitive optokinetische Stimulation (R-OKS) zur Behandlung des multimodalen Neglects. *Neurol. Rehabil.*, 7: 179–184.

Levine, D.N., Warach, J.D., Benowitz, L. and Calvanio, R. (1986) Left spatial neglect: effects of lesion size and premorbid brain atrophy on severity and recovery following right cerebral infarction. *Neurology*, 36: 362–366.

Lin, K.C., Cermak, S.A., Kinsbourne, M. and Trombly, C.A. (1996) Effects of left-sided movements on line bisection in unilateral neglect. *JINS*, 2: 404–411.

Mattingley, J.B., Bradshaw, J.L. and Bradshaw, J.A. (1994) Horizontal visual motion modulates focal attention in left unilateral spatial neglect. *J. Neurol. Neurosurg. Psychiatry*, 57: 1228–1235.

Pantano, P., Di Piero, V., Fieschi, C., Judica, A., Guariglia, C. and Pizzamiglio, L. (1992) Pattern of CBF in the rehabilitation of visuospatial neglect. *Int. J. Neurosci.*, 66: 153–161.

Paolucci, S., Traballesi, M., Giallloretti, L.E., Pratesi, L., Lubich, S., Antonucci, G. and Caltagirone, C. (1998) Changes in functional outcome in inpatient stroke rehabilitation resulting from new health policy regulations in Italy. *Eur. J. Neurol.*, 5: 17–22.

Pizzamiglio, L., Frasca, R., Guariglia, C., Incoccia, C. and Antonucci, G. (1990) Effect of optokinetic stimulation in patients with visual neglect. *Cortex*, 26: 535–540.

Pizzamiglio, L., Vallar, G. and Magnotti, L. (1996) Transcutaneous electrical-stimulation of the neck muscles and hemineglect rehabilitation. *Rest. Neurol. Neurosci.*, 10: 197–203.

Pizzamiglio, L., Perani, D., Cappa, S.F., Vallar, G., Paolucci, S., Grassi, F., Paulesu, E. and Fazio, F. (1998) Recovery of neglect after right hemispheric damage — H2(15)0 positron emission tomographic activation study. *Arch. Neurol.*, 55: 561–568.

Remy, P., Zilbovicius, M., Degos, J.-D., Bachoudlevi-Lévi, A.-C., Rancurel, G., Cesaro, P. and Samson, Y. (1999) Somatosensory cortical activations are suppressed in patients with tactile extinction. A PET study. *Neurology*, 52: 571–577.

Riddoch, M.J. and Humphreys, G.W. (1983) The effect of cueing on unilateral neglect. *Neuropsychologia*, 21: 589–599.

Robertson, I.H. (1999) Cognitive rehabilitation: attention and neglect. *Trends Cogn. Sci.*, 3: 385–393.

Rode, G., Charles, N., Perenin, M.-T., Vighetto, A., Trillet, M. and Aimard, G. (1992) Partial remission of hemiplegia and somatoparaphrenia through vestibular stimulation in a case of unilateral neglect. *Cortex*, 28: 203–208.

Rode, G., Tiliket, C., Charlopain, P. and Boisson, D. (1998) Postural asymmetry reduction by vestibular caloric stimulation in left hemiparetic patients. *Scand. J. Rehabil. Med.*, 30: 9–14.

Rode, G., Pisella, L., Rossetti, Y., Farnè, A. and Boisson, D., 2003. Bottom-up transfer of sensory-motor plasticity to recovery of spatial cognition: visuomotor adaptation and spatial neglect. In: C. Prablanc, D. Pélisson and Y. Rossetti (Eds.), *Neural Control of Space Coding and Action Production. Progress in Brain Research*, Vol. 142. Elsevier, Amsterdam, pp. 257–271 (this volume).

Rossetti, Y., Rode, G., Pisella, L., Farné, A., Boisson, D. and

Perenin, M.-T. (1998) Prism adaptation to a rightward optical deviation rehabilitates left hemispatial neglect. *Nature*, 98: 166–169.

Schindler, I. and Kerkhoff, G. (1997) Head and trunk orientation modulate visual neglect. *NeuroReport*, 8: 2681–2685.

Schindler, I., Kerkhoff, G., Karnath, H.-O., Keller, I. and Goldenberg, G. (2002) Neck muscle vibration induces lasting recovery in spatial neglect. *J. Neurol. Neurosurg. Psychiatry*, 73: 412–419.

Smania, N., Martini, M.C., Gambina, G., Tomelleri, G., Palamara, A., Natale, E. and Marzi, C.A. (1998) The spatial distribution of visual attention in hemineglect and extinction patients. *Brain*, 121: 1759–1770.

Stone, S.P., Wilson, B., Wroot, A., Halligan, P.W., Lange, L.S. and Marshall, J.C. (1991) The assessment of visuo-spatial neglect after acute stroke. *J. Neurol. Neurosurg. Psychiatry*, 54: 345–350.

Tiliket, C., Rode, G., Rossetti, Y., Pichon, J., Li, L. and Boisson, D. (2001) Prism adaptation to rightward optical deviation improves postural imbalance in left-hemiparetic patients. *Curr. Biol.*, 11: 1–5.

Vallar, G. (1993) The anatomical basis of spatial neglect in humans. In: I.H. Robertson and J. Marshall (Eds.), *Unilateral Neglect: Clinical and Experimental Studies*. Lawrence Erlbaum Associates, Hove, pp. 27–53.

Vallar, G., Guariglia, C. and Rusconi, M.L. (1997) Modulation of the neglect syndrome by sensory stimulation. In: P. Thier and H.-O. Karnath (Eds.), *Parietal Lobe Contributions to Orientation in 3D Space*. Springer, Berlin, pp. 555–578.

Vallar, G., Bottini, G. and Sterzi, R. (2003) Anosognosia for left-sided motor and sensory deficits, motor neglect and sensory hemiinattention: is there a relationship? In: C. Prablanc, D. Pélisson and Y. Rossetti (Eds.), *Neural Control of Space Coding and Action Production. Progress in Brain Research*, Vol. 142. Elsevier, Amsterdam, pp. 289–301 (this volume).

C. Prablanc, D. Pélisson and Y. Rossetti (Eds.)
Progress in Brain Research, Vol. 142
© 2003 Elsevier Science B.V. All rights reserved

CHAPTER 17

Bottom-up transfer of sensory-motor plasticity to recovery of spatial cognition: visuomotor adaptation and spatial neglect

Gilles Rode [1,2,3,*], Laure Pisella [1,3], Yves Rossetti [1,2,3], Alessandro Farnè [4] and Dominique Boisson [1,2,3]

[1] *Espace et Action, Institut National de la Santé et de la Recherche Médicale, Unité 534, 16 avenue Lépine, Case 13, 69676 Bron, France*
[2] *Service de Rééducation Neurologique, Hôpital Henry Gabrielle, Hospices Civils de Lyon et Université Claude Bernard, Lyon, France*
[3] *Institut Fédératif des Neurosciences de Lyon, Lyon, France*
[4] *Dipartimento di Psicologia, Università di Bologna, Viale Berti Pichat 5, 40127 Bologna, Italy*

Abstract: A large proportion of right-hemisphere stroke patients show hemispatial neglect, a neurological deficit of perception, attention, representation, and/or performing actions within their left-sided space, inducing many functional debilitating effects on everyday life, and responsible for poor functional recovery and ability to benefit from treatment. This spatial cognition disorder affects the orientation of behavior with a shift of proprioceptive representations toward the lesion side. This shift is similar to that produced by psychophysical manipulations as a wedge-prism exposure in normal healthy subjects. In both subjects, one major compensatory effect of short-term prism adaptation is a shift of proprioceptive representations, demonstrated by a shift in manual straight-ahead pointing in the dark, in a direction opposite to the visual shift. In neglect patients, prism adaptation involves the shift of proprioceptive representations to the left with a reduction of rightward bias observed in neglect patients in visuo-manual tasks as line-bisection, line-cancellation or copy drawing. Improvement of neglect is also observed in no visuo-manual tasks as mental imagery, auditory extinction or posture. This generalization of prism adaptation effects at different neglect level symptoms suggests that the process of prism adaptation may activate brain functions related to multisensory integration and higher spatial representations. Moreover the positive effects found for both sensorimotor and more cognitive spatial functions lasted for at least two or more hours after prism removal. Unlike reduction of neglect through sensory stimulations, the long-lasting improvement of neglect after prism adaptation suggests the activation of short-term plasticity of brain functions related to coordinate transformations and space representations. Lastly, the duration of these effects could be useful in rehabilitation programs, as suggested by the effects of prism adaptation on disabling neglect symptoms as wheelchair driving, posture or writing.

Neglect, an oriented-space-behavior disorder

Hemispatial neglect is defined as the patient's failure to report, respond to, or orient toward novel and/or meaningful stimuli presented to the side opposite to the brain lesion (Heilman et al., 1985). Chronic neglect is most frequently consecutive to the damage of the right brain hemisphere. For example, neglect patients can forget to read the left part of a journal or a book, omit to eat the left half of a plate, forget to shave the left hemiface, or hit obstacles on the left. Associated with contralesional hemiplegia, hemianesthesia and hemianopia, chronic neglect worsens the severity of these motor-

* Correspondence to: G. Rode, Service de Rééducation Neurologique, Hôpital Henry Gabrielle, Hospices Civils de Lyon and Université Claude Bernard, route de Vourles, BP 57, F-69565 St Genis-laval, France. Tel.: +33-478-86-50-23; Fax: +33-478-86-50-30; E-mail: gilles.rode@chu-lyon.fr

or sensory-associated deficits inducing many functionally debilitating effects on everyday life, and is responsible for poor functional recovery and ability to benefit from treatment (Denes et al., 1982; Fullerton et al., 1986; Halligan et al., 1989; see also Vallar et al., 2003, this volume) (Fig. 1).

For these reasons, many attempts have been made in the last 20 years to rehabilitate neglect. Different approaches have been proposed relying mainly on passive physiological stimulations or active training (see review in Rossetti and Rode, 2002). The main goal of these methods is to favor the re-orientation of the motor behavior toward the neglected side and the first difficulty is to obtain a generalization of the effects at a functional level.

Hemispatial neglect is a disorder of spatial orientation in which the behavior is biased to the side of the lesion. This bias may be demonstrated by the clinical observation of patients or by simple tests such as a line bisection task. It may also be illustrated in patients by the shift of straight-ahead pointing in the dark, and has been even interpreted as an impairment of the transformation of sensory input into motor output (Jeannerod and Biguer, 1987). This hypothesis, also called 'egocentric reference', is compatible with current knowledge about the crucial role of the parietal cortex in coordinate transformation (reviews: Jeannerod and Rossetti, 1993; Andersen, 1995; Milner and Goodale, 1995; Pisella and Rossetti, 2000; Rossetti and Pisella, 2002). The prediction made by Jeannerod and Biguer (1987) was that unilateral lesions "produce an illusory 'rotation' of the egocentric reference, somewhat as if the subject felt being constantly rotated toward the lesion side." This idea has been recently revisited by Karnath (1997) and Vallar et al. (1997), who proposed that the coordinate transformation system was biased by an internal constant error with a translation or a rotation of the egocentric spatial frame. It has also been challenged by several recent observations (Farnè et al., 1998; Bartolomeo and Chokron, 1999; Pisella et al., 2002).

Shift of proprioceptive representations after prism adaptation

It is interesting that a similar shift in manual straight-ahead pointing may be produced by psychophysical manipulations in normal healthy subjects (Jeannerod and Rossetti, 1993). For example, exposure to an optical alteration of the visual field is known to produce an initial disorganization of visuo-motor behavior, which can be corrected through visuo-motor adaptation. Such adaptation has been widely used to demonstrate the plasticity of coordinate transformations involved in multisensory and sensorimotor integration. One major compensatory effect of short-term wedge-prism exposure is a shift of proprioceptive representations, which can be demonstrated by a shift in manual straight-ahead pointing in the dark, in a direction opposite to the visual shift produced by the prisms. This shift appears similar to that showed by neglect patients and one may therefore wonder whether the egocentric reference of patients with spatial neglect could be altered by prism adaptation, and whether a hypothetical shift can be accompanied by an improvement of other neglect symptoms.

Reduction of egocentric reference shift after prism adaptation in neglect

The adaptability of neglect patients to a right lateral shift of visual field (induced by a simple target-pointing task with base-left wedge prisms) was thus evaluated (for details see Rossetti et al., 1998a,b) with the measure of manual body-midline demonstration. Patients produced 10 straight-ahead pointing trials before and after a short period of adaptation. A group of five healthy control subjects was also tested in the same conditions. The amount of visual displacement was set at 10 degrees, chosen as being the best compromise between a significant shift, required to generate adaptation, and visual comfort

---

Fig. 1. Hemispatial neglect is a disorder of spatial cognition. (a) Drawing from memory, (b) drawing by copy of a scene with five items (Gainotti et al., 1972) showing a space- and object-centered neglect, and (c) apple-tart performed by right-damaged patients with neglect. These examples show a neglect of the object side located to the contralesional side as well as constructive modifications consecutive to alteration of spatial cognition. They also revealed the functional consequence of hemispatial neglect in daily life.

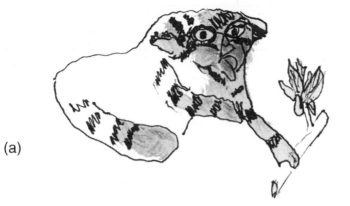

(a)

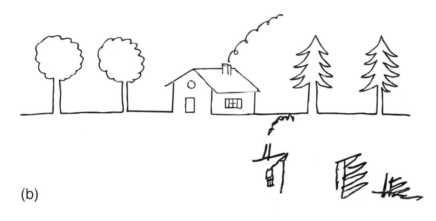

(b)

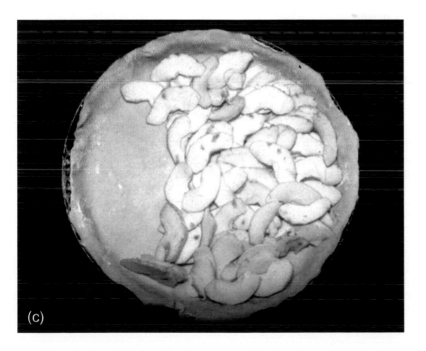

(c)

(stronger displacement being responsible for curvature distortion and color fringes). The procedure used to generate the adaptation was simply to require the patients to perform 60 pointing movements to visual targets presented in front of them. Attention was paid to keeping the head straight throughout the testing and the adaptation procedure, and to prevent any view of the hand at its starting position. Patients were then always tested without the prismatic goggles.

As in several previous studies, the patient's mean straight-ahead was initially shifted to the right. Following the adaptation, both patients and controls demonstrated relative straight-ahead shifts to the left. These results demonstrated that neglect patients can easily adapt to a lateral shift of the visual field to the right, and that prism adaptation, acting against the rightward bias of straight-ahead demonstration allows these patients to show a close-to-normal post-test performance. Moreover the results showed also that the amount of the prism after-effect was about twice that of normals (Fig. 2a).

Recent studies have shown that this and other prism adaptation after-effects can be sustained over several days in patients (Farnè et al., 2002; Frassinetti et al., 2002; Pisella et al., 2002) (Fig. 2b).

Improvement of neglect symptoms after prism adaptation

The main question was whether the straight-ahead shift to the left produced by prism adaptation may be associated to a reduction of rightward bias observed in neglect patients in visuo-manual tasks.

Line bisection (Schenckenberg et al., 1980), copy drawing (Gainotti et al., 1972), line cancellation (Albert, 1973), daisy drawing, and text reading were compared in two groups of five patients who were exposed to a similar pointing procedure. The test group wore prismatic goggles while the control group wore neutral goggles. Patients were tested prior to the pointing procedure, immediately upon goggle removal and again 2 h after. A multiple analysis of variance showed that the prism group was significantly improved but not the control group and, to our surprise, that the improvement was sustained for at least the 2-h follow-up period (Fig. 3a). On average all tests exhibited better values after adaptation. Interestingly, aspects of object-based neglect and space-based neglect were equally improved by the adaptation procedure (Rossetti et al., 1998a) (Fig. 3b).

It would seem logical that the effects of prism adaptation should be restricted to, or best for, visuo-motor tasks, because they have more common features with the visuo-manual adaptation procedure. In the original study, we observed that the best improvement was observed for the Schenckenberg bisection test (6/6 patients markedly improved), whereas the weakest improvement was obtained for text reading (2/6 patients markedly improved). Therefore other tests of neglect were investigated (Table 1).

Rode et al. (1998, 2001a) explored the effect of prism adaptation on visual imagery and found a clear-cut improvement in two patients who could initially not evoke cities on the western half of an internally generated map of France (Fig. 4a). This result strongly suggested that the after-effects of vi-

---

Fig. 2. Shift of straight-ahead pointing after prism adaptation. (a) Comparison of the amplitude of the immediate after-effects in a group of neglect patients and a control group. Blindfolded subjects were required to point straight ahead while their head was kept aligned with the body's sagittal axis. Ten pointing trials were run in the pre-test (without goggles) and in the post-test (immediately upon the 10° prism (white arrow) removal). As expected, the midline demonstrations made by the neglect group were initially shifted to the right, whereas control subjects pointed to their actual straight-ahead. Patients were more affected by the adaptation than controls (black arrows), and the magnitude of this effect was less variable in patients (arrow whiskers). (from Rossetti et al., 1998a). (b) Longitudinal study of the evolution of the straight-ahead after prism adaptation in two neglect patients: temporal evolution of the performance of two neglect patients (SA and PE) in a straight-ahead pointing task. Blindfolded subjects were required to point straight ahead while their head was kept aligned with the body's sagittal axis. Ten pointing trials were run in the pre-test (without goggles) and in the post-test (immediately upon the 10° prism removal) and late-tests (Day 2–Day 4). Positive values correspond to right deviations, and negative ones to left deviations. The shadowed area represents the pretesting period gathering the two sessions realized by the patients before a single prism adaptation procedure. The x-axis zero corresponds to the experimental testing performed just after adaptation (upon prism removal). In the late-tests, the performance of patient PE seemed to be stabilized around the normal value. By contrast, patient SA did not show a long-term improvement with respect to the demonstration performed prior to prism adaptation. (From Pisella et al., 2002.)

suo-manual adaptation can no longer be considered to be restricted to visual and motor parameters (Rossetti et al., 1999a).

Farnè et al. (2002) compared visuo-motor tasks (including line and bell cancellation tests, and two sub-tests taken from the Behavioral Inattention Test (B.I.T) battery, namely letter cancellation and line bi-section) with visuo-verbal tasks (the visual scanning test, also taken from the B.I.T. (Wilson et al., 1987), requiring a verbal description of the objects depicted on a colored picture; an object-naming task with 30 Snodgrass pictures of familiar objects intermingled with geometric shapes as distracters; word and non-word reading), in six patients. They observed that

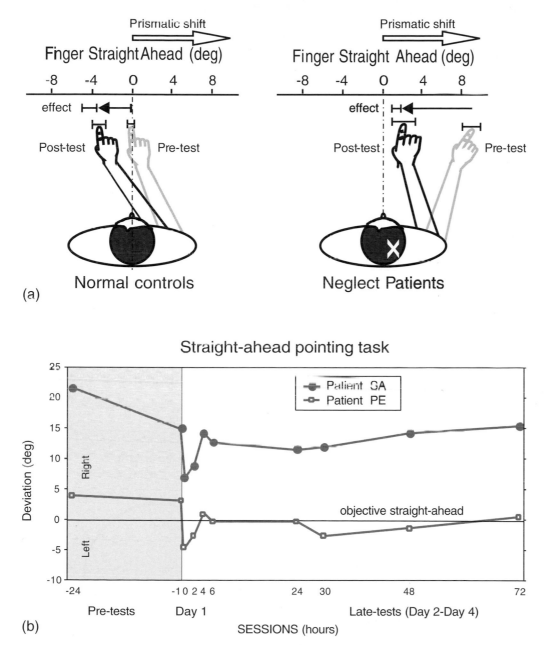

(a)

Finger Straight Ahead (deg)

Normal controls — Neglect Patients

(b)

Straight-ahead pointing task

TABLE 1

Different symptoms of hemispatial neglect alleviated by prism adaptation and duration of improvement

Symptoms of neglect	Duration of improvement
Visuo-spatial neglect [a,b,c,d,f,g,h,j,l,n]	≥ 2 h
Object-centered neglect [a]	≥ 2 h
Space-centered neglect [a,b,c,d,f,g,h,j]	≥ 2 h
Personal neglect [a]	≥ 2 h
Representational neglect [b,j]	immediate
Subjective straight-ahead shift [a,b,c,d,f,g,k]	96 h
Motor reaction time [e]	immediate
Left auditory extinction [k]	immediate
Haptic neglect [h,l]	≥ 2 h
Ocular scanning [m]	≥ 2 h
Functional disabilities	
Wheelchair driving [c]	≥ 96 h
Postural instability [i]	immediate
Reading [a,g,h,n]	≥ 2 h
Writing (unpublished results)	≥ 2 h

[a] Rossetti et al., 1998a,b.
[b] Rode et al., 1998.
[c] Jacquin et al., 1998.
[d] Luauté et al., 2000.
[e] Rode et al., 2000.
[f] Pisella et al., 2002.
[g] Farnè et al., 2002.
[h] McIntosh et al., 2002.
[i] Tilikete et al., 2001.
[j] Rode et al., 2001a,b.
[k] Courtois-Jacquin et al., 2001.
[l] Toutounji et al., 2001.
[m] Dijkerman et al., 2002.
[n] Frassinetti et al., 2002.

the two groups of tasks followed a strictly parallel improvement, which lasted for at least 24 h.

The fact that other sensory modalities can be improved [haptic circle centering (McIntosh et al.,

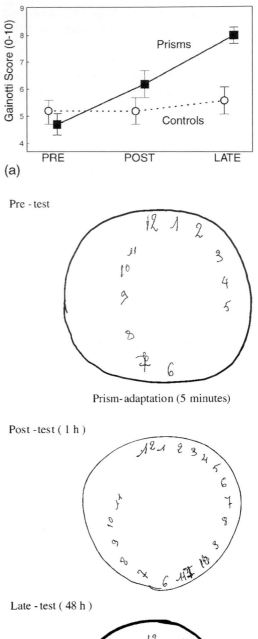

Pre-test

Prism-adaptation (5 minutes)

Post-test (1 h)

Late-test (48 h)

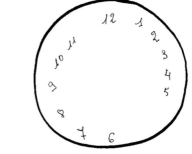

(b)

Fig. 3. Effect of prism adaptation on hemispatial neglect assessed by visuo-motor tasks. (a) Copying test (Gainotti et al., 1972) performed by a patient group exposed to prism adaptation and a control group. The figure shows the mean number of items drawn symmetrically (± s.e.m.) in the two groups. The score is improved in the 'prisms' group and the performance increases between the post-test and the late-test. (Derived from Rossetti et al., 1998a.) (b) Drawing from memory. Effect of prism adaptation on free drawing of object (clockwise) in a neglect patient (M.G.) prior to prism exposure (pre-test) and after a delay of about 1 h (post-test) and 48 h (late-test).

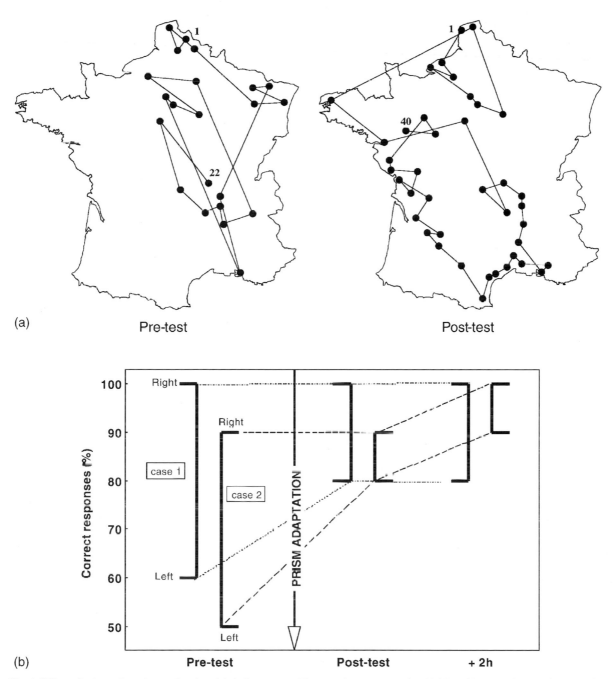

Fig. 4. Effect of prism adaptation on hemispatial neglect assessed by non-visuo-motor tasks. (a) Mental imagery. Maps of France plotted from the mental evocation of the patient prior to a prism exposure (pre-test) and immediately after removing the goggles (post-test). The filled circles indicate the geographical loci of the different responses and the bold number indicates the total number of responses. (From Rode et al., 2001a,b.) (b) Auditory extinction. Improvement of left auditory extinction assessed by dichotic listening test after prism adaptation in two neglect patients. The difference of correct responses percentage between the right and the left ear is dramatically reduced after the prism adaptation period, suggesting that a simple visuo-manual adaptation task may influence the orientation of attention in other sensory modalities. (From Courtois-Jacquin et al., 2001.)

2002), dichotic listening (Courtois-Jacquin et al., 2001), haptic object recognition (Toutounji et al., 2001)] and that several non-manual tasks [postural control (Tilikete et al., 2001), wheelchair driving (Jacquin et al., 1998; Rossetti et al., 1999b), imagery (Rode et al., 1998, 2001b), verbal reports in a Temporal Order Judgement task (Pisella and Mattingley, 2003)] were also improved suggests that the effects of prism adaptation are not restricted to visuo-manual parameters as they are known to be in normal subjects. These results strongly suggest that adaptation to wedge prisms somehow affects the very core of hemispatial neglect (see also Michel et al., 2003).

Possible explanations of prism adaptation action on neglect

If prism adaptation can improve numerous aspects of neglect, then the possible mechanisms of this improvement are worth investigating because they could help us develop a comprehensive description of neglect physio-pathology and hence facilitate the development of more refined methods of rehabilitation. One obvious candidate would be the effect of prisms on the patient's egocentric reference, as it provided the rationale for initiating this series of experiments. However, Pisella et al. (2002) showed that there was no significant correlation between the effect of prisms on manual straight-ahead pointing and on line bisection performance. Furthermore they reported that these two parameters could be affected in contrasting ways by prism adaptation, such that a dynamic double dissociation could be observed in the long-term effects. This result not only confirmed the dissociability between the egocentric reference frame and other aspects of neglect (Farnè et al., 1998; Bartolomeo and Chokron, 1999), but they also excluded a possible direct causal role of the sensory-motor after-effects of prisms on the general spatial deficit exhibited by the patients.

Another explanation for the effects of adaptation on the patients' deficits would be the existence of possible cross-talk or synergy between the short-term plasticity mechanisms involved in the adaptation, and the longer-term plasticity mechanisms involved in recovery. This hypothesis was explored by Luauté et al. (2000) who compared the effects of left- versus right-deviating prisms. Because the

sensory-motor after-effects produced by these two types of wedge prisms are symmetrical in normals, one might predict that they should generate a similar amount of plasticity and thus affect hemispatial neglect in the same way. However, adaptation to left-sided visual displacement did not improve a group of five patients. As for the question of specificity, this result also demonstrated that non-lateralized parameters such as arousal could not account for the effect of adaptation (Rossetti and Rode, 2002). Moreover, the lack of effect on spatial cognition in conditions of pointing with neutral goggles (Rossetti et al., 1998a) or passive exposure to prisms (Colent et al., 2000) reinforced the idea of a specific effect of prism adaptation on neglect.

Prism adaptation in normal subjects produces visual after-effects of similar amplitudes, regardless of the left or the right direction of the prismatic shift (e.g. Welsch, 1986; Redding and Wallace, 1992). Therefore, the asymmetrical after-effects observed on line bisection tasks cannot simply be explained away as the product of symmetrical visual after-effects. Moreover, visual after-effects are known to occur in the same direction as the prismatic deviation (e.g. Welsch, 1986; Redding and Wallace, 1992), whereas the perceptive and cognitive after-effects are observed in the opposite direction (rightward prisms allow neglect patients to explore further to the left space).

Lastly, in one left neglect patient, an improvement of leftward ocular scanning was evidenced following prism adaptation without correlated reduction of the size underestimation of the left stimulus (Dijkerman et al., 2002). These preliminary results suggest that the effects of prism adaptation on spatial cognition may not be mediated by a modification of ocular scanning but rather by higher-level effects.

The last candidate mechanism is obviously associated with the attentional theory of neglect. Preliminary results from Pisella et al. (unpublished data) suggested that the strong left–right attentional gradient observed in neglect patients could be reduced following prism adaptation. Another pure attentional deficit as sensory extinction could also be improved after prism adaptation. In six right-brain damaged patients with left visuo-spatial neglect and auditory extinction, prism adaptation involved an improvement of both visuo-spatial deficit and auditory extinction

TABLE 2

Effect of prism adaptation on intentional disturbance of two neglect patients (values in ms)

Cases	LRT		RRT	
	before	after	before	after
HAC	584	381	523	438
HAY	629	481	521	587

Two left neglect patients (cases HAC and HAY) were asked to reach and grasp an object (tennis ball) placed on their sagittal axis and then throw it in a left or a right basket; they were slower to initiate their movement to the left side as compared to the right. These results suggest that anticipation of the ultimate goal of an action led to a retrograde transfer of neglect onto action elements which have no left-right component by themselves. No comparable effect was found in two left brain-damaged patients and two control subjects. Abbreviations: LRT, left reaction time; RRT, right reaction time.

(Fig. 4b). These results suggest thus that the calibration of sensory-motor transformations induced by prism adaptation, which directly affects visual space representation and action, may also alter the orientation of attention in other sensory modalities (Courtois-Jacquin et al., 2001).

Moreover intentional disturbance showed by neglect patients may be also improved after prism

adaptation. These disturbances may be illustrated by the fact that preparation of a movement sequence ending to the left is longer than a movement sequence ending to the right in neglect patients (Rode et al., 2000). In two neglect patients we tested the effect of a prism adaptation period on this parameter and showed that the initial increase in reaction time for movements ending to the left was reversed after the adaptation (Table 2), suggesting that prism adaptation can produce an effect on higher-level control of action which are linked to intention to act to the right or to the left (Rossetti and Pisella, 2002).

However, further investigations are required to confirm whether prism adaptation mechanisms alter the brain mechanisms for the spatial distribution of attention or intention, as there is no suggestion of such a link in the classical prism adaptation literature.

Prism adaptation and neural structures involved

An intriguing question is to know whether prism adaptation favors the spontaneous recovery of neglect or facilitates the occurrence of selective compensation mechanisms. This question refers either to the cerebral plasticity naturally involved after the

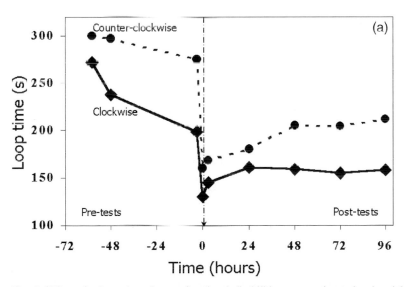

Fig. 5. Effect of prism adaptation on functional disabilities consecutive to hemispatial neglect. (a) Wheelchair driving. A patient was repeatedly tested prior to and following a short prism adaptation session for his ability to make one tour of the medical unit (either clockwise or anti-clockwise). An abrupt improvement was produced by prism adaptation and partly sustained over the 96 h of the follow-up. (From Courtois-Jacquin et al., 1999.)

Pre-test

Prism-adaption (5 minutes)
Post-test (1 h)

Late-test (48 h)

(b)

Fig. 5 (continued). (b) Writing. Writing under dictation and free drawing from memory (daisy) prior to prism exposure (pre-test), and after a delay of about 1 h (post-test) and 48 h (late-test) in a neglect patient (R.R.O.) with neglect dysgraphia. Before adaptation, writing showed a neglect of the left part of the sheet, a rightward shift of beginning of line and oblique slope of lines. These abnormalities are reduced after prism adaptation. The patient used the entirety of sheet space, the lines are horizontal and the legibility of text was improved.

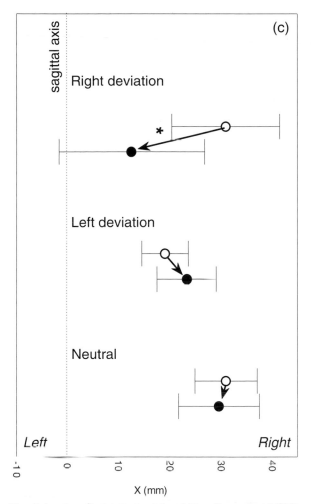

Fig. 5 (continued). (c) Postural instability. Comparison of effects of prism adaptation period shifting the visual field to the right or the left and neutral prisms in three groups of five right-brain-damaged patients on postural imbalance assessed by a statokinesimetric platform. The figure indicates that only an adaptation to rightward-shifting prisms reduces significantly the displacement of the center of pressure. (From Tilikete et al., 2001.)

cerebral damage or to the cerebral plasticity specifically activated by the visuo-motor adaptation task. In normal subjects, neural structures considered to be involved in prism adaptation have long been restricted to the cerebellar region (Jeannerod and Rossetti, 1993), as shown by the inability of adaptation of patients with focal olivocerebellar lesion (Weiner et al., 1983; Martin et al., 1996). The posterior parietal cortex contralateral to the acting hand might

be activated during adaptation to a prism-induced shift of the visual field (Clower et al., 1996). The reciprocal connections between the deep cerebellar structures and the posterior parietal cortex provide an anatomical substrate that may support the cerebellar participation also in high-order processing (Schmahmann, 1998; Rossetti et al., 2000). Lastly, one may also suppose that the motor component of the visuo-motor adaptation task (pointing movements of the ipsilesional hand) may also favor the implication of the ipsi- and contralateral frontal areas in recovery of neglect following prism exposure. Imagery studies show that these areas are involved in natural recovery of neglect. The reciprocal connections between the cerebellum support of motor control and adaptation and the frontal lobe support of action and intention may be activated following prism adaptation (Rode et al., 2001b).

Duration of improvement

One of the side effects of questions about basic mechanisms is that they should help us to answer the intriguing question of why the effects of prism adaptation last for so long in the patients, whereas the after-effects observed in normals in the same conditions resolve within a few minutes (see Table 1).

The main interest of prism adaptation is that the effects produced by a single 5-min session of adaptation last for much longer than any other method. Two group studies showed fully sustained effects after at least 2 h (Rossetti et al., 1998a,b), and 1 day (Farnè et al., 2002), respectively. Case studies reported even more prolonged improvements, lasting for about 4 days (Jacquin et al., 1998; Pisella et al., 2002). Although a recent group study found no sustained improvement of neglect one week after the adaptation session (Farnè et al., 2002), it is possible that some patients are improved for a longer period than others (McIntosh et al., 2002). But the best prospect for rehabilitation purposes is to repeat adaptation sessions. Recently a treatment with prismatic lenses in twice-daily sessions over a period of 2 weeks was applied in a group of seven neglect patients compared with a control group. The results showed an improvement in the experimental patient's performance after prism adaptation, which was maintained during a 5-week period after treat-

284

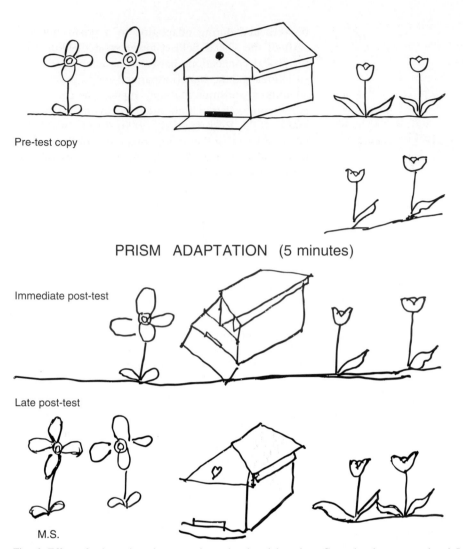

Pre-test copy

PRISM ADAPTATION (5 minutes)

Immediate post-test

Late post-test

M.S.

Fig. 6. Effect of prism adaptation on resistant hemispatial neglect. Copy drawing was explored 5 years after the stroke in a case of persistent hemispatial neglect. The patient was a 72-year-old, right-handed female who suffered from a severe left hemiplegia with left hemi-anesthesia, hemianopia and neglect following a large hematoma of the right cerebral hemisphere. The patient had benefited from specific active training for neglect and caloric vestibular stimulation during the first year post-stroke. Before prism exposure (pre-test), she copied only the most rightward parts of the drawing, showing an associated object-centered neglect. In the immediate post-test, two items were added to the patient's drawing; in the late-test (after 2 h), all items are drawn, the object-centered neglect was reduced (limited to the bee-hive) and the constructive apraxia had also improved.

ment. This long-term improvement of neglect symptoms was found in standard as well as in behavioral tests and in all spatial domains (Frassinetti et al., 2002). We have investigated the effects of a daily session of adaptation and found no further improvement in the days following the initial exposure to prisms. Controlled clinical trial has to be initiated with a longer between-sessions period. In addition,

the functional outcome for the patients will need to be investigated carefully. So far only a few measures have been provided (e.g. wheelchair driving, writing or postural control) (Fig. 5a–c).

Another of the crucial questions raised by the observation of a strong and sustained improvement of hemispatial neglect by a single short adaptation session is whether this plastic effect is restricted to the acute phase of the deficit. In our original study patients were tested between 3 weeks and 14 months post-stroke (Rossetti et al., 1998a). We have now collected data on a group of patients who were exposed to the adaptation procedure between 5 and 12 years post-stroke and surprisingly found the same amount of improvement. Fig. 6 shows the example of a patient who benefited from prism adaptation 5 years after her stroke.

Neglect-like syndrome after prism adaptation in healthy subjects

One of the most striking aspects of prism exposure in neglect patients is that, in strong contrast to healthy subjects, they exhibit a reduced awareness of the optical effects of the prisms. Most patients performed accurate pointing movements with the prisms on, which implies that their initially misdirected pointing trajectories are corrected during the course of the movement. Nevertheless they do not report that the goggles are responsible for any visual shift, even when specifically questioned. In a way, they show a kind of 'hypernosognosia', as if they had been so used to missing things on the left side that they over-attribute the prism-induced errors to themselves. This hypothesis would also explain why they develop more adaptation than healthy individuals in identical prism exposure conditions.

Conclusion

Taken as a whole, investigations of the effects of prism adaptation on hemispatial neglect have been very frustrating in terms of the difficulty in providing plausible theoretical accounts for the strong positive effects produced. These effects can by no means be compared with the classical knowledge about prism adaptation in healthy individuals, for whom both the duration and the generalization of the adaptation after-effects are extremely restricted. However, two interesting perspectives have emerged from these studies. The theoretical perspective is that it seems possible to emulate hemispatial neglect in healthy individuals (Colent et al., 2000; Michel et al., 2002; N. Berberovic and J.B. Mattingley, pers. commun., 2002). The practical perspective is that the long duration of the improvement produced by prism adaptation should give rise to clinical studies proposing routine protocols for the rehabilitation of patients.

Acknowledgements

This work was supported by INSERM (PROGRES) and ACI Plasticité. The authors wish to thank Jean-Louis Borach for his technical assistance and M. Rossetti for his art of bees.

References

Albert, M.L. (1973) A simple test for visual neglect. *Neurology*, 23: 658–664.

Andersen, R.A. (1995) Encoding of intention and spatial location in the posterior parietal cortex. *Cereb. Cortex*, 5: 457–469.

Bartolomeo, P. and Chokron, S. (1999) Egocentric frame of reference: its role in spatial bias after right hemisphere lesions. *Neuropsychologia*, 37: 881–894.

Berberovic, N. and Mattingley, J.B. (2003) Effects of prismatic adaptation on judgements of spatial extent in peripersonal and extrapersonal space. *Neuropsychologia*, in press.

Clower, D.M., Hoffman, J.M., Votaw, J.R., Fabert, T.L., Woods, R. and Alexander, G.E. (1996) Role of posterior parietal cortex in the recalibration of visually guided reaching. *Nature*, 383: 618–621.

Colent, C., Pisella, L., Bernieri, C., Rode, G. and Rossetti, Y. (2000) Cognitive bias induced by visuo-motor adaptation to prisms: a simulation of unilateral neglect in normal individuals? *Neuroreport*, 11: 1–4.

Courtois-Jacquin, S., Rossetti, Y., Rode, G., Fischer, C., Michel, C., Allard, C. and Boisson, D. (2001) Effect of prism adaptation on auditory extinction: an attentional effect? *International Symposium on Neural Control of Space Coding and Action Production*. Lyon, March 22–24, 2001.

Denes, G., Semenza, C., Stoppa, E. and Lis, A. (1982) Unilateral spatial neglect and recovery from hemiplegia. A follow-up study. *Brain*, 105: 543–552.

Dijkerman, H.C., McIntosh, R.D., Milner, A.D., Rossetti, Y., Tilikete, C. and Roberts, R.C. (2002) The effects of prism adaptation on perceptual size distortion and ocular scanning in spatial neglect. Submitted.

Farné, A., Ponti, F. and Ladavas, E. (1998) In search for biased egocentric reference frames in neglect. *Neuropsychologia*, 36: 611–623.

Farné, A., Rossetti, Y., Toniolo, S. and Làdavas, E. (2002) Ameliorating neglect with prism adaptation: visuo-manual vs. visuo-verbal measures. *Neuropsychologia*, 40: 718–729.

Frassinetti, F., Angeli, V., Meneghello, F., Avanzi, S. and Ladavas, E. (2002) Long-lasting amelioration of visuospatial neglect by prism adaptation. *Brain*, 125: 608–625.

Fullerton, K.J., McSherry, D. and Stout, R.W. (1986) Albert's test: a neglected test of perceptual neglect. *Lancet*, 327: 430–432.

286

Gainotti, G., Messerli, P. and Tissot, R. (1972) Qualitative analysis of unilateral spatial neglect in relation to laterality of cerebral lesions. *J. Neurol. Neurosurg. Psychiatry*, 35: 545–550.

Halligan, P.W., Marshall, J.C. and Wade, D.T. (1989) Visuospatial neglect: underlying factors and test sensitivity. *Lancet*, 2: 908–911.

Heilman, K.M., Watson, R.T. and Valenstein, E. (1985) Neglect and related disorders. In: K.M. Heilman and E. Valenstein (Eds.), *Clinical Neuropsychology*. Oxford University Press, New York, NY, pp. 243–293.

Jacquin, S., Luauté, J., Li, L., Rode, G., Rossetti, Y. and Boisson, D. (1998) Amélioration de la conduite en fauteuil roulant après adaptation prismatique chez le patient héminégligent. *Ann. Réadaptation Méd. Phys.*, 41: 320–321.

Jeannerod, M. and Biguer, B. (1987) The directional coding of reaching movements. A visuo-motor conception of spatial neglect. In: M. Jeannerod (Ed.), *Neurophysiological and Neuropsychological Aspects of Spatial Neglect*. North-Holland, Amsterdam, pp. 87–113.

Jeannerod, M. and Rossetti, Y. (1993) Visuomotor coordination as a dissociable function: experimental and clinical evidence. In: C. Kennard (Ed.), *Visual Perceptual Defects. Baillère's Clinical Neurology, International Practise and Research*. Ballière Tindall, London, pp. 439–460.

Karnath, H.O. (1997) Spatial orientation and the representation of space with parietal lobe lesions. *Philos. Trans. R. Soc. Lond.*, 352: 1411–1419.

Luauté, J., Rode, G., Jacquin-Courtois, S., Pisella, L., Boisson, D. and Rossetti, Y. (2000) Improvement of left spatial neglect after prismatic adaptation: lateralized warning signal or cerebral plasticity? *European Conference on Cognitive and Neural Bases of Spatial Neglect*. Como, 14–17 Sept. 2000.

Martin, T.A., Keating, J.G., Goodkin, H.P., Bastian, A.J. and Thatch, W.T. (1996) Throwing while looking through prisms, I. Focal olivocerebellar lesions impair adaptation. *Brain*, 119: 1183–1198.

McIntosh, R.M., Rossetti, Y. and Milner, A.D. (2002) Prism adaptation improves chronic visual and haptic neglect. *Cortex*.

Michel, C., Pisella, L., Halligan, P., Luauté, J., Rode, G., Boisson, D. and Rossetti, Y. (2003) Simulating unilateral neglect using prism adaptation: implications for theory. *Neuropsychologia*, 41: 25–39.

Milner, A.D. and Goodale, M.A. (1995) *The Visual Brain in Action, Oxford Psychology Series 27*. Oxford University Press, New York, NY, 248 pp.

Pisella, L. and Mattingley, J. (2003) Prism adaptation improves temporal order judgement in neglect patients. In preparation.

Pisella, L. and Rossetti, Y. (2000) Interaction between conscious identification and non-conscious sensori-motor processing: temporal constraints. In: Y. Rossetti and A. Revonsuo (Eds.), *Beyond Dissociation: Interaction Between Dissociated Implicit and Explicit Processing*. Benjamins, Amsterdam, pp. 129–151.

Pisella, L., Rode, G., Farnè, A., Boisson, D. and Rossetti, Y. (2002) Dissociated long lasting improvements of straight-ahead pointing and line bisection tasks in two hemineglect patients. *Neuropsychologia*, 40: 327–334.

Redding, G. and Wallace, B. (1992) Effects of pointing rate and availability of visual feedback on visual and proprioceptive components of prism adaptation. *J. Motor Behav.*, 24: 226–237.

Rode, G., Rossetti, Y., Li, L. and Boisson, D. (1998) The effect of prism adaptation on neglect for visual imagery. *Behav. Neurol.*, 11: 251–258.

Rode, G., Rossetti, Y., Farnè, A., Boisson, D. and Bisiach, E. (2000) The motor control of a movement sequence ending to the left is altered in unilateral neglect. *European Conference on Cognitive and Neural Bases of Spatial Neglect*. Como, 14–17 Sept. 2000.

Rode, G., Rossetti, Y. and Boisson, D. (2001a) Prism adaptation improves representational neglect. *Neuropsychologia*, 39: 1250–1254.

Rode, G., Rossetti, Y., Badan, M. and Boisson, D. (2001b) Rôle de l'action dans la rééducation du syndrome d'héminégligence (Role of action in the rehabilitation of hemineglect syndromes). *Rev. Neurol. (Paris)*, 157: 497–505.

Rossetti, Y. and Pisella, L. (2002) Several 'vision for action' systems: a guide to dissociating and integrating dorsal and ventral functions. In: W. Prinz and B. Hommel (Eds.), *Attention and Performance XIX; Common Mechanisms in Perception and Action*. Oxford University Press, New York, NY, pp. 62–119.

Rossetti, Y. and Rode, G. (2002) Reducing spatial neglect by visual and other sensory manipulations: non-cognitive (physiological) routes to the rehabilitation of a cognitive disorder. In: H.-O. Karnath, A.D. Milner and G. Vallar (Eds.), *The Cognitive and Neural Bases of Spatial Neglect*. Oxford University Press, New York, NY, pp. 375–396.

Rossetti, Y., Rode, G., Pisella, L., Farnè, A., Li, L. and Boisson, D. (1998a) Prism adaptation to a rightward optical deviation rehabilitates left hemispatial neglect. *Nature*, 395: 166–169.

Rossetti, Y., Rode, G., Cheikh-Rouhou, M., Farnè, A., Pisella, L., Li, L. and Boisson, D. (1998b). Amélioration durable des symptômes de la négligence par adaptation prismatique: quels arguments pour les théories référentielle, attentionnelle et intégrationnelle? In: D. Perennou, V. Brun and J. Pélissier (Eds.), *Les Syndromes de Négligence Spatiale*. Masson, Paris, pp. 299–310.

Rossetti, Y., Rode, G., Pisella, L., Farne, A., Li, L. and Boisson, D. (1999a) Sensorimotor plasticity and cognition: prism adaptation can affect various levels of space representation. In: M. Grealy and J.A. Thomson (Eds.), *Studies in Perception and Action*. Lawrence Erlbaum Associates, Mahwah, pp. 265–269.

Rossetti, Y., Rode, G. and Boisson, D. (1999b) Sensori-motor plasticity and the rehabilitation of hemispatial neglect (Plasticité sensori-motrice et récupération fonctionnelle: les effets thérapeutiques de l'adaptation prismatique sur la négligence spatiale unilatérale). *Médecine/Sciences*, 15: 239–245.

Rossetti, Y., Pisella, L., Colent, C., Rode, G., Tilikete, C., Vighetto, A., Boisson, D. and Pelisson, D. (2000) A cerebellar therapy for a parietal deficit? (abstract). In: P.H. Weiss (Ed.), *Action and Visuo-Spatial Attention. Neurobiological Bases and Disorders*. Life Sciences, Reihe Lebenswissenschaften, Forschungszentrum Jülich GmbH, Jülich, Germany, p. 21.

Schenckenberg, T., Bradford, D.C. and Ajax, E.T. (1980) Line bisection with neurologic impairment. *Neurology*, 30: 509–517.

Schmahmann, J.D. (1998) Dysmetria of thought: clinical consequences of cerebellar dysfunction on cognition and affect. *Trends Cogn. Sci.*, 2: 362–371.

Tilikete, C., Rode, G., Rossetti, Y., Li, L., Pichon, J. and Boisson, D. (2001) Prism adaptation to rightward optical deviation improves postural imbalance in left hemiparetic patients. *Curr. Biol.*, 11: 524–528.

Toutounji, N., Michel, C., Luauté, J., Rode, G., Boisson, D. and Rossetti, Y. (2001) Prism adaptation improves haptic object recognition in hemispatial neglect. Société de Neuropsychologie de Langue Française, Paris, 2001.

Vallar, G., Guariglia, C. and Rusconi, M.L. (1997) Modulation of the neglect syndrome by sensory stimulation. In: P. Their and H.-O. Karnath (Eds.), *Parietal Lobe Contribution to Orientation in 3D Space*. Springer, Heidelberg, pp. 555–579.

Vallar, G., Bottini, G. and Sterzi, R. (2003) Anosognosia for left-sided motor and sensory deficits, motor neglect and sensory hemiinattention: is there a relationship? In: C. Prablanc, D. Pélisson and Y. Rossetti (Eds.), *Neural Control of Space Coding and Action Production. Progress in Brain Research*, Vol. 142. Elsevier, Amsterdam, pp. 289–301 (this volume).

Weiner, M.J., Hallett, M. and Funkenstein, H.H. (1983) Adaptation to lateral displacement of vision in patients with lesions of the nervous system. *Neurology*, 33: 766–772.

Welsch, R.B. (1986) Adaptation of space perception. In: K.R. Boff, L. Kaufman and J.P. Thomas (Eds.), *Handbook of Perception and Human Performance, Vol. 1. Sensory Process and Perception*. Wiley, New York, NY, pp. 241–245.

Wilson, B., Cokburn, J. and Halligan, P. (1987) Development of a behavioral test of visuospatial neglect. *Arch. Phys. Med. Rehabil.*, 68: 98–102.

C. Prablanc, D. Pélisson and Y. Rossetti (Eds.)
Progress in Brain Research, Vol. 142
© 2003 Elsevier Science B.V. All rights reserved

CHAPTER 18

Anosognosia for left-sided motor and sensory deficits, motor neglect, and sensory hemiinattention: is there a relationship?

Giuseppe Vallar [1,*], Gabriella Bottini [2,3] and Roberto Sterzi [4]

[1] *Dipartimento di Psicologia, and Laboratorio di Neuroimmagini Cognitive e Cliniche, Università degli Studi di Milano-Bicocca, Milan, Italy*
[2] *Dipartimento di Psicologia, Università degli Studi di Pavia, Pavia, Italy*
[3] *Laboratorio di Neuropsicologia, Dipartimento di Scienze Neurologiche, Ospedale Niguarda Cà Granda, Milan, Italy*
[4] *Divisione Neurologica, Ospedale S. Anna, Como, Italy*

Abstract: In recent years, research on unilateral spatial neglect has focussed on dissociations between different aspects of the clinical syndrome, which is now considered by many students as a multi-componential disorder. Notwithstanding this leading view, there is at least one empirical argument which supports a unitary interpretation of the disorder. This is based on the observation, now replicated many times, that a variety of sensory stimulations (vestibular, optokinetic, transcutaneous mechanical vibration and nervous electrical, visual prism adaptation) involving a lateral change (left–right asymmetry) in the input pattern, affect in a very similar fashion virtually *all* manifestations of the syndrome, including: visuo-spatial neglect; hemianaesthesia (somatosensory hemi-inattention); extinction, hemiparesis, hemiplegia, and anosognosia for these motor disorders; somatoparaphrenia. These effects may be accounted for with reference to a spatial medium, articulated in a number of specific components, which is modulated by sensory input in a fundamentally similar fashion. Recent investigations concerning the neural bases of some of these stimulations support this view. In this chapter the case of the co variation of the effects of vestibular stimulation on motor deficits and on anosognosia for hemiplegia is considered. The suggestion is made that one mechanism underlying anosognosia for hemiplegia is unawareness of a deficit of intention, or movement planning component, rather than, or in addition to, unawareness of a primary motor deficit. Temporary remission of anosognosia after vestibular stimulation may represent recovery from this neglect related component, of which, as of other manifestations of the syndrome, patients are typically unaware. The recovered intention to move may allow the detection by the patient of the presence of a residual primary motor deficit, through a feedback mechanism.

Anosognosia for left hemiplegia. A specific monitoring deficit

In the second half of the 19th century, clinical neurologists concerned with the investigation of cognitive disorders associated with cerebral lesions noted in individual cases that the patient may be unaware of the neurological deficit (review in Papagno and Vallar, 2002).

Constantin von Monakow (1885), professor of neurology in the University of Zürich (Switzerland), described a patient with cortical blindness and word

---

* Correspondence to: G. Vallar, Dipartimento di Psicologia, and Laboratorio di Neuroimmagini Cognitive e Cliniche, Università degli Studi di Milano-Bicocca, Milan, Italy. Tel.: +39-02-64-48-68-10; Fax: +39-02-64 48-67-06; E-mail: giuseppe.vallar@unimib.it

deafness who did not see obstacles in front of him, was unable to find the food when he had to eat, did not blink when a fist was shown in front of his eyes and looked as a blind man. The patient did not seem to be aware of his deficit, thinking that the environment was dark. Von Monakow also noticed that intellectual functions were not disproportionately impaired. The cortico-subcortical bilateral lesions involved the occipital gyri of both sides of the brain and the temporal areas of the left hemisphere.

Gabriel Anton (1893), professor of neurology in the University of Graz (Austria), a few years later reported a patient who, after a road accident, exhibited a somatosensory impairment, involving both superficial and deep (the patient was unable to evaluate the position of his limbs) sensation. Although a confusional state was present, preventing a complete examination, Anton briefly mentioned that the patient was not aware of his left-sided paralysis. The patient's lesion involved the right cerebral cortex from the temporo-parietal to the occipital area, including the white matter and the optic thalamus. Anton (1899) reported two additional patients, one with word deafness and another with cortical blindness. The latter, according to Anton, suffered from a *Seelenblindheit* (psychic blindness) for the symptom, namely: the patient did not notice her massive and later complete loss of her ability to see. Anton noticed that this symptom was relatively frequent in lesions of the occipital cortex. He mentioned Dufour, a Swiss physician, who thought that patients with hemianopia had lost also the sense of their half-field defect (*'hemianopsie nulle'*). According to Dufour, this symptom could be used to differentiate between *central* (cortical) and *peripheral* (ocular, subcortical) damage to the visual pathways. The latter type of lesion brought about *'vision noire'* (visual blackness), a deficit of which the patient was aware. Anton (1898) mentioned two kinds of patients showing unawareness of neurological deficits: (1) patients with a loss of deep (proprioceptive) sensation, with or without paralysis, who tried anyway to walk; (2) patients with word deafness and cortical blindness. According to Anton, unawareness of neurological disease could not be easily explained as an impairment of intellectual functions. In sum, Anton made a brief mention of the symptom of *Nichtbewußtsein* (non-awareness) of hemiparesis, but his main inter-

est concerned unawareness of word deafness and of cortical blindness. The main points he drew attention to were the possible correlations with somatosensory deficits, and the frequent absence of an intellectual impairment.

Arnold Pick, 1898 (pp. 168–185), professor of psychiatry in the University of Prague, described a 31-year-old patient, Adolf W., who, after an acute accident, developed a severe left hemiparesis, of which he was not aware, and a left homonymous hemianopia. No associated somatosensory deficits were present. The patient, reading a newspaper, consistently omitted the first (left-sided) word of each line, showing left neglect dyslexia. A post-mortem examination showed a lesion in the left temporal lobe (3 years after the initial observation the patient developed also language disturbances) and in the right optic thalamus.

The clinical reports of Anton and Pick include three main features of *non-awareness* (*Nichtbewußtsein*) of hemiplegia. First, *a general mental deterioration* was not a main aspect of the impairment of these patients, and could not, therefore, constitute the main underlying deficit. Also in von Monakow's (1885) patient, who was unaware of his cortical blindness, intellectual functions were not disproportionately impaired. Both Anton's and Pick's patients, however, were confused and disoriented. Second, a somatosensory impairment was not necessarily associated with non-awareness of motor deficits (Pick, 1898), and, as mental deterioration, could not entirely account for the disorder. Third, in the two patients described by Anton and Pick unawareness of the motor deficit concerned the *left side* of the body. No particular significance was attached to this fact, however. Pick's patient showed also left neglect dyslexia.

In 1914 the French neurologist Josef François Babinski, head of the service at the 'Hôpital de la Pitié' in Paris, presented before the 'Société de Neurologie de Paris' the cases of two stroke patients showing unawareness of hemiplegia. The communication of Babinski (1914) was specifically devoted to this issue and he suggested a neologism to design this pathological behaviour (*anosognosia*). For hemiplegic patients who, without ignoring the existence of their paralysis, did not seem to attach much importance to it, as if it was a minor disease, Babinski suggested the term *anosodiaphoria* (adiaphoria, indifference).

Babinski was apparently not aware of the cases previously reported by von Monakow, Anton and Pick, but he mentioned a previous observation by Barat (1912, quoted by Babinski): the case of a patient with a left hemiplegia and blindness, who despite being not intellectually impaired, was not aware of her paralysis. The patient was, however, mentally confused, totally disoriented in time and space, and had visual hallucinations. Babinski's interpretation of his findings was cautious. He seems not to favour the hypothesis of malingering. He also considered that this denial of illness may have provided to the patient a mean to cope better with the disease. As to specific neurological factors, Babinski suggested that deficits of sensation apparently played an important role, and noted the lateralization of the disorder, suggesting a possible association with damage to the right hemisphere. In the discussion which followed Babinski's report, the most distinguished French neurologists of the time took part. Apparently, other cases had been observed. Souques (quoted by Babinski) briefly reported the case of a colleague who, probably after a stroke, developed a left hemiplegia with total hemianaesthesia, but no apparent intellectual deterioration. Henry Meige (quoted by Babinski), in addition to confirming that some patients with hemiplegia exhibit a sort of indifference towards the deficit, remarked that, after strength has recovered, patients may persist in their inert state and do not execute movements, even though these have become again possible. Meige mentioned that 10 years earlier (*Septième Congrès de médicine interne*, Paris, 1904) he had proposed the existence of '*amnésies motrices fonctionnelles*' (motor functional amnesias) in hemiplegic patients, who appear to have forgotten the function of their paralysed limbs. Meige concluded his comment, suggesting an interpretation of Babinski's cases in terms of '*anosognosie par amnésie motrice fonctionnelle*' (anosognosia for motor functional amnesia). Four years later, Babinski (1918), in a brief communication, recapitulated the main features of anosognosia, stressing the role of the associated deficit of deep sensation (position sense), which, in his view, was likely to be a necessary condition, though not the complete explanation.

In the following years Babinski's observations were confirmed by other French neurologists. The clinical observations by Babinski and other French neurologists, published in the *Revue Neurologique* between 1914 and 1924 (Babinski, 1923; Barré et al., 1923; Joltrain and Babinski, 1924), comprised five main features of unawareness of hemiplegia, in addition to the novel names assigned to the varieties of the disorder (*anosognosia and anosodiaphoria*): (1) general mental deterioration, confusional state, impairment of memory functions or malingering could not explain anosognosia; (2) anosognosia for hemiplegia was not a manifestation of a more general unawareness of disease (for example, when she was asked about her present problem, Babinski's (1914) patient #2 answered that she suffered from an old phlebitis, which was indeed the case); (3) somatosensory deficits, with particular reference to the associated impairment of position sense, were likely to play an important, though not exclusive, role; (4) in all the reported patients anosognosia concerned left hemiplegia, and was therefore associated with damage to the right cerebral hemisphere; (5) the manifestations of the disorder could differ in degree, ranging from anosognosia (complete unawareness or denial of hemiplegia) to *anosodiaphoria* (emotional indifference towards hemiplegia, which could be admitted without concern).

In the following years these observations were confirmed by many investigators. In series of patients with unilateral brain lesions an association between damage to the right hemisphere and anosognosia for left hemiplegia was found, with some left brain-damaged patients showing anosognosia for right hemiplegia. The frequent association between somatosensory deficits (cutaneous sensation and position sense) and anosognosia was also confirmed (Von Hagen and Ives, 1937; Nathanson et al., 1952; Cutting, 1978). Studies performed in large series of right-brain-damaged patients provided however evidence to the effect that anosognosia for left hemiplegia may occur with no associated deficits in sensation for both touch (Cutting, 1978; Willanger et al., 1981a; Bisiach et al., 1986b) and position sense (Willanger et al., 1981a; Small and Ellis, 1996), confirming Pick's (1898) early observations. Conversely, patients with left-sided defects for touch and position sense may acknowledge the motor disorder, suggesting that a somatosensory impairment is neither a necessary nor a sufficient condition for anosognosia to occur. Anosognosia is also double-dissociated from extra-personal visuo-spatial unilateral neglect (Willanger et al., 1981b; Bisiach et al., 1986b). Similarly, personal neglect or hemiasomatognosia is an independent disorder, which may occur in isolation, even though its association with anosognosia is frequent (Bisiach et al., 1986b; Berti et al., 1996; Berti et al., 1998; Meador et al., 2000). Anosognosia for hemiplegia cannot therefore be interpreted as a manifestation of a more general disorder of the internal representation (image or schema) of the body (Nielsen, 1946; Sandifer, 1946; Roth, 1949; Critchley, 1953; Hécaen and Albert, 1978, pp. 303–307). The early clinical observations in individual patients that anosognosia for left hemiplegia may occur in the absence of general intellectual impairment or confusion (Gilliatt and Pratt, 1952) have been confirmed in series of right-brain-damaged patients, investigated through psychometric batteries (Levine et al., 1991; Berti et al., 1996; Small and Ellis, 1996). The selectivity of the manifestations of the disorder was unequivocally revealed by observations such as patient #3 of Von Hagen and Ives (1937), who recognized that she was paralysed in the left upper limb, but always denied paralysis of the lower limb. Similarly, Anton's (1899) patient Ursula Mercz, denied blindness, but was aware of her mild dysphasia. One patient described by Gassel and Williams (1963) was aware of right hemiplegia, but not of right homonymous hemianopia.

More recently, these findings from studies in patients with permanent unilateral hemispheric damage have been confirmed and extended through a different experimental paradigm, the temporary dysfunction of one cerebral hemisphere produced by intracarotid barbiturate injection (Wada test). Gilmore et al. (1992) reported that eight patients did not recall their left motor weakness after injection of amytal into their right carotid artery, but recalled their right hemiparesis and aphasia after left-sided injection. The authors concluded that the patients' defective memory for left-sided weakness was due to their never having been aware of it (see also Durkin et al., 1994). This study, however, differs from the clinical reports mentioned earlier in that awareness of hemiparesis was not assessed *during*

hemispheric inactivation and the actual presence of the motor deficit. Under these conditions anosognosia could then reflect a memory deficit, rather than unawareness. Adair et al. (1995a) found however that the vast majority of their subjects, questioned during and after right-hemisphere anaesthesia, demonstrated anosognosia for left hemiparesis in both assessments (24 out of 28 patients, 86%), concluding that defective recall of left-sided weakness reflected a failure of awareness of disease, rather than a memory disorder. Converging evidence was obtained in a series of 31 patients by Carpenter et al. (1995), who also found that a general memory impairment could not constitute the factor underlying anosognosia for left hemiparesis. In nine patients they assessed awareness for arm weakness during left hemiparesis, finding anosognosia in five cases (related evidence in Adair et al., 1995a,b). Finally, three out of the four other patients aware of left weakness following right hemisphere inactivation by amytal could not subsequently recall it. This suggests that the right hemisphere has a specific mnestic function for weakness of the contralateral arm, in addition to the gnostic function.

The specificity of the disorder was also further confirmed. Amytal injection into the patient's left carotid artery may bring about anosognosia for right weakness, for dysphasia, or for both deficits (Breier et al., 1995). In many patients anosognosia for left hemiplegia is not associated with personal neglect (Adair et al., 1995b). Anosognosia for left hemiplegia induced by the left-sided amytal injection is not systematically related to factors such as age, general intelligence, hemisphere of seizure focus, or temporal lobe pathology (Adair et al., 1995b; Carpenter et al., 1995).

The clinical and experimental studies in neurological patients with both unilateral lesions and temporary hemispheric dysfunctions concur to suggest that anosognosia for left hemiplegia is a deficit of a specific right-hemisphere-based monitoring function. Explanations in terms of a mode of adaptation to the stress caused by the disease (Schilder, 1935; Weinstein and Kahn, 1955), and of associated somatosensory (proprioceptive) and intellectual impairments (Levine, 1990; Levine et al., 1991) are made unlikely by a number of facts: (1) there is a hemispheric asymmetry for anosognosia for hemiplegia, which is more frequent after dysfunction of the right cerebral hemisphere; (2) in some patients anosognosic phenomena are selective (e.g., unawareness of hemiplegia, but not of aphasia and vice versa); (3) anosognosia on the one hand, and the putatively associated responsible factors (general cognitive impairment, somatosensory deficits, hemiasomatognosia or personal neglect) on the other, do not necessarily co-occur; (4) vestibular stimulation, a manoeuvre which may temporarily improve a number of manifestations of the syndrome of spatial unilateral neglect (Vallar et al., 1997c), ameliorates also anosognosia for left hemiplegia (Cappa et al., 1987; Vallar et al., 1990; Rode et al., 1992, 1998).

These latter observations, showing that the neural processes defective in anosognosia for left motor weakness, and in other aspects of the syndrome of spatial unilateral neglect, are modulated in a similar fashion by specific sensory inputs, provide a case for a fundamentally unitary account of the syndrome of spatial unilateral neglect (Bisiach and Vallar, 2000; Vallar et al., 2002).

These empirical observations support interpretations of anosognosia in terms of the dysfunction of specific monitoring processes, which may produce unawareness for neurological disorders such as hemiplegia and hemianopia (Bisiach and Geminiani, 1991; Berti et al., 1996, 1998). According to a different, though related, view, damage to a 'posterior' (inferior parietal) conscious awareness system (CAS) may bring about anosognosia for perceptual and motor deficits, while disconnections of this CAS from particular input modules may result in specific forms of anosognosia (McGlynn and Schacter, 1989, and Berti et al., 1998, for a critical discussion of the CAS hypothesis). An early neurologically based hypothesis had been put forward by Geschwind (1965), in the more general context of his account of many neuropsychological disorders as disconnection syndromes. Anosognosic phenomena would be due to a disconnection from the speech areas of the left hemisphere: in the case of anosognosia for left hemiplegia, a right–left inter-hemispheric disconnection. However, manoeuvres such as placing the left arm in the unaffected right half-space, where sensory processing is mainly performed by the left hemisphere, do not consistently induce a remission of anosognosia (Adair et al., 1995a, 1997). Accounts of anosognosia for left hemiplegia in terms of interruption of the flow of information to the left hemisphere do not appear at present supported by the available empirical evidence.

Anosognosia of what? Left hemiplegia vs. a motor neglect disorder

Starting from the seminal early observations by von Monakow, Anton and Pick, and the succinct but clear definition of the phenomenon by Babinski (with a name — anosognosia — referring to this specific disorder), a comprehensive consideration of the clinical features of unawareness of hemiplegia indicates that the disorder reflects the impairment of a specific monitoring system, rather than being produced by a combination of associated somatosensory (particularly proprioceptive) and widespread cognitive deficits. The more recent and experimentally controlled investigations of anosognosia for hemiplegia support this view.

Current accounts of anosognosia share the assumption that the deficit of awareness of disease (be it a disorder of a specific monitoring process, or one manifestation of a more widespread cognitive deterioration) concerns a primary motor disorder: hemiplegia.

In the 1914 discussion of the report by Babinski, Henry Meige made a comment, which diverges from this widely accepted view. Meige, as noted in the previous section, had proposed the existence of 'amnésies motrices fonctionnelles' in hemiplegic patients, who appear to have forgotten the function of their paralysed limbs and, even after strength has recovered, persist in their inert state and do not execute movements, though these have become again possible. This is an early description of the 'motor neglect' ('négligence motrice' in the French neurological literature) component deficit of the neglect syndrome, whereby patients fail to execute movements with the contralesional limbs, though strength is not disproportionately reduced (Garcin et al., 1938; Critchley, 1953; Castaigne et al., 1970, 1972; Heilman et al., 1993; Mark et al., 1996, for a terminological discussion of this complex and multi-componential deficit). Motor neglect, as anosognosia, is more frequent following damage to the right hemisphere (Barbieri and De Renzi, 1989; Coslett and Heilman, 1989).

Heilman and his coworkers (Heilman, 1991; Gold et al., 1994, for an empirical verification) proposed an interpretation of anosognosia for hemiplegia as a loss of motor intention. According to their feed-forward hypothesis, because patients with anosognosia for hemiplegia do not attempt to move their paretic limbs (motor neglect), there is no expectancy of movement and no mismatch between expectation and actual performance, resulting in unawareness of the motor deficit. This hypothesis resembles Meige's account in that, according to both views, patients with anosognosia for left motor deficits are reluctant to move their left limbs, due to a higher-order, non-primarily motor, disorder: 'motor functional amnesia' in Meige's terminology, 'defective motor intention' according to Heilman and his coworkers.

Three recent studies have shown that the left-sided motor weakness of right-brain-damaged patients is temporarily improved by optokinetic (Vallar et al., 1997b) and vestibular (Rode et al., 1992, 1998) stimulations, as other components of the neglect syndrome (Vallar et al., 1997c; Rossetti and Rode, 2002). These results provide empirical support to Meige's early suggestion that a non-primarily motor disorder, which may be provisionally referred to as a manifestation of 'motor neglect', or as a deficit of 'intention' or 'premotor' planning, contributes to the left-sided weakness (see Kerkhoff, 2003, and Rode et al., 2003, this volume). The contribution of this neglect-related motor deficit to the manifestations of contralesional hemiparesis and hemiplegia is clinically relevant. In a community-based epidemiological survey, Sterzi et al. (1993) found that left-sided motor deficits were more frequent than right-sided deficits, namely: damage to the right cerebral hemisphere brought about contralesional disorders more often that damage to the left hemisphere.

Rode et al. (1992) assessed in the same patients the effects of vestibular stimulation on both anosognosia for hemiplegia and hemiplegia itself. Caloric vestibular stimulation (i.e., the irrigation of the left external ear canal with cold water) temporarily improved left-sided motor deficits in seven out of nine right-brain-damaged patients. Neglect for the left side of the body (personal neglect) fully recovered in eight patients, and improved in one patient. All patients had exhibited anosognosia in the acute post-stroke stage, but the deficit was still present at the time of the vestibular stimulation study in six out of nine patients. Anosognosia completely recovered in five out of these six patients. In one patient (#6) neither anosognosia nor the motor deficit recovered. Rates of recovery from anosognosia for the left-sided motor deficits, from the motor deficits themselves, and from personal neglect showed no correlation, although it should be noted that the range of the scores for the motor deficit (0 to 130, maximum deficit) on the one hand, and for anosognosia and personal neglect on the other (0 to 3, maximum deficit) were very different. With reference to the multi-component nature of the clinical entity 'motor neglect', Rode et al. (1998) mention that in two patients with a type of 'motor neglect' which was improved by verbal command (Laplane and Degos, 1983; Laplane, 1990) and was not associated with spatial sensory neglect, vestibular stimulation was not effective. By contrast, in the nine patients whose motor deficit was improved by vestibular stimulation, and in whom other manifestations of the neglect syndrome were present, it was the verbal command to be ineffective.

The observation by Rode et al. (1998) that vestibular stimulation may temporarily improve both left-sided motor deficits and anosognosia for them was replicated in four right-brain-damaged patients, examined within 24 h after stroke onset. All patients had a left homonymous hemianopia and hemianaesthesia, and exhibited a severe visuo-spatial extra-personal unilateral neglect, as assessed by bisection and cancellation tasks. Patient #1 (Fig. 1) had a cortico-subcortical lesion in the vascular territory of the middle cerebral artery, involving mainly the frontal and temporal regions. Three patients had subcortical lesions: patient #2 had an ischaemic lesion in the right internal capsule (not available for mapping); patient #3 an haemorrhagic lesion involving the genu and the posterior limb of the internal capsule, the posterior insula and the periventricular subcortical white matter (Fig. 2); patient #4 an haemorrhagic lesion involving the basal ganglia (putamen and pallidum), the posterior limb of the internal capsule, and the white matter (Fig. 3).

Muscle strength was assessed by a standardized exam (based on Côté et al., 1986), which assessed the following movements: (1) upper limb (arm raising, flexion at the elbow, finger flexion and extension; (2) lower limb (flexion and extension at the hip

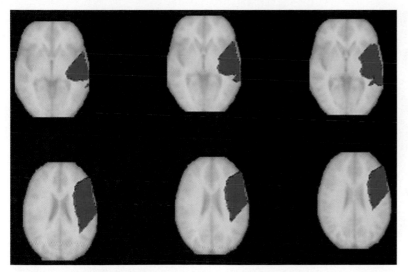

Fig. 1. Right-hemispheric lesion in patient #1.

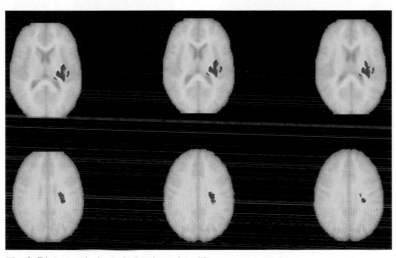

Fig. 2. Right-hemispheric lesion in patient #3.

joint, flexion and extension of the toes). For each movement the following scores were given: 0 (no movement), 1 (palpable contraction), 2 (movement not involving gravity), 3 (movement against gravity, but not against resistance), 4 (normal movement). The total maximum motor scores were 12 for the upper limb and 8 for the lower limb.

Anosognosia was assessed by a standard interview (based on the scale by Bisiach et al., 1986b), providing a 4-point scale: 0 (the patient reports the contralesional motor deficit after a *general* question about his or her health), 1 (the patient reports the

contralesional motor deficit after a *specific* question about his or her upper/lower limbs), 2 (the patient reports the contralesional motor deficit after a *specific* question about his or her *left* upper/lower limbs), 3 (the patient reports the contralesional motor deficit only after demonstration through the neurological examination), 4 (the patient does not report the contralesional motor deficit).

Personal neglect was assessed by a 3-point scale (Bisiach et al., 1986a). The patient is required by a verbal command to touch the left contralesional hand with the right unaffected hand: 0 (the patient

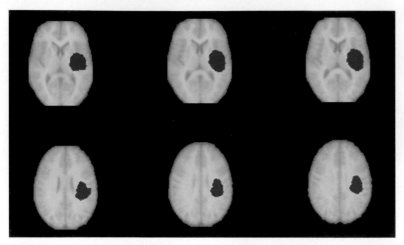

Fig. 3. Right-hemispheric lesion in patient #4.

touches the left hand rapidly, and without hesitation or search), 1 (the patient touches the left hand with hesitation and search), 2 (the patient does not reach the left hand), 3 (the patient does not make any movement).

Table 1 summarizes the effects of vestibular stimulation on muscle strength in the left limbs, on anosognosia for left hemiplegia, and on personal neglect. All four patients had a severe motor deficit in the upper limb, which was temporarily improved by vestibular stimulation. In patients #2 (who had no motor impairment of the lower limb) and #4 the improvement of muscle strength was confined to the upper limb. In all four patients temporary recovery of the muscle strength deficit paralleled recovery from anosognosia. In patient #4 neither the strength deficit in the lower limb nor anosognosia recovered after vestibular stimulation. In the series of nine

right-brain-damaged patients of Rode et al. (1998), in one patient (#6) neither the motor deficit nor anosognosia recovered after vestibular stimulation; in another patient (#5) in that series anosognosia, but not the motor deficit, recovered. Personal neglect appears to be unrelated to anosognosia for the left-sided motor deficit, being present in only two out of four patients (see also Adair et al., 1995b). Finally, the present study confirms the temporal pattern of the effects of vestibular stimulation (Cappa et al., 1987; Vallar et al., 1990, 1993b). 30 min after the treatment all scores (motor deficit, anosognosia, personal neglect) were comparable to the baseline assessment.

The available empirical data show that vestibular stimulation may temporarily improve both anosognosia for motor deficits and the motor deficits themselves. This association of positive effects leads to

TABLE 1

Effects of caloric vestibular stimulation in four right-brain-damaged patients with left-sided motor deficits and anosognosia

Patient (age/sex)	Motor deficit			Anosognosia for motor deficit			Personal neglect		
	Pre	Post	Post 30 min	Pre	Post	Post 30 min	Pre	Post	Post 30 min
#1 (82/F)	4–3	**9–6**	4–4	4–4	**0–0**	4–4	–	–	–
#2 (42/M)	4–8	**8–8**	4–8	4–0	**0–0**	4–0	–	–	–
#3 (82/F)	0–0	**3–2**	0–0	4–4	**0–0**	4–4	3	1	3
#4 (75/F)[a]	1–0	**4–0**	1–0	4–4	**2–4**	4–4	3	3	3

The scores (x–x) refer to the upper–lower limbs. – indicates deficit absent. Improvement after vestibular stimulation is marked bold. Motor deficits were assessed first, followed by anosognosia, and personal neglect.
[a] The complete assessment was repeated six times, yielding similar results.

the somewhat counterintuitive conclusion that patients become aware of the motor deficits when these become less severe, due to the positive effects of the stimulation. Secondly, the temporary regression of the contralesional motor deficits after vestibular stimulation suggests that they have a non-primarily motor component. This conclusion is supported by the observation that the sensory stimulations which temporarily improve contralesional motor deficits have non-symmetrical effects, related to the side of the lesion. Both optokinetic (Vallar et al., 1997b) and vestibular (Rode et al., 1992, 1998) stimulations temporarily improve left-sided motor deficits, but have no effects on right-sided motor disorders produced by right-brain damage. Positive effects on right-sided motor and somatosensory deficits have been reported in a few left-brain-damaged patients with evidence of right spatial unilateral neglect (Vallar et al., 1993b, patients #30 and 31; Vallar et al., 1996, patient #11; Rode et al., 1998, patient #17). This hemispheric asymmetry, which is similar to the one which characterizes the syndrome of spatial unilateral neglect, provides an argument against the view that optokinetic and vestibular stimulations exert their temporary positive effects on a primary motor disorder. Were this the case, the effects of sensory stimulations should not differ according to the side of the hemispheric lesion.

The observation that vestibular stimulation improves both hemiplegia and anosognosia of it may be explained by the hypothesis that anosognosia does not concern a primary motor deficit, but a higher-order neglect-related disorder, such as a defective intention to execute movements with the contralesional arm. Anosognosia may be therefore considered as an intrinsic component of the patients' intentional or 'motor neglect' disorder. Seen in this perspective, patients may be unaware of their defective intention to execute movements with the contralesional limbs, rather than of a primary motor deficit per se, in the same way as they are unaware of their personal (hemiasomatognosia) or extra-personal (e.g., visuo-spatial) unilateral neglect. As Henry Meige put it in the 1914 discussion, the patients may suffer from 'anosognosie par *amnésie motrice fonctionnelle*'. In addition, as Heilman and his colleagues suggest, a defective intention to execute motor acts (or a 'motor amnesia') would pre-

vent the activation of the motor system, as well as the probing of its normal or disordered (in patients with left motor weakness) function. Accordingly, a primary motor disorder would not be detected by monitoring processes. In other patients, however, in whom the motor neglect component (as revealed, for instance, by sensory stimulation) is comparatively minor, anosognosia for hemiplegia may result mainly from the disordered operation of a system specifically devoted to the monitoring of motor function.

The present conclusion that anosognosia for hemiplegia is, at least in part, unawareness of a higher-order deficit of motor intention or planning, which is an intrinsic component part of the neglect syndrome, rather than unawareness of a primary motor disorder (hemiplegia), may account for a number of findings, which result from the studies by Rode and his coworkers (1992, 1998), as well as from the present findings. First, in the right-brain-damaged patients mentioned previously the motor disorder is temporarily and in part improved by vestibular stimulation, which also ameliorates, with the same temporal pattern, other components of the neglect syndrome. This suggests the existence of a higher-order component of the motor deficit, of which patients, similar to the case of other manifestations of the neglect syndrome, are usually not aware. Second, the conclusion that anosognosia is an intrinsic feature of a deficit of motor planning or intention may readily explain the hemispheric asymmetry of the disorder, in terms similar to the interpretations which account for the whole syndrome of spatial unilateral neglect. The right hemisphere possesses a bilateral representation of personal and extra-personal space. After damage to this cerebral hemisphere, the relevant spatial representation underpinning motor planning by the left-sided limbs is disrupted, with no, or minimal, compensation by the undamaged left hemisphere, because this is mainly concerned with the contralateral right side (Bisiach and Vallar, 2000; Mesulam, 2002; Vallar et al., 2002).

This interpretation of anosognosia as defective motor intention, of which (as of other manifestations of the neglect syndrome) the patient is not aware, may also account for the finding that, after vestibular stimulation, recovery from motor deficits parallels recovery from anosognosia. When the neglect-related component of the motor disorder temporarily improves, patients may attempt at utilizing the contralesional arms, realizing that a primary deficit is present (Heilman, 1991; Gold et al., 1994). This interpretation also implies that contralesional motor deficits in right-brain-damaged patients include both a primary motor component and a higher-order, neglect-related, deficit. In line with this view, in all the studies discussed earlier vestibular (Rode et al., 1992, 1998) and optokinetic (Vallar et al., 1997b) stimulations bring about a recovery which is sometimes dramatic, but never complete.

In Rode et al.'s (1998) study, vestibular stimulation improved muscle strength in three patients who had no longer anosognosia for hemiplegia at the time of the stimulation, suggesting a dissociation between the deficit of motor planning or intention, characterized by unawareness, and anosognosia for the motor disorder. In these three patients, however, some residual movements were possible. In the context of the present interpretation, this might have been sufficient to allow monitoring of the presence of a primary motor deficit.

Conclusion

To summarize, the view that unawareness of motor neurological deficits contralateral to a hemispheric lesion involves, at least in some patients, a higher-order, neglect-related, disorder, rather than a primary motor impairment, accounts for the observation that vestibular stimulation improves, in a number of reported patients, both anosognosia for hemiplegia and hemiplegia itself. Furthermore, the view that unawareness is an intrinsic feature of a higher-order disorder of motor planning or intention accounts for the hemispheric asymmetry of anosognosia for motor deficits in a similar fashion to the case of the right-hemispheric lateralization of other components of the neglect syndrome. Recovery from anosognosia for hemiplegia after vestibular stimulation results from the regression of the motor planning deficit, which itself contributes to the clinical manifestations of hemiparesis or hemiplegia (Rode et al., 1992, 1998; Sterzi et al., 1993; Vallar et al., 1997b): patients, attempting at moving their left--sided limbs, may become aware of a primary motor deficit, which too has improved, due to the tem-

porary reduction of the neglect-related component. Similarly, in the process of spontaneous recovery, remission of anosognosia for the motor disorder may reflect the improvement of the associated disorder of motor planning or intention.

The present interpretation is compatible with a multi-component view of anosognosia: in patients with no deficit in motor planning or intention, anosognosia for left hemiplegia may represent a specific deficit of monitoring of a primary motor function. A combination of both pathological mechanisms may contribute to shape the spectrum of the clinical manifestations of the disorder (see Heilman et al., 1998, for a discussion of the manifold pathological factors contributing to anosognosia).

Finally, the hypothesis that unawareness of hemiplegia should be conceived (in some patients) as anosognosia for a neglect-related disorder (defective motor planning or intention) may be extended to other pathological phenomena of defective awareness for putatively primary neurological contralesional disorders. It has long been known that right-brain-damaged patients with left unilateral neglect may be unaware of left-sided visual-field deficits (hemianopia) (Bisiach et al., 1986b) and left-sided somatosensory deficits (hemianaesthesia) (Heilman et al., 1993). As for left-sided motor impairments (as well as for other manifestations of spatial unilateral neglect), there is evidence that vestibular (Vallar et al., 1990, 1991a, 1993b), optokinetic (Vallar et al., 1993a, 1995, 1997a), and electrical transcutaneous nervous (Vallar et al., 1996) stimulations may temporarily improve left-sided somatosensory and proprioceptive (position sense) deficits. Secondly, in right brain-damaged patients manoeuvres which manipulate the egocentric frames of reference, so that the somatosensory or visual stimulus is presented in the preserved right side of space (even though its position is still left-sided in somatotopic or retinotopic coordinates) improve stimulus detection (Kooistra and Heilman, 1989; Aglioti et al., 1999). This suggests that neglect-related deficits (somatosensory and visual contralesional inattention) may masquerade as hemianaesthesia and hemianopia. The contribution of these higher-order spatial disorders to the frequency and severity of neurological hemisyndromes contralateral to a hemispheric lesion is clinically relevant. Not only hemiplegia, but also hemianopia and hemianaesthesia are more frequent after damage to the right cerebral hemisphere (Sterzi et al., 1993).

In one study (Vallar et al., 1991b), three right-brain-damaged patients with spatial unilateral neglect, and left hemianopia, hemianaesthesia or both disorders, revealed by a behavioural standard neurological assessment, showed preserved visual and somatosensory evoked potentials to stimuli they were unable to report (see also Angelelli et al., 1996). This dissociation between a preserved analysis (demonstrated by electrophysiological techniques) and a defective report provides evidence for an interpretation of some aspects of spatial unilateral neglect in terms of processing without awareness and defective access to conscious experience (Vallar et al., 1991a; Berti and Rizzolatti, 1992). All three patients were also entirely unaware of the behaviourally assessed hemianopia and hemianaesthesia, showing denial of these disorders. As for the case of hemiplegia, denial of what? The electrophysiological evidence indicates that these patients were unaware of a disorder arising at higher-order levels of processing of the visual input, for which the clinical neuropsychological terms of somatosensory and visual hemiinattention may be used. As for hemiplegia, the patient's unawareness of the inability to detect and report contralesional sensory stimuli (anosognosia for hemianopia and hemianaesthesia) may be, in some patients, an intrinsic component of a spatial neglect-related disorder, rather than a specific deficit of monitoring of a primary sensory impairment.

Acknowledgements

Supported in part by a MIUR-Cofin 2001 grant to G.V. Dr. Martina Gandola mapped the patients' lesions.

References

Adair, J.C., Gilmore, R.L., Fennell, E.B., Gold, M. and Heilman, K.M. (1995a) Anosognosia during intracarotid barbiturate anesthesia: unawareness or amnesia for weakness. *Neurology*, 45: 241–243.

Adair, J.C., Na, D.L., Schwartz, R.L., Fennell, E.M., Gilmore, R.L. and Heilman, K.M. (1995b) Anosognosia for hemiplegia: test of the personal neglect hypothesis. *Neurology*, 45: 2195–2199.

Adair, J.C., Schwartz, R.L., Na, D.L., Fennell, E., Gilmore, R.L. and Heilman, K.M. (1997) Anosognosia: examining the disconnection hypothesis. *J. Neurol. Neurosurg. Psychiatry*, 63: 798–800.

Aglioti, S., Smania, N. and Peru, A. (1999) Frames of reference for mapping tactile stimuli in brain-damaged patients. *J. Cogn. Neurosci.*, 11: 67–79.

Angelelli, P., De Luca, M. and Spinelli, D. (1996) Early visual processing in neglect patients: a study with steady-state VEPs. *Neuropsychologia*, 34: 1151–1157.

Anton, G. (1893) Beiträge zur klinischen Beurteilung und zur Lokalisation der Muskelsinnstörungen im Grosshirne. *Z. Heilkd.*, 14: 313–348.

Anton, G. (1898) Über Herderkrankungen des Gehirnes, welche vom Patienten selbst nicht wahrgenommen werden. *Wiener Klin. Wochenschr.*, 11: 227–229.

Anton, G. (1899) Über die Selbstwahrnehmung der Herderkrankungen des Gehirns durch den Kranken bei Rindenblindheit und Rindentaubheit. *Arch. Psychiatrie Nervenkrankh.*, 32: 86–127.

Babinski, J. (1914) Contribution à l'étude des troubles mentaux dans l'hémiplégie organique cérébrale. *Rev. Neurol. (Paris)*, 27: 845–848.

Babinski, J. (1918) Anosognosie. *Rev. Neurol. (Paris)*, 31: 365–367.

Babinski, J. (1923) Sur l'anosognosie. *Rev. Neurol. (Paris)*, 39: 731–732.

Barbieri, C. and De Renzi, E. (1989) Patterns of neglect dissociation. *Behav. Neurol.*, 2: 13–24.

Barré, J.A., Morin, L. and Kaiser, A. (1923) Etude clinique d'un nouveau cas d'anosognosie. *Rev. Neurol.*, 39: 500–503.

Berti, A. and Rizzolatti, G. (1992) Visual processing without awareness: Evidence from unilateral neglect. *J. Cogn. Neurosci.*, 4: 345–351.

Berti, A., Làdavas, E. and Della Corte, M. (1996) Anosognosia for hemiplegia, neglect dyslexia and drawing neglect: Clinical findings and theoretical considerations. *J. Int. Neuropsychol. Soc.*, 2: 426–440.

Berti, A., Làdavas, E., Stracciari, A., Giannarelli, C. and Ossola, A. (1998) Anosognosia for motor impairment and dissociations with patients' evaluation of the disorder: theoretical considerations. *Cogn. Neuropsychiatry*, 3: 21–44.

Bisiach, E. and Geminiani, G. (1991) Anosognosia related to hemiplegia and hemianopia. In: G.P. Prigatano and D.L. Schacter (Eds.), *Awareness of Deficit After Brain Injury*. Oxford University Press, New York, pp. 17–39.

Bisiach, E. and Vallar, G. (2000) Unilateral neglect in humans. In: F. Boller, J. Grafman and G. Rizzolatti (Eds.), *Handbook of Neuropsychology, Vol. 1*. Elsevier, Amsterdam, pp. 459–502.

Bisiach, E., Perani, D., Vallar, G. and Berti, A. (1986a) Unilateral neglect: personal and extrapersonal. *Neuropsychologia*, 24: 759–767.

Bisiach, E., Vallar, G., Perani, D., Papagno, C. and Berti, A. (1986b) Unawareness of disease following lesions of the right hemisphere: anosognosia for hemiplegia and anosognosia for hemianopia. *Neuropsychologia*, 24: 471–482.

Breier, J.I., Adair, J.C., Gold, M., Fennell, E.B., Gilmore, R.L.

and Heilman, K.M. (1995) Dissociation of anosognosia for hemiplegia and aphasia during left-hemisphere anesthesia. *Neurology*, 45: 65–67.

Cappa, S., Sterzi, R., Vallar, G. and Bisiach, E. (1987) Remission of hemineglect and anosognosia during vestibular stimulation. *Neuropsychologia*, 25: 775–782.

Carpenter, K., Berti, A., Oxbury, S., Molyneux, A.J., Bisiach, E. and Oxbury, J.M. (1995) Awareness of and memory for arm weakness during intracarotid sodium amytal testing. *Brain*, 118: 243–251.

Castaigne, P., Laplane, D. and Degos, J.-D. (1970) Trois cas de négligence motrice par lésion rétro-rolandique. *Rev. Neurol. (Paris)*, 122: 234–242.

Castaigne, P., Laplane, D. and Degos, J.-D. (1972) Trois cas de négligence motrice par lésion frontale pré-rolandique. *Rev. Neurol. (Paris)*, 126: 5–15.

Coslett, H.B. and Heilman, K.M. (1989) Hemihypokinesia after right hemisphere stroke. *Brain Cogn.*, 9: 267–278.

Côté, R., Hachinski, V.C., Shurvell, B.L., Norris, J.W. and Wolfson, C. (1986) The Canadian Neurological Scale: A preliminary study in acute stroke. *Stroke*, 17: 731–737.

Critchley, M. (1953) *The Parietal Lobes*. Hafner, New York.

Cutting, J. (1978) Study of anosognosia. *J. Neurol. Neurosurg. Psychiatry*, 41: 548–555.

Durkin, M.W., Meador, K.J., Nichols, M.E., Lee, G.P. and Loring, D.W. (1994) Anosognosia and the intracarotid amobarbital procedure (Wada test). *Neurology*, 44: 978.

Garcin, R., Varay, A. and Hadji-Dimo (1938) Document pour servir à l'étude des troubles du schéma corporel (sur quelques phénomènes moteurs, gnosiques et quelques troubles de l'utilisation des membres du côté gauche au cours d'un syndrome temporo-pariétal par tumeur, envisagés dans leurs rapports avec l'anosognosie et les troubles du schéma corporel). *Rev. Neurol. (Paris)*, 69: 498–510.

Gassel, M.M. and Williams, D. (1963) Visual function in patients with homonymous hemianopia. Part III. The completion phenomenon; insight and attitude to the defect; and visual functional efficiency. *Brain*, 86: 229–260.

Geschwind, N. (1965) Disconnexion syndromes in animals and man, part II. *Brain*, 88: 585–644.

Gilliatt, R.W. and Pratt, R.T.C. (1952) Disorders of perception and performance in a case of right-sided cerebral thrombosis. *J. Neurol. Neurosurg. Psychiatry*, 15: 264–271.

Gilmore, R.L., Heilman, K.M., Schmidt, R.P., Fennell, E.M. and Quisling, R. (1992) Anosognosia during Wada testing. *Neurology*, 42: 925–927.

Gold, M., Adair, J.C., Jacobs, D.H. and Heilman, K.M. (1994) Anosognosia for hemiplegia: an electrophysiologic investigation of the feed-forward hypothesis. *Neurology*, 44: 1804–1808.

Hécaen, H. and Albert, M.L. (1978) *Human Neuropsychology*. John Wiley, New York.

Heilman, K.M. (1991) Anosognosia: Possible neuropsychological mechanisms. In: G.P. Prigatano and D.L. Schacter (Eds.), *Awareness of Deficit After Brain Injury*. Oxford University Press, New York, pp. 53–62.

Heilman, K.M., Watson, R.T. and Valenstein, E. (1993) Neglect and related disorders. In: K.M. Heilman and E. Valenstein (Eds.), *Clinical Neuropsychology*. Oxford University Press, New York, pp. 279–336.

Heilman, K.M., Barrett, A.M. and Adair, J.C. (1998) Possible mechanisms of anosognosia: a defect in self-awareness. *Philos. Trans. R. Soc. Lond. B Biol. Sci.*, 353: 1903–1909.

Joltrain, E. and Babinski, J. (1924) Un nouveau cas d'anosognosie. *Rev. Neurol.*, 42: 638–640.

Kerkhoff, G. (2003) Modulation and rehabilitation of spatial neglect by sensory stimulation. In: C. Prablanc, D. Pélisson and Y. Rossetti (Eds.), *Neural Control of Space Coding and Action Production. Progress in Brain Research*, Vol. 142. Elsevier, Amsterdam, pp. 257–271 (this volume).

Kooistra, C.A. and Heilman, K.M. (1989) Hemispatial visual inattention masquerading as hemianopia. *Neurology*, 39: 1125–1127.

Laplane, D. (1990) La négligence motrice: a-t-elle un rapport avec la négligence sensorielle unilatérale? *Rev. Neurol.*, 146: 635–638.

Laplane, D. and Degos, J.D. (1983) Motor neglect. *J. Neurol. Neurosurg. Psychiatry*, 46: 152–158.

Levine, D.N. (1990) Unawareness of visual and sensorimotor defects: a hypothesis. *Brain Cogn.*, 13: 233–281.

Levine, D.N., Calvanio, R. and Rinn, W.E. (1991) The pathogenesis of anosognosia for hemiplegia. *Neurology*, 41: 1770–1781.

Mark, V.W., Heilman, K.M. and Watson, R. (1996) Motor neglect: What do we mean? *Neurology*, 46: 1492–1493.

McGlynn, S.M. and Schacter, D.L. (1989) Unawareness of deficits in neuropsychological syndromes. *J. Clin. Exp. Neuropsychol.*, 11: 143–205.

Meador, K.J., Loring, D.W., Feinberg, T.E., Lee, G.P. and Nichols, M.E. (2000) Anosognosia and asomatognosia during intracarotid amobarbital inactivation. *Neurology*, 55: 816–820.

Mesulam, M.-M. (2002) Functional anatomy of attention and neglect: from neurons to networks. In: H.-O. Karnath, A.D. Milner and G. Vallar (Eds.), *The Cognitive and Neural Bases of Spatial Neglect*. Oxford University Press, Oxford, in press.

Nathanson, M., Bergman, P.S. and Gordon, G.G. (1952) Denial of illness. *Arch. Neurol. Psychiatry*, 68: 380–387.

Nielsen, J.M. (1946) *Agnosia, Apraxia, and their Value in Cerebral Localization*. Hafner, New York.

Papagno, C. and Vallar, G. (2002) Anosognosia for left hemiplegia: Babinski's (1914) cases. In: C. Code, C.-W. Wallesch, Y. Joanette and A.R. Lecours (Eds.), *Classic Cases in Neuropsychology, Vol. 2*. Psychology Press, Hove, East Sussex, in press.

Pick, A. (1898) Über allgemeine Gedächtnisschwäche als unmittelbare Folge cerebraler Herderkrankung. Beiträge zur Pathologie und Pathologische Anatomie des Centralnervensystems mit Bemerkungen zur normalen Anatomie desselben. Karger, Berlin.

Rode, G., Charles, N., Perenin, M.T., Vighetto, A., Trillet, M. and Aimard, G. (1992) Partial remission of hemiplegia and somatoparaphrenia through vestibular stimulation in a case of unilateral neglect. *Cortex*, 28: 203–208.

Rode, G., Perenin, M.T., Honoré, J. and Boisson, D. (1998) Improvement of the motor deficit of neglect patients through vestibular stimulation: evidence for a motor neglect component. *Cortex*, 34: 253–261.

Rode, G., Pisella, L., Rossetti, Y., Farnè, A. and Boisson, D. (2003) Bottom-up transfer of sensory-motor plasticity to recovery of spatial cognition: visuomotor adaptation and spatial neglect. In: C. Prablanc, D. Pélisson and Y. Rossetti (Eds.), *Neural Control of Space Coding and Action Production. Progress in Brain Research*, Vol. 142. Elsevier, Amsterdam, pp. 273–287 (this volume).

Rossetti, Y. and Rode, G. (2002) Reducing spatial neglect by visual and other sensory manipulations: non-cognitive (physiological) routes to the rehabilitation of a cognitive disorder. In: H.-O. Karnath, A.D. Milner and G. Vallar (Eds.), *The Cognitive and Neural Bases of Spatial Neglect*. Oxford University Press, Oxford, in press.

Roth, M. (1949) Disorders of the body image caused by lesions of the right parietal lobe. *Brain*, 72: 89–111.

Sandifer, P.H. (1946) Anosognosia and disorders of body scheme. *Brain*, 69: 122–137.

Schilder, P. (1935) *The Image and Appearance of the Human Body*. International Universities Press, New York.

Small, M. and Ellis, S. (1996) Denial of hemiplegia: an investigation into the theories of causation. *Eur. Neurol.*, 36: 353–363.

Sterzi, R., Bottini, G., Celani, M.G., Righetti, E., Lamassa, M., Ricci, S. and Vallar, G. (1993) Hemianopia, hemianaesthesia, and hemiplegia after left and right hemisphere damage: a hemispheric difference. *J. Neurol. Neurosurg. Psychiatry*, 56: 308–310.

Vallar, G., Sterzi, R., Bottini, G., Cappa, S. and Rusconi, M.L. (1990) Temporary remission of left hemianaesthesia after vestibular stimulation. *Cortex*, 26: 123–131.

Vallar, G., Bottini, G., Sterzi, R., Passerini, D. and Rusconi, M.L. (1991a) Hemianesthesia, sensory neglect and defective access to conscious experience. *Neurology*, 41: 650–652.

Vallar, G., Sandroni, P., Rusconi, M.L. and Barbieri, S. (1991b) Hemianopia, hemianesthesia and spatial neglect. A study with evoked potentials. *Neurology*, 41: 1918–1922.

Vallar, G., Antonucci, G., Guariglia, C. and Pizzamiglio, L. (1993a) Deficits of position sense, unilateral neglect, and optokinetic stimulation. *Neuropsychologia*, 31: 1191–1200.

Vallar, G., Bottini, G., Rusconi, M.L. and Sterzi, R. (1993b) Exploring somatosensory hemineglect by vestibular stimulation. *Brain*, 116: 71–86.

Vallar, G., Guariglia, C., Magnotti, L. and Pizzamiglio, L. (1995) Optokinetic stimulation affects both vertical and horizontal deficits of position sense in unilateral neglect. *Cortex*, 31: 669–683.

Vallar, G., Rusconi, M.L. and Bernardini, B. (1996) Modulation of neglect hemianesthesia by transcutaneous electrical stimulation. *J. Int. Neuropsychol. Soc.*, 2: 452–459.

Vallar, G., Guariglia, C., Magnotti, L. and Pizzamiglio, L. (1997a) Dissociation between position sense and visual–spatial components of hemineglect through a specific rehabilitation treatment. *J. Clin. Exp. Neuropsychol.*, 19: 763–771.

Vallar, G., Guariglia, C., Nico, D. and Pizzamiglio, L. (1997b) Motor deficits and optokinetic stimulation in patients with left hemineglect. *Neurology*, 49: 1364–1370.

Vallar, G., Guariglia, C. and Rusconi, M.L. (1997c) Modulation of the neglect syndrome by sensory stimulation. In: P. Thier and H.-O. Karnath (Eds.), *Parietal Lobe Contributions to Orientation in 3D Space*. Springer, Heidelberg, pp. 555–578.

Vallar, G., Bottini, G. and Paulesu, E. (2002) Neglect syndromes: the role of parietal cortex. In: A. Siegel, R. Andersen, H.-J. Freund and D. Spencer (Eds.), *The Parietal Lobe*. Lippincott, Williams and Wilkins, Philadelphia, PA, in press.

Von Hagen, K.O. and Ives, E.R. (1937) Anosognosia (Babinski), imperception of hemiplegia. *Bull. Los Angeles Neurol. Soc.*, 2: 95–103.

Von Monakow, C. (1885) Experimentelle und pathologisch–anatomische Untersuchungen über die Beziehungen der sogenannten Sehsphäre zu den infracorticalen Opticuscentren und zum N. opticus. *Arch. Psychiatrie Nervenkrankh.*, 16: 151–199.

Weinstein, E.A. and Kahn, R.L. (1955) *Denial of Illness. Symbolic and Physiological Aspects*. Charles C. Thomas, Springfield, IL.

Willanger, R., Danielsen, U.T. and Ankerhus, J. (1981a) Denial and neglect of hemiparesis in right-sided apoplectic lesions. *Acta Neurol. Scand.*, 64: 310–326.

Willanger, R., Danielsen, U.T. and Ankerhus, J. (1981b) Visual neglect in right-sided apoplectic lesions. *Acta Neurol. Scand.*, 64: 327–336.

Subject Index

Abducens nucleus, 35, 36, 38, 40, 42
Action, 233, 281
Adaptation, 21, 206, 210, 215, 216, 219, 276
   disconjugate, 32
   monocular, 21
   phoria, 20, 21
      horizontal, 26
      vertical, 26, 32
   tropia, 21
   visuo-manual, 277
Anosognosia, 290 294, 296–298
   (for) hemianopia, 290, 298, 299
   (for) hemiplegia, 289 294, 296–298
Aphasia, 292
Arm
   movement, 173, 178, 180, 214
   simulation, 214
   trajectory, 175
Arm–hand coordination, 186
   body distal part, 183
   body proximal part, 183
Automatic pilot, 167
Awareness, 159, 160, 292

Basal ganglia, 133, 180
Brain (cerebral) damage, 243, 283
Brainstem, 55, 61, 74
   paramedian pontine reticular formation (PPRF),
      35
      burst neuron, 40, 46
   reticular formation, 82
   superior colliculus (SC), 35, 37, 42, 44, 46, 47,
      51, 65, 71, 82, 115, 117, 120, 239, 240
      buildup neuron (BUN), 62, 92, 103
      burst neuron (BN), 62
      deep (dSC), 80
      deep layers, 92, 93, 157
      electrical stimulation, 60, 82
      fixation cells, 157
      fixation neuron (SCFN), 62, 92, 94, 95, 102,
      103
      intermediate layer, 92, 93
      motor map, 61, 66, 72, 80, 81, 93
      moving hill hypothesis, 62
      saccadic neuron, 96
      stimulation, 115, 117
      superficial layer, 93
      visual map, 93

Cat, 62, 66, 74
   head unrestrained, 78
Cell
   movement field, 44
   rate code, 37
   scales of measurement, 40
   synchronous firing, 245
Cerebellum, 83, 133, 180, 185, 210, 216, 283
   anterior, 181, 183, 185
   deep (cerebellar) nuclei, 72, 73
   fastigial nucleus, 19, 20, 76
      cFN, 75, 77
   lesion, 32
   medio posterior (MPC), 70, 73, 75, 82
   superior, 183, 186
   vermis, 19, 20, 29, 30, 32, 70, 73, 74, 75
      dorsal vermis (lobules V–VII), 19
      lobules VI VII, 19, 74
      vermal lesions, 21, 29
Cerebral cortex, cortex, 5, 120, 186
   dorsolateral prefrontal, 8
   frontal cortex, 103, 115, 116, 240
      frontal eye field (FEF), 5, 103, 259
      supplementary eye field (SEF), 5, 103
   gyrus
      fusiform, 249
      inferior posterior temporal, 249
      lingual, 249
      superior frontal, 132
   prefrontal cortex, 129
   premotor cortex, 225
      dorsal (PMd), 128, 129, 131
      ventral (PMv), 128, 133
Compensation, 281
Coordinate system, 110, 111, 117, 141
   canal-like, 119
   Fick, 112, 120

Listing, 112
Coordinates
 egocentric, 238
 transformation, 274

Deafferented, 206, 209–211, 215, 217, 219
Degrees of freedom, 110, 186
Double step, 156
 unconscious, 158, 168
Dual task, 168

Efference (efferent) copy, 29, 156, 163, 167, 171,
  210
EMG, 158, 211, 213, 214
Equilibrium point hypothesis (EPH), 158
Eye, 142, 209
 alignment (phoria), 20, 21, 23, 26, 28
  horizontal, 32
  vertical, 32
 centered map, 115
 direction, 149
 direction change, 142
 disparity, 20
 displacement, 60
 Donders' law, 112, 113, 117
 latency, 146, 147
 Listing's plane, 112, 113, 118
 orbital position, 50
 path, 144
 position, 73, 75, 76
 simulation, 214
 torsion, 110
 tracking, 147, 210
  interaction with hand tracking, 147
  latency, 147
  speed, 147
 trajectory, 145
Eye movement, 3, 49, 141, 214, 252
 binocular, 19, 20
 conjugate, 20
 direction, 146
 horizontal, 32
 lesions, 19
 monocular, 20
 ocular alignment, 19, 21
 ocular tracking, 142
 pursuit, 19
 saccadic, 72

 smooth pursuit, 147
  speed, 147, 149
  speed change, 142
 vergence, 19, 20, 23, 29
  convergence, 23
  disparity-induced, 29
  divergence, 23
Eye–arm co-ordination, 208–210, 217
Eye–hand co-ordination, 156, 186, 208, 210
Eye–head co-ordination, 79, 117

Feedback, 167
 proprioceptive, 178, 189, 195
Feedforward, 167
Flexibility, 160, 162
Frontal lobe, 283
Functional imaging, 132, 178
 functional magnetic resonance imaging (fMRI),
  176, 185
  event-related, 130, 132
 positron emission tomography (PET), 130, 132,
  162
Functional visual imaging, *see* Functional imaging

Gaze, 55, 155
 accuracy, 57
 direction, 73
 displacement, 61
 dynamics, 79, 80
 dysmetria, 79
 feedback, 57
 feedback control, 59
 feedback loop, 57
 kinematics, 112
 latency, 79
 metrics, 80
 movement, 78
 position, 143, 145, 149, 151
 position error (GPE), 55, 62, 65
 saccadic, 83
 shift, 49, 76, 78, 80, 83, 109, 120
  cat, 63
  human, 63
  monkey, 63
 trajectory, 62, 145
 velocity, 145
Grasp, grasping, 131, 132, 136, 155, 160, 161, 178
 delayed real, 229

immediate, 227, 232
immediate real, 229
pantomimed, 227, 229
Gravity, 189
Grip, 130, 226
 aperture, 228
 force, 172, 175, 178, 180, 183
 pantomime, 226
 size, 226
Grip force–load force coupling, 173, 175, 177, 183,
 185, 186

Hand
 configuration, 178
 posture, 173
 trajectory, 176
Head
 displacement, 60
 free, 115
 mechanical perturbation, 57
 movement, (motion), 57, 71, 78, 79
 restrained, 72, 78
 torsion, 110
 unrestrained, 74, 77, 78, *see* free
Hemianaesthesia, 273, 291, 299
Hemianopia, 273
Hemineglect, *see* Unilateral neglect
Hemiplegia, 273

Ideomotor apraxia (IM), 134
 delay, 135
 pantomime, 135
Impedance, 206, 217
Inactivation, 46, 61, 82, 292
 muscimol, 29
Intention, 253, 283, 297
Internal model, 164, 165, 203, 204, 206, 208, 217
 forward model, 171, 172, 175, 176, 185, 186,
  205, 217
 inverse dynamic model (IDM), 173, 175, 176
 inverse model, 171, 204, 205, 217
 learning rate, 176
 MOSAIC structure, 173
Interstitial nucleus of Cajal (INC), 117
 stimulation, 119

Kinematics, 163

Lateral inhibition, 103
Limb representation, 129
Load force, 172

Magnetic misreaching, 239
Magnetic reaching, 160
Matching, 228, 229
Memory, 292
 in dorsolateral prefrontal cortex (DLPFC), 3
 medium term, 11
 short term, 9, 14
 spatial, 5 subitem working, 226
Model, 115, 196, 199, 208, 210, 217
 gaze feedback, 60
 separate comparator, 61
 simulation, 198, 211
 vision, 250
Modularity, 173
Monkey, 66, 115, 210
 head-unrestrained, 66
Monkey electrophysiology, 133
Motivation, 5, 13
Motor, 208, 210, 297, 298
 adaptation, 204
 apparatus, 208
 behavior, 209
 command, 173, 204, 209, 211, 215
 control, 204
 error, 130, 164
 latency, 162
 learning, 206
 planning, 297
 program, 206
 program cancellation, 167
 skill, 204
 system, 204, 206, 208, 209, 216
Movement (motricity), 5, 159, 162, 180, 181, 295
 acceleration, 159, 160
 control, 158
 deactivation, 185
 deceleration, 159
 duration, 167
 end part, 158
 onset, 158–160
 peak velocity, 160
 planning, 158, 162
 velocity profile, 232
Multisensory integration, 189

Neural integrator, 119
Neural network, 120, 220
Neuron
    coarse coding, 35, 38, 46, 50
    movement field, 46, 97
    place code, 46, 51
    preferred direction, 102
    purely saccadic, 94
    purely visual, 94
    rate code, 46, 50
    receptive field (RF), 105
        tactile, 133
    scales of measurement, 37, 44
    sparse coding, 35, 38, 42, 50
    spike density, 94
    spike frequency, 97
    visual saccadic, 94

Object, *see also* Tool
    acting on, 128, 134, 136
    acting with, 128, 134
    manipulation, 136, 173
    transport, 180
    width, 226
Ocular scanning, 280
Oculomotor, 155
    system, 209–211
On-line correction, 160, 162, 239, *see also* Double
    step, Automatic pilot
Optic ataxia, 133, 163, 225, 227, 233, 238
    grasping
        delayed, 226
        immediate, 226
        pantomimed, 226
    pointing
        delayed, 235
        immediate, 235
        real, delayed, 236
    reaching
        congruent, 236
        delayed, 236, 238, 240
        immediate, 236, 238, 240
        incongruent, 236
Overshoot, 147

Parietal cortex, 247, 274
    anterior intraparietal (AIP), 128, 131, 132
    bilateral damage, 227, 246

    inferior parietal cortex, 240
    inferior parietal lobule (IPL), 128, 129
    intraparietal sulcus (IPs), 128, 130, 226, 227
    lateral intraparietal (LIP), 105, 128, 227
    medial intraparietal (MIP), 128, 131
    parietal eye field (PEF), 5, 14
    parietal reach region, 141
    parietofrontal, 129, 136
    posterior parietal cortex (PPC), 128, 162, 167,
        225, 232, 239, 283
    superior parietal lobule (SPL), 128, 129, 133
    ventral intraparietal (VIP), 128, 129, 133
Perception
    anti-extinction, 251
    attention, 244, 249, 251–253
    binding, 243, 244, 245, 251
        background, 246
        edge, 249
        foreground, 246
        form, 245, 248, 250
        shape, 245, 246, 248, 249
        surface, 246, 248–250
        temporal, 244, 251, 252
    boundary contour system, 250
    color, 244
    conscious, 243
    consciousness, 253
    depth, 246
    extinction, 248
    feature, 244
        competition, 250
        contour system (FCS), 250
        exchange, 248
        integration theory, 250
    form, 244
    grouping, 245, 248, 253
    illusory conjunction, 247, 248
    location, 244
    motion, 244
    segmentation, 245, 250
    unitary, 243
Perceptual stability, 113
Perturbation, 159, 160, 167, 214, 215, 217
    amplitude, 159
    force field, 162
    orientation, 161
    positional, 161
    visual, 162

Plasticity, 274, 281
  synaptic, 171
Pointing, 129, 155, 225
  accuracy, 157, 158, 227
  straight-ahead, 274
Postural control, 200, 280
  center of mass (COM), 191
    angular displacement, 192
    gain, 193, 194
    phase, 194
  center of pressure (COP), 193
    displacement, 192
    gain, 194
    phase, 195
  set point, 196, 198, 200
Prism, 161
  adaptation, 30, 274
  after-effect, 276
Proprioception, 29, 162, 195, 206, 208–210, 215,
    216
  ankle, 195
  muscle spindle, 214
Proprioceptive, 190, 217, 219, 298
  representation, 274
Purkinje cells, 29, 74

Reaching, 129, 131, 131, 136, 160, 161, 225, 228,
    232, 240
Reaction time, 167
Reference frame, 110, 111, 117, 298
  transformation, 120
Refractory period, 91, 156
Rehabilitation, 257

Saccade (saccadic), 19, 20, 70, 75, 167, 91, 210
  accuracy, 30
  amplitude, 46, 93
  antisaccade, 8
  conjugate, 30
  corrective, 156, 157
  direction, 46, 93, 148, 149, 150, 151
  disconjugate, 30
  double step, 9, 92, 94, 96
    onward, 97, 99
    reverse, 97, 99
  dynamics, 76
  dysmetria, 75–77
  express, 92, 104, 157

gaze shifts, 72
inhibition, 8
intentional, 8
latency, 76, 148, 149, 156
memorized, 103
memory-guided, 9
metrics, 70, 74
peak velocity, 159
phoria, 30
primary, 156, 159
primary amplitude, 157
reaction time, 91, 94, 99
reflexive, 3, 8, 14
secondary, 167
single step, 92, 94, 95
suppression, 130
undershoot, 156
velocity, 30
Schema, 206
Schemata, 131, 134
Sensor fusion, 196
Sensory–motor system, 204, 208, 210
Sensory–motor control, 172
Sequential, 158
Simulation, 210, 217
Simultanagnosia, 227
Size–contrast illusion, 232
Smooth pursuit, 151, 208–211, 214–216
Somatosensory, 195, 292, 298
Space representation, 281
Spatial coding, 233
  context-relative, 233
Subcortical system, 240
Substantia nigra (SNpr), 104
Synchronization, 151, 209, 211, 214, 216, 219
Synergic, 158

Target
  direction, 159
  direction change, 144, 145
  peripheral, 238
  velocity, 142, 208
Thalamus, 180
Tool (tool use), 128, 133, 136
Top-down mechanism, 253
Tracking, 144, 151, 152, 206, 208, 209, 214
  hand (manual), 142, 147, 151
    acceleration, 143, 146, 147

deceleration, 147
direction, 142
latency, 146, 147
movement, 141
position error, 143
smooth pursuit, 142, 147
ocular (eye), 209, 215
oculomotor and manual (eye and hand)
coupling, 143, 152
interaction, 143, 144, 147, 217
similarity, 144, 152
latency, 147
speed, 147
Transcranial magnetic stimulation (TMS), 74, 130,
162, 167, 269
Transport, 178, 180, 181

Unawareness, 159, 160, 290, 293, 298, 299, *see also*
Anosognosia
Unilateral neglect, 259, 261, 273, 292, 294, 295,
297–299
anatomy, 258
anosodiaphoria, 291
attentional theory, 280
auditory, 265
awareness, 268, 285
caloric stimulation, 259, 294
cueing, 261, 266
definition, 257
dichotic, 280
drug treatment, 257
dyslexia, 265, 290
egocentric reference, 233, 274
extinction, 262, 266, 280
frequency, 258
magnetic stimulation, 266, 268
metabolic activity, 259
motor, 293, 294, 297
neck vibration, 261, 265, 269
optokinetic stimulation, 259, 264, 265, 269
optokinetic, 297, 298

pharmacological treatment, 263
prism adaptation, 266, 269
recovery, 258
rehabilitation, 263, 264, 269, 280, 283, 285
sensory stimulation, 257, 262
stimulation, 298
transcutaneous electroneural stimulation
(TENS), 262
Velocity profile, 176
Vestibular
stimulation, 296–298
Vestibular system, 190
canal–otolith interaction, 197
loss, 190, 199
otolith, 190
semicircular canal, 61, 190
stimulation, 294
vestibulo-ocular reflex, 47, 49
Vibration, 214, 215, 219
Vision, visual, 210, 217, 233
attention
disengagement, 240
central, 163
central sparing, 240
fixation
disengagement, 240
foveal, 163
illusion, 240
peripheral, 163, 290
stream
dorsal, 225, 226, 227, 238, 240
ventral, 226, 233
suppressed, 159
binding, 244
imagery, 276
reafference, 157, 161
Visuomotor psychophysics, 162

Weighted linear contrast, 178
Wheelchair driving, 280